PACES for the
MRCP

The Blackpool, Fylde & Wyre
Health Library

This book is due for return on or before the last date shown below
to avoid overdue charges.
Books may be renewed (twice only) unless required by other readers.
Renewals may be made in person or by telephone, quoting reader number
and the number on the barcode below.

For Catriona and my family

Commissioning Editor: Laurence Hunter
Project Development Manager: Siân Jarman
Project Manager: Frances Affleck
Designer: George Ajayi
Illustrator: MTG

PACES for the
MRCP

Tim Hall MB ChB (Aberdeen) MRCP(UK) MRC GP

Specialist Registrar in General Internal Medicine and
Geriatric Medicine, South Western Deanery
formerly General Practitioner, Aberdeen and
formerly Medical Registrar,
Fremantle Hospital,
Western Australia

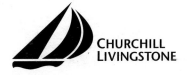
CHURCHILL
LIVINGSTONE

EDINBURGH LONDON NEW YORK PHILADELPHIA ST LOUIS SYDNEY TORONTO 2003

CHURCHILL LIVINGSTONE
An imprint of Elsevier Science Limited

© 2003, Timothy Hall

First published 2003

ISBN 0-443-07190-X

British Library Cataloguing in Publication Data
A catalogue record for this book is available from the British Library

Library of Congress Cataloging in Publication Data
A catalog record for this book is available from the Library of Congress

Notice
Medical knowledge is constantly changing. Standard safety precautions must be
followed, but as new research and clinical experience broaden our knowledge,
changes in treatment and drug therapy may become necessary or appropriate.
Readers are advised to check the most current product information provided by
the manufacturer of each drug to be administered to verify the recommended
dose, the method and duration of administration, and contraindications. It is the
responsibility of the practitioner, relying on experience and knowledge of the
patient, to determine dosages and the best treatment for each individual
patient. Neither the publisher nor the author assumes any liability for any injury
and/or damage to persons or property arising from this publication.

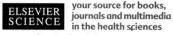

ELSEVIER
SCIENCE
your source for books,
journals and multimedia
in the health sciences
www.elsevierhealth.com

The
publisher's
policy is to use
**paper manufactured
from sustainable forests**

Printed in China by RDC Group Limited

PREFACE

Without the right facts, an enormous amount of time can be wasted. When I was preparing for the MRCP clinical exam, I wanted an all-inclusive text containing everything that I needed to know, no more and no less. Of course, it didn't exist.

The remit of cases and examiners' questions in PACES is far reaching, and candidates generally ask how to *prepare* for PACES and not how to *cram* for PACES. The problem with many exam aids is that they are too brief – books of lists which neither explain difficult concepts nor securely prepare candidates with sufficient information. *PACES for the MRCP* is not just a revision aid for the final days before the exam. *PACES for the MRCP* is a systematic text, teaching exactly what PACES tests:

- The ability to examine patients
- The ability to recognise and interpret physical signs
- The ability to apply sound history taking skills
- The ability to apply sound communication skills and an ethical framework
- The ability to discuss cases

When preparing for PACES there is no substitute for practising communication, history taking and examination skills with a wide range of patients, and this book is best used as a ward 'adjunct'. It has been carefully designed to complement day-to-day experience and steer candidates safely through the broad remit of the exam.

There is certainly more, rather than less, information than is needed to pass PACES in *PACES for the MRCP*. But candidates who know more usually pass!

This is the book I would have wanted for PACES. I hope it helps you pass an exam that you can easily pass with the right guidance.

T.H.
Aberdeen, 2003

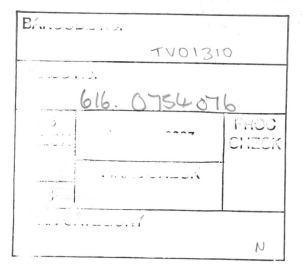

NOTES

References

References in *PACES for the MRCP* have been kept to a minimum. In no way is this meant to dismiss the sources of medical knowledge. Many commonly accepted facts were once research projects, before becoming accepted as established wisdom and used as substrates for further research in the continuously evolving world of evidenced-based medicine. Most of the information in this book is 'commonly accepted medical knowledge', a distillate of information gleaned from many years of tutorials, lectures, grand rounds, courses and literature reading, disassembled and reassembled into a method the author has found helpful in teaching candidates. To quote every paper, report, review and editorial read is not possible. Most of these have been indirect sources of help. Where, however, a particular book or journal article has a more direct bearing on what appears in this book, it is acknowledged. Key guidelines produced by national or international guideline organisations and specialist societies are also referenced with website addresses.

Disclaimer

The teaching approaches in *PACES for the MRCP* have been developed in tight accordance with the aims of PACES and in conjunction with many Royal College of Physicians (RCP) members, fellows and examiners. However, *PACES for the MRCP* is not a document of RCP policy about PACES.

Note for medical students

This book can serve as a medical text for final MB. The knowledge base for final MB and MRCP is not dissimilar. The difference is that at the stage of final MB most medical students do not have the clinical experience to complement all that they are taught, and consequently much of what is taught is not retained. Cases in final MB may be very similar to those in this book but unlike MRCP are marked more leniently.

ACKNOWLEDGEMENTS

I am very grateful to the following for reading and commenting on sections of the text: Dr Christopher M. Bellamy, Consultant Cardiologist, Glan Clwyd Hospital, UK; Professor Peter W. Brunt, retired Consultant Physician and Gastroenterologist, Aberdeen Royal Infirmary, UK; Professor James A. R. Friend, Consultant in Thoracic Medicine, Aberdeen Royal Infirmary, UK; Dr Rod D. Harvey, Consultant Physician, Raigmore Hospital, Inverness, UK; Professor Tony (R. A.) Hope, Professor of Medical Ethics, University of Oxford, UK; Dr Kevin Jennings, Consultant Cardiologist, Aberdeen Royal Infirmary, UK; Dr David Kluth, Consultant Nephrologist, Aberdeen Royal Infirmary, UK; Dr W. Knezevic, Consultant Neurologist, Fremantle Hospital, Western Australia; Dr John A. Olson, Consultant in Medical Ophthalmology, Aberdeen Royal Infirmary, UK; Dr Anthony D. Ormerod, Consultant Dermatologist, Aberdeen Royal Infirmary, UK; Dr J. A. Norris Rennie, Consultant Rheumatologist, Aberdeen Royal Infirmary, UK; Dr Richard N. M. Stitson, Specialist Registrar in Histopathology, Leicester Royal Infirmary, UK.

I am also very grateful to the following for their kind permission to reproduce photographs of their patients (and of course to the patients who gave kind consent to appear in the book): Mr Peter Ayliffe, Dr John Bevan, Professor Sir Graeme Catto, Dr Clifford Eastmond, Dr Rod Harvey, Dr John Hewitt, Dr Lilian Murchison, Dr Tony Ormerod, Dr Donald Pearson, Professor Andy Rees, Dr C Christopher Smith, Dr Marion White. I am grateful to many others who agreed to help with photographs, but whose patients, for varying reasons, were not in the end selected.

I am especially grateful to Dr John Olson for permission to reproduce retinal images from the Eye Department in Aberdeen, and to the eye photographers Alison Farrow and Sandra McKay for retrieving excellent slides.

I am indebted to Keith Duguid, Head of Aberdeen's Department of Medical Illustration, and his team, for their many hours of help in selecting and preparing images for publication. Keith's advice about image quality and procedures was much appreciated. I also thank Grampian University Hospitals Trust for granting permission to reproduce all images.

Permission to reproduce some images from Mir, *Atlas of Clinical Diagnosis*, 1995, Saunders, London, is also gratefully acknowledged.

I am also indebted to Dr Neil Edward and Dr Conal Daly, whose supportive comments on early drafts of the manuscript paved the way to acceptance for publication.

Special thanks to Dr Mike Taylor, Director of Postgraduate General Practice Education in Aberdeen, and to Holburn Medical Group, Aberdeen, for kindly (and very patiently!) supporting this project. I am especially grateful to Drs Alison Glenesk, Dorothy Lynch, Stuart Scott, Chris Milburn, Andrew Hay and Cameron Munro, and Ms Donna Dickson. I am also very grateful for the support of Great Western Road Medical Group, Aberdeen.

Enormous thanks to Frances Kelly (my agent), Laurence Hunter (Commissioning Editor at Elsevier Science), and Siân Jarman (Project Development Manager). These, and all who made the manuscript into a book, endured my many suggestions and questions and handled them superbly.

Thanks also to Rev. Bill Anderson, Seonaidh Cotton, Alice Gavin and Abigail Blyth for additional comments and support. I am also indebted to the many medical mentors in Western Australia who sparked my interest in clinical medicine.

Most importantly, thank you to Catriona and my family for their enduring patience and support whilst I hid myself away to write this book.

FOREWORD

Ensuring that doctors are up to date and fit for practice has become an important concept for the public and the profession. How doctors perform in practice is influenced by the knowledge and skills they acquire—and that in turn depends on appropriate assessment procedures. Over the last few years the Royal Colleges of Physicians have radically revised the way that they assess candidates for the MRCP (UK) making the examinations more clearly clinically relevant. This book reflects the new clinical examination through its history taking and examination cases, and its questions and answers help to explore the candidates understanding of both the underlying science and clinical medicine.

Gaining experience of this new examination method helps the candidates improve their understanding of common medical conditions and so is of direct benefit to patient care. The principal purpose of this book is to help candidates prepare for the PACES examination. The real achievement, however, is to produce a text that meets that objective and at the same time is lucid and interesting to read. Candidates and patients have reason to welcome this book, written by a young physician with an interest in medicine for the MRCP.

Sir Graeme Catto
President
General Medical Council

Contents

STATION 4: COMMUNICATION SKILLS AND ETHICS   363

STATION 5: SKIN, LOCOMOTOR SYSTEM, EYES, ENDOCRINE SYSTEM 419

8. SKIN 421

9. LOCOMOTOR SYSTEM 474

1. INTRODUCTION

THE PRACTICAL ASSESSMENT OF CLINICAL EXAMINATION SKILLS (PACES)

PACES comprises five clinical stations:

Station 1:

Respiratory system (10 minutes)
Abdominal system (10 minutes).

Station 2:

History taking skills (14 minutes, then 1 minute for thought gathering, followed by 5 minutes for discussion).

Station 3:

Cardiovascular system (10 minutes)
Central nervous system (10 minutes).

Station 4:

Communication skills and ethics (15 minutes, followed by 5 minutes for discussion).

Station 5:

Skin (5 minutes)
Locomotor (5 minutes)
Eyes (5 minutes)
Endocrine (5 minutes).
At each system candidates are given a brief written instruction. These instructions are not set by the MRCP Examining Board but 'in house' by the local examination centre hosting patients.

Stations 1, 3 and 5, in the words of the MRCP (UK) Policy Committee, are 'similar in objective to the short cases in the former MRCP (UK) clinical examination', namely to assess the candidate's ability to 'examine the patient, interpret physical signs and discuss the case'.

Station 2 assesses the ability to gather and assimilate information from a patient and then discuss the case. Candidates are observed for 15 minutes taking the history, and then there are 5 minutes for discussion (after the patient has left the station).

Station 4 assesses the ability to guide and organise an interview with a subject (e.g. a patient, relative or health care worker), provide information and emotional support, and discuss further management. Candidates are observed for 15 minutes while they are communicating with the subject, and then there are 5 minutes for discussion (after the subject has left the station).

At each station there are two examiners. The compulsory eight systems with written instructions and time limits are designed to provide a more standardised and objective assessment of a candidate's skills. Further information on PACES procedures and how examiners mark each station may be found at www.rcplondon.ac.uk or www.mrcpuk.org.

PACES FOR THE MRCP

PACES for the MRCP follows the format of the PACES exam and has been carefully designed to maximise efficiency in preparing for PACES and maximise performance on the day.

Stations 1, 3, 5: the Clinical Examination Cases

The clinical examination cases should reflect everyday clinical medicine, with less emphasis these days on esoteric conditions. However, an *important difference between these cases and real practice is that these cases bypass history taking and focus on clinical examination:*

- The ability to *examine* systems
- The ability to *recognise* signs
- The ability to *interpret* those signs
- The ability to *discuss* matters arising from the case.

To help you prepare for stations 1, 3 and 5, the cases in *PACES for the MRCP* follow a consistent approach. This approach is designed to structure your knowledge and sharpen your clinical skills to directly meet the needs of the PACES exam. The approach can also be used on the wards in preparation for PACES so that you are 'primed' for using it in the exam.

Examination of systems

Whilst candidates might be expected to be very good at examining the major systems in everyday clinical practice, the truth is that most candidates struggle with clinical examination before PACES, particularly when under pressure, and need help in developing this skill.

A comprehensive examination scheme is given at the start of each system (respiratory, abdominal, cardiac, nervous, skin, locomotor, eyes, endocrine).

Careful coverage is given to aspects of clinical examination which candidates find consistently difficult, such as the jugular venous pulse, neurological examination and regional locomotor examination.

The examination schemes are written in such a way as to be easily modified according to the instruction. They may be followed from start to finish, or fragments (such as the jugular venous pulse and praecordium) may be spliced out if asked to specifically examine these.

You should become so familiar with the clinical examination schemes that you do not need to think about what to do next, concentrating instead on the recognition and interpretation of signs. Relegating examination technique to this more subconscious level is achievable by practising the stepwise schemes given in this book.

Instruction: *An example of the type of written instruction for candidates is given for each case within each system.*

Individual cases follow the Recognition–Interpretation–Discussion (RID) format:

RECOGNITION

You are accustomed *in practice to converging upon diagnoses through history taking, examination and investigations. In PACES, examination skills are paramount in eliciting diagnoses and patients tend to have diagnoses that are readily disclosed by examination.* This is not always so in practice, and in some ways PACES requires the reverse of your approach in practice.

The first thing to do in the exam case is to work out what it is that you are being asked to look at. This book describes (in a form which can be easily recited to the examiners) the *clinical signs* which help you to decide this.

You will be looking at one of two broad abnormalities:

1. *A specific diagnosis* (e.g. rheumatoid arthritis)
2. *A pattern of signs for which there may be numerous differential diagnoses* (e.g. lung consolidation, chronic liver disease, Horner's syndrome, spastic paraparesis).

INTERPRETATION

Recognising the abnormality is your first goal. To comfortably pass you must then attempt to further interpret your initial findings. You should *know what to do next before presenting your initial findings* and *decide how you are going to present all of your findings* to the examiners.

The important extra information to gather next and a framework for presenting it all (Box 1.1) is organised within one or more of seven headings:

Box 1.1   Notes on 'Interpretation'

You will not have time to examine for all of the features given under the 'Interpretation' headings in this book. Many of the features can merely be reported to examiners as ones you would look for in practice. Most important is having a framework to guide you through examining and presenting.

It may seem artificial to separate signs under the headings 'Recognition' and 'Interpretation'. For example, you may have recognised aortic stenosis and during your initial examination elicited signs of severity. The 'Interpretation' section serves merely to organise these signs into a checklist which aids thought gathering and subsequent presentation.

Further, 'Interpretation' in this book *does not always mean actively examining*. Time may be more wisely spent demonstrating your wide knowledge than examining. The classic signs of acromegaly may be instantly recognisable, and a good candidate may proceed to check the blood pressure but find it more productive to tell the examiners that she/he would be alert to the risks of glucose intolerance, bitemporal hemianopia, obstructive sleep apnoea and colorectal cancer than spend all of her/his time examining the visual fields.

Confirm the diagnosis

This is important if there is *diagnostic ambiguity*. For example, examining the elbows in a patient with 'rheumatoid hands' for nodules or psoriatic plaques may confirm or revise your initial impression.

Assess other systems

This may be important in cases where you have recognised a *specific diagnosis*. For example, if you diagnose rheumatoid hands you should consider the possible extra-articular features of rheumatoid disease. There would not be time to examine for all of them, but this book outlines those your examiners would expect you to know. You might look briefly for one or two and mention some others.

Look for/consider causes

This may be important in cases in which you have recognised a *pattern of signs for which there could be numerous differential diagnoses*. An example is to look for or tell your examiners that you would look for signs of a Pancoast's tumour if you find Horner's syndrome.

Assess severity

In many cases it is important to determine if there are signs associated with increased morbidity and mortality. An example is aortic stenosis, for which there are established signs indicating severe disease.

Evidence of decompensation (organ failure)

It may be important to look specifically for signs of decompensation, such as for signs of hepatocellular failure in chronic liver disease.

Assess function

Awareness of the possible effects of a diagnosis on your patient's functional status is very important. For example, a patient with rheumatoid arthritis may have marked difficulty with grip and a patient with chronic lung disease may be housebound.

Look for/consider associated diseases

Occasionally, there may be time to contemplate associated diseases to which your patient may be at increased risk. This is particularly relevant in autoimmune disease.

DISCUSSION

The key to impressing examiners is in ever striving 'to go further'. Examiners prefer candidates who spontaneously present their findings and thoughts. Examiners are less certain of candidates from whom information has to be 'dragged'.

From an examiners' perspective you do two things in each case. Firstly you *examine* your patient. Secondly you *present* your findings. From your perspective you are doing a lot more. Whilst examining you are looking for signs, deciding how to further interpret your findings and thinking about how you might present them. The recognition and interpretation framework in this book should aid both your examination of patients and presentation to examiners. By adopting this framework of *diverging* from your initially recognised findings and reporting more information to the examiners spontaneously, you will perform well. The examiners can interrupt at any point with questions but are less likely to do so early if you appear to have a structured approach. At some stage, however, examiners will ask you questions, and your presentation will merge into a discussion.

The discussion sections of each case in this book provide, through questions and answers, revision of important areas of 'MRCP medicine' you might be expected to discuss. You are expected to have a working knowledge of the causes, underlying pathophysiology, symptoms, investigation and further management of the wide range of conditions that you could encounter in PACES.

Questions and answers tend to be a more effective way of learning information than straight text. It is very easy to skim through pages of text thinking 'I know this' without really knowing it at all! Questions, on the other hand, make you think. The answers given in this book are sometimes quite long, often covering more than the examiners would expect (especially in the short time available) but have been designed to maximise your understanding of each disease. Remember that the emphasis in PACES is on common conditions, and that you even know which system you are being examined on. Recognising common conditions may not be especially discriminating. Rather, the examiners will be testing your wider knowledge about these common conditions.

For more information on examining and presenting, read '100 Tips for Passing PACES' in the Appendix.

Station 2: History Taking Skills

History taking skills
History taking *skills* are at the core of history taking. They are, simply, the techniques you use to obtain the information you need.

Good history taking skills underlie any history taking case, and are far more than a clerking checklist. Since the competent demonstration of such skills is pivotal to performing well at this station, this book explores them in depth.

History taking cases
In PACES you must apply these skills to a specific case. Station 2 of this book covers a broad range of cases to which you might

2. RESPIRATORY SYSTEM

EXAMINATION: RESPIRATORY SYSTEM

Inspection

1. Introduce yourself, ensure that your patient is sitting comfortably at 45°, then stand back! Placing your hands behind your back is a good way to show that you remember how important inspection is.
2. Look around, at bedside lockers, for example, for *cigarettes, metered dose inhalers, nebulisers* and *sputum* pots.
3. Note any *cachexia*.
4. Count the *respiratory rate* (*tachypnoea* is often the first sign of respiratory or haemodynamic compromise) and note whether the patient is breathless at rest or when moving.
5. *Listen to* the *breathing* with unaided ears, noting:
   (i) If expiration is longer than in-spiration (normally the reverse)
   (ii) *Expiratory wheeze* (obstructive air-ways disease affects small airways)
   (iii) *Inspiratory stridor* (obstruction of upper airways from mediastinal masses, bronchial carcinoma, etc.)
   (iv) *Clicks* (bronchiectasis)
   (v) *Gurgling noises* (airway secretions). Strictly the term *stridor* refers to airway noise which may be purely *expiratory* (bronchial airways), *inspiratory* (larynx) or *biphasic* (trachea). *Stertor* refers to noisy breathing arising above the larynx as in severe tonsillitis.

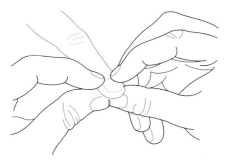

Fig. 2.1 *Fluctuation at the nail base in early clubbing (see also page 443)*

6. Briefly inspect the *hands* for *tar staining, clubbing* (Fig. 2.1), *peripheral cyanosis or wasting*. Feel the *pulse* to ascertain if it is bounding and note any flapping or fine tremor.
7. Briefly look at the *face* for any *central cyanosis* (best seen at the tongue) or *pursed lip breathing* or an obvious *Horner's syndrome*.
8. Look at the jugular venous pulse (JVP). The *JVP is raised and pulsatile* in cor pulmonale but *fixed* in superior vena cava obstruction (SVCO). SVCO characteristically causes marked venous distension in the neck and may also result in distension of veins in the hands, the underside of the tongue and upper chest wall.
9. Whilst looking at the neck, look for any phrenic nerve crush scars in the supraclavicular fossae.
10. Look at the *shape of the chest*, and note any *thoracotomy scars, radiotherapy field markings/telangiectasia* or *muscle wasting*.

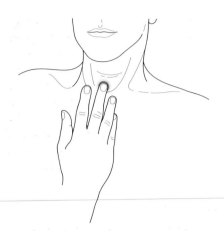

Fig. 2.2 *Determining the position of the trachea*

11. Look at *chest wall movement* (*upwards* in emphysema, *asymmetrical* in fibrosis, collapse, pleural effusion or pneumothorax). Note the use of *accessory muscles*, including abdominal or scalene muscles, or *intercostal indrawing*.

Palpation

12. Feel the *trachea* for *deviation* (using the middle finger as the exploring finger and the index and ring fingers resting on the manubriosternum either side—Fig. 2.2) and *cricoid-suprasternal notch distance*, decreased in hyperinflation.
13. Feel for cervical, supraclavicular and axillary lymph nodes, always from behind using flat fingers and not poking with fingertips.

Examination is now confined to the chest and you may start at the front or back (you are more likely to find signs at the back) but complete all of the front or back before you move to the other. Remember that the lower lobes occupy most of the posterior chest and the upper lobes the anterior chest (Fig. 2.6)!

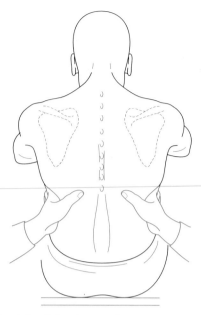

Fig. 2.3 *Palpating respiratory movements of the lower ribs posteriorly*

14. Examine *chest expansion*. For the inframammary area and for the back of the chest use a 'bucket handle' approach with your fingers in the intercostal spaces at either side of the chest and your thumbs floating in the midline (Fig. 2.3). This allows the ribs to move outwards. For the supramammary area, where the ribs move predominantly upwards, place your hands on the chest wall with thumbs meeting.
15. Tactile vocal fremitus gives the same information as vocal resonance. The author and most examiners think tactile vocal fremitus can be omitted.

Percussion

16. Percuss the supraclavicular areas, clavicles and chest on both sides (Fig. 2.4). More than four or five levels of percussion is time consuming as a screen but percuss further to delineate

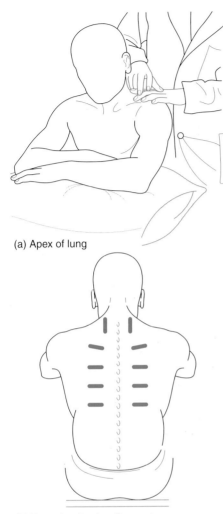

(a) Apex of lung

(b) Posterior chest wall

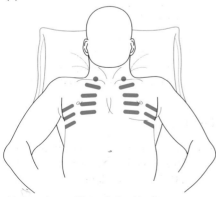

(c) Anterior and lateral chest wall

Fig. 2.4 *Percussion sites*

any abnormality you find. Always compare right with left and superior with inferior (left → right at same level → right inferiorly → left at same level → left inferiorly → right at same level and so on). Ensure that the finger applied to the chest is applied firmly; the percussing finger should tap lightly, springing away after contact, to elicit signs effectively.

Auscultation

Auscultate the supraclavicular areas, axillae, and upper, middle and lower chest for:

17. *Breath sounds*, which may be normal *vesicular* or *bronchial*, the latter having equal inspiratory and expiratory components. Bronchial breathing resembles the sound you would hear when applying your stethoscope to the neck.
18. Added sounds:
    (i) *Early inspiratory crackles* (COPD, asthma)
    (ii) *Late inspiratory crackles* (fibrosing alveolitis, pulmonary oedema)
    (iii) *Fine crackles* (fibrosing alveolitis, pulmonary oedema)
    (iv) *Coarse crackles* (pneumonia, pulmonary oedema)
    (v) Early and mid inspiratory crackles and recurring in expiration or changing with coughing (bronchiectasis)
    (vi) *Wheeze*
    (vii) *Pleural rub*, which does not change with coughing.
19. *Vocal resonance*. Sound transmission is enhanced through solid tissue (*consolidation*) and attenuated through fluid (*pleural effusion*) compared to transmission through air (normal).

Mention that you would perform ward spirometry as part of your examination.

CASE STUDY	2.1 CHRONIC OBSTRUCTIVE PULMONARY DISEASE (COPD)

Instruction: *This 62-year-old man has been troubled with cough, wheeze and shortness of breath. Please examine his chest and discuss your findings.*

RECOGNITION

There may be *tar-stained fingers, central cyanosis, pursed lip breathing* and a generally *plethoric* appearance.

There are signs of hyperinflation (Box 2.1).

There may be a monophonic *expiratory wheeze*. Inspiratory crackles would suggest superimposed infection.

A *bounding pulse* and *flapping* tremor suggest CO_2 retention.

Box 2.1   Signs of Hyperinflation

- *Increased anteroposterior (AP) chest diameter*
- *Indrawing* of the *intercostal muscles* and *supraclavicular fossae*
- *Flattening* of the *subcostal angle*
- A *shortened cricoid-notch distance* (normally greater than 3 finger breadths)
- *Decreased chest expansion*
- *Attenuation of heart and liver dullness* (with *liver descent*)
- *Hyperresonance*

INTERPRETATION

Look for/consider causes

- Smoking is by far the commonest cause. Look for *tar-stained* fingers.

- Alpha-1 antitrypsin deficiency, characterised by lower zone emphysema.

Box 2.2   Sequence of Signs in Pulmonary Hypertension

1. *Loud* (and later palpable) pulmonary component of second heart sound (*P2*)
2. *Pulmonary regurgitation* (*early diastolic murmur* louder in *inspiration*, sometimes called a 'Graham Steel' murmur)
3. Right ventricular overload and a *right ventricular heave* (and sometimes a prominent 'a' wave in the JVP—page 222)
4. *Tricuspid regurgitation* (*pansystolic murmur* louder in *inspiration*)
5. '*V*' *wave* in JVP (page 222)
6. Tender, pulsatile *hepatomegaly*
7. Sacral and peripheral *oedema*

Assess other systems

Consider *cor pulmonale*: pulmonary hypertension, triggered by hypoxia (which also causes central cyanosis and polycythaemia), sets up a cascade of backward pressure events (Box 2.2, Fig. 2.5) leading to right heart failure.

Evidence of decompensation

● Signs of cor pulmonale ● Signs of CO_2 retention.

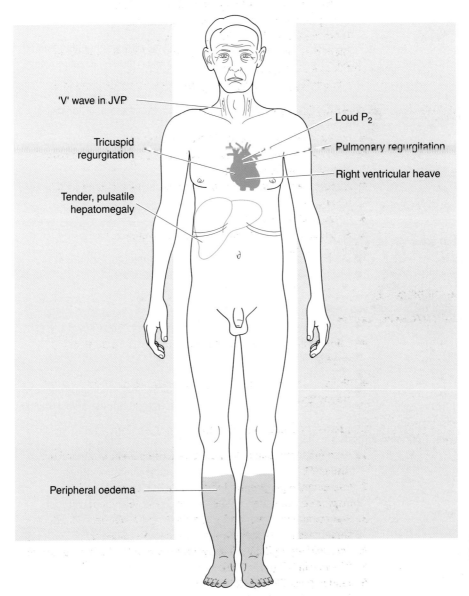

Fig. 2.5   *Sequence of signs in pulmonary hypertension*

DISCUSSION

What do you understand by the term chronic obstructive pulmonary disease (COPD)?

COPD is a chronic, progressive disease characterised by signs of airflow obstruction and obstructive lung disease on spirometry. There tends to be minimal reversibility with bronchodilators. It affects about 5% of the population over the age of 45.

✓ *Chronic bronchitis* is defined clinically as chronic, productive cough for at least 3 months of two consecutive years in the absence of other diseases causing sputum production.

✓ *Emphysema* is defined pathologically as permanent enlargement of airways distal to the terminal bronchiole. There is accompanying destruction of their walls without obvious fibrosis. Emphysema may be predominantly centriacinar (especially associated with smoking and affecting the upper lobes), panacinar, paraseptal or localised around scars.

See page 118 for definitions of COPD severity.

What is meant by one smoking pack year?

The duration and quantity of smoking is very important in COPD. One pack year is equivalent to smoking 20 cigarettes a day for one year.

List some causes of COPD other than smoking

- Alpha-1 antitrypsin deficiency ● Environmental (pollution)
- Occupational (coal workers, cadmium workers).

What tests would you consider?

- Spirometry ($FEV_1 < 80\%$, $FEV_1/FVC < 70\%$—pages 113–117)
- Full blood picture (polycythaemia)
- Arterial blood gases (ABGs)
- Sputum culture
- Chest X-ray (hyperinflation, bullae, prominent pulmonary vessels)
- ECG (p pulmonale, right axis deviation, right bundle branch block).

What treatment options are there in COPD?

- Smoking cessation strategies (willpower, self help literature, GP/physician advice, smoking cessation clinics, nicotine replacement, bupropion).
- Advice on regular exercise if not in a pulmonary rehabilitation programme.
- Weight reduction if overweight.
- Inhaled bronchodilators are the cornerstone of treatment. Long-acting inhaled antimuscarinic therapy is now available as add-on therapy to inhaled β-agonists. There is little data supporting the role of nebulisers over high dose inhalers.

- Evidence for regular inhaled glucocorticoids remains inconclusive.
- Antibiotics for infective exacerbations.
- Long-term oxygen therapy (LTOT).
- Pulmonary rehabilitation, which involves exercise, smoking cessation, nutritional assessment, education and empowering patients to take more interest in, and control of, their condition. Depression is common in COPD patients and should be considered as a cause of poor compliance.
- Lung volume reduction surgery for severe bullae.
- Annual influenza vaccination; pneumococcal vaccination every 5–10 years.

How can we assess treatment response in COPD?

There is often minimal improvement in spirometry. Symptomatic improvement may include reduced breathlessness, increased exercise capacity and improved sleep.

What are the indications for LTOT?

- Po_2 on air < 7.3 kPa (55 mmHg) or 7.3–8.0 kPa (55–60 mmHg) if there is pulmonary hypertension or nocturnal hypoxaemia
- FEV_1 < 1.5 litres.

ABGs should be measured when clinically stable and on two occasions at least 3 weeks apart. Po_2 should rise above 8 kPa without unacceptable hypercapnia. Oxygen is administered via nasal cannulae at 2–4 L/min via a concentrator for at least 15 hours a day. Patients must not smoke!

What do you know about non-invasive positive pressure ventilation (NIPPV) in COPD?

NIPPV, unlike conventional PPV via an endotracheal tube or tracheostomy, is delivered via a tightly fitting nasal or face mask and has been used increasingly in the management of exacerbations of COPD with acute respiratory failure.

What is alpha-1 antitrypsin deficiency?

Alpha-1 antitrypsin is a protease inhibitor (Pi) enzyme which inhibits neutrophil elastase. Low levels of the enzyme, determined by various genotypes (PiZZ the most severe), fail to protect the lung from proteolytic attack. This results in basal, panlobular emphysema, accelerated in smokers, and cirrhosis.

What is cor pulmonale?

Right ventricular enlargement and failure occurring secondary to lung/chest wall/pulmonary circulatory disease.

Central to the development of cor pulmonale is pulmonary hypertension.

CASE STUDY   **2.2 CONSOLIDATION (PNEUMONIA AND LUNG CANCER)**

Instruction: *This 65-year-old man has an unresolving cough. Please examine his respiratory system and discuss your findings.*

RECOGNITION

The patient may be *tachypnoeic*. There may be *reduced expansion on the affected side* but the *trachea is central*. There is *dullness* to percussion over one or more lobes (Fig. 2.6). There are *bronchial breath sounds (± coarse crackles)* and *vocal resonance is increased* over the affected lobe(s). There may be *whispering pectoriloquy* and a *pleural friction rub.*

INTERPRETATION

Confirm the diagnosis

● In *collapse*, the *trachea deviates towards* the *affected side*.
● In a *pleural effusion*, there is *stony dullness* to percussion with *reduced breath sounds* and *reduced vocal resonance*.

Look for/consider causes

The common causes are *pneumonia* and *bronchial carcinoma*.
Look for other signs of *lung cancer:*

● Cachexia
● Clubbing
● Lymphadenopathy
● Radiation marks

Fig. 2.6 *Surface markings of the various lobes*

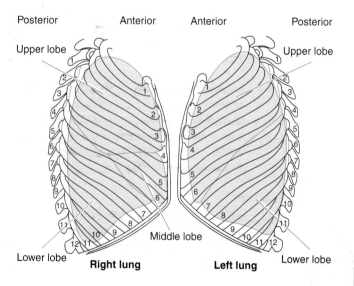

Posterior   Anterior   Anterior   Posterior

Upper lobe   Upper lobe

Middle lobe

Lower lobe
Right lung   **Left lung**   Lower lobe

- Previous thoracotomy
- Pleural effusion
- Pancoast's syndrome (page 280)
- Horner's syndrome (Case study 6.8)
- Wasting of the small muscles of the hand (Case study 6.26)
- Hypertrophic pulmonary osteoarthropathy (HPOA), which causes periostitis (seen on X-ray), arthritis and gross finger clubbing. It is most commonly associated with squamous cell carcinoma and involves the long bones.

Tell the examiners that you would ask about:

- *Endobronchial symptoms* (cough, dyspnoea, haemoptysis)
- *Constitutional symptoms* (weight loss, anorexia)
- *Pain* (Pancoast's syndrome, for example, is painful if there is infiltration of the brachial plexus; metastatic bone pain)
- Hormonal/metabolic symptoms (page 20).

DISCUSSION

What types of lower respiratory tract infection (LRTI) can occur?
1. Cough with sputum (acute bronchitis)
2. Acute exacerbation of COPD
3. Community acquired pneumonia (CAP)
4. Atypical pneumonia.

When might you treat acute bronchitis with antimicrobial therapy?

Acute bronchitis is common after upper respiratory tract infection and usually self-limiting. Pathogens are similar to those in CAP. Antimicrobials, although often prescribed, are indicated if there is clinical deterioration or if focal chest signs develop. There is no evidence that antimicrobials prevent complications secondary to acute bronchitis.

When might you treat an acute exacerbation of COPD with antimicrobial therapy?

An acute exacerbation of COPD may be defined as increased cough, sputum and dyspnoea without focal signs. The pathogen is usually viral. The British Thoracic Society recommends antimicrobials if two or more of worsening dyspnoea, increased sputum purulence or increased sputum volume are present.

What is pneumonia?

Pneumonia is an inflammatory, usually infectious, disease of the lung parenchyma. Most pneumonia is managed in primary care. In over half of those patients referred to hospital or investigated no organism is isolated.

What are the common pathogens in community acquired pneumonia (CAP)?

Streptococcus pneumoniae is by far the commonest pathogen, followed by *Haemophilus influenzae* and *Moraxella catarrhalis*. Other pathogens include atypical organisms (page 19), *Staphylococcus aureus* and viruses.

What are the clinical features of streptococcal pneumonia?

Streptococcal pneumonia is more common in winter. It is characterised by its abrupt onset and often causes high fever and rigors. Lobar consolidation is typical. Herpetic cold sores may be associated. In elderly patients it may cause confusion. Vaccination is recommended for high risk patients.

Which organism commonly supersedes influenza infection?

Staphylococcus aureus.

What do you know about prognostic indicators in pneumonia?

British Thoracic Society guidelines identify, in addition to age and the presence of coexisting disease, three core adverse prognostic features:

- Respiratory rate > 30
- Confusion
- Blood pressure < 90 mmHg systolic or < 60 mmHg diastolic.

Other adverse features include multilobar/bilateral involvement, leucopenia or high leucocytosis, raised blood urea concentration, hypoxia and bacteraemia.

What are the possible complications of pneumonia?

- Respiratory failure (page 120) ● Pleural effusion (common)
- Empyema (less common) ● Lung abscesses (rare) ● Cavitation
- Fibrosis.

Empyema (pus in the pleural space) is usually associated with persistent fevers, malaise and weight loss. It may cause clubbing.

List some differential diagnoses of unresolving pneumonia

- Bronchial carcinoma ● Empyema ● Pulmonary oedema ● Fibrotic lung disease ● Pulmonary emboli.

Which organisms tend to cause cavitation?

Staphylococcus aureus, Klebsiella pneumoniae, Mycobacterium tuberculosis. Other causes of cavitation include carcinoma, lung abscesses, pulmonary infarction and Wegener's granulomatosis.

What would be your empirical first antibiotic choice for community acquired pneumonia?

Amoxicillin remains the first choice for patients without penicillin hypersensitivity. A macrolide such as clarithromycin or a fluoroquinolone are alternatives.

Box 2.3	**Extrapulmonary Features of Atypical Pneumonia**

- Arthralgias and myalgias
- Autoimmune haemolytic anaemia (usually mild) due to cold agglutinins is common in *Mycoplasma* infection
- Maculopapular rash, erythema multiforme, Stevens Johnson syndrome, erythema nodosum
- Bullous myringitis (*Mycoplasma*)
- Sterile meningitis, meningoencephalitis, transverse myelitis, cranial neuropathies, peripheral mononeuropathies, acute demyelinating inflammatory polyneuropathy
- Myocarditis and pericarditis
- Hepatitis

How does atypical pneumonia present?

There are no diagnostic features, but atypical pneumonia:

- Often affects young adults and there is frequently a travel history.
- Tends to produce insidious constitutional symptoms and a paucity of respiratory symptoms after a 10–20 day incubation period. Despite this, chest signs may be present and chest radiography may be impressive, often with bilateral infiltrates.
- Often produces extrapulmonary features (Box 2.3).
- Causes a spectrum of disease ranging from asymptomatic infection to severe hypoxic respiratory failure requiring ventilatory support.

Which organisms cause atypical pneumonia?

- *Mycoplasma pneumoniae*, which tends to occur in epidemics every few years. A non-productive cough (paroxysms of coughing are very common) is invariable, usually associated with a paucity of signs in comparison with symptoms and chest X-ray findings.
- *Chlamydia pneumoniae*, which tends to affect an older age group than *Mycoplasma pneumoniae*. Extrapulmonary features are less common.
- *Chlamydia psittaci*, which is classically transmitted from birds (which may be very sick), and often presents with severe headache.
- *Legionella pneumophila*, a gram negative bacillus which proliferates in stagnant water and which causes Pontiac fever (an acute self-limiting febrile illness) and Legionnaire's disease (which commonly produces diarrhoea, abdominal pain, abnormal liver function and headaches before respiratory symptoms). Peripheral blood cytopenias and renal failure may occur. Legionnaire's disease is more prevalent in patients with pre-existing lung disease.
- *Coxiella burnettii*, usually transmitted from farm animals, causing the rare Q fever which ranges from asymptomatic infection to severe pneumonia or extrapulmonary features.

What are the causes of lung cancer?

- Smoking, implicated in > 90% of cases. The risk is cumulative.
- Environmental/occupational exposure to asbestos, silicosis, arsenic, nickel, chromium, aromatic hydrocarbons and radon.
- The incidence is also increased in various medical disorders including cryptogenic fibrosing alveolitis and dermatomyositis.

How is lung cancer classified?

Lung cancer is the commonest cause of cancer death in the UK.

1. About 20% is small cell lung cancer (SCLC).
2. About 80% is non-small cell lung cancer (NSCLC), of which there are three main types:
   - (i) Squamous cell, the primary disease often being in the main bronchus
   - (ii) Adenocarcinoma, often peripheral
   - (iii) Large cell.

List some contraindications to surgery in NSCLC?

- Poor lung function (generally, FEV_1 should be > 1 litre to consider a lobectomy and > 1.5 litres to consider a pneumonectomy)
- Left laryngeal nerve palsy (right does not necessarily imply mediastinal involvement)
- Malignant effusion
- Dysphagia due to oesophageal obstruction by lymph nodes or tumour
- Mediastinal (e.g. subcarinal) lymph node involvement. Generally, nodes < 1 cm are probably normal, those 1–3 cm may require biopsy and nodes > 3 cm are likely to be malignant
- Superior vena cava obstruction (SVCO)
- Phrenic nerve palsy (raised hemidiaphragm)
- Rib or distant metastases.

What are the common sites of metastasis?

- Bone ● Liver ● Brain and spinal cord.

What paraneoplastic associations do you know of?

- Squamous cell carcinoma may produce parathroid hormone related peptide (PTHrp) causing hypercalcaemia. Hypercalcaemia is, however, mostly a consequence of bone metastases.
- SCLC, which is neuroendocrine derived, may cause ectopic secretion of numerous hormones including ACTH (Cushing's syndrome – page 554) and antidiuretic hormone (SIADH – page 554).
- Gynaecomastia.
- Eaton–Lambert syndrome.

What do you know about lung cancer prognosis?

Prognosis for both NSCLC and SCLC is poor, with only around a third being potentially localised at presentation. In a 1995 Scottish lung cancer audit the median survival for SCLC was 3.6 months. For NSCLC, 5-year survival may be up to 60% for small tumours without nodal involvement, but drops rapidly for more extensive disease. Overall, 6–7% of patients are alive at 5 years.

What diagnostic tests are available in lung cancer?
● Sputum cytology ● Bronchoscopy and biopsy ● CT-guided biopsy (for more peripheral lesions) ● Pleural fluid analysis.

What treatments are there for NSCLC?
1. *Surgery* offers the best chance of cure and is considered for fit patients with early disease (stages IA – T1N0M0; IB – T2N0M0; IIA – T1N1M0, especially if peripheral), and involves lobectomy or pneumonectomy. Segmentectomy recurrence rates are higher.
2. Radical *radiotherapy*, which is potentially curative, is considered in patients unfit for surgery or patients with mediastinal node involvement. Fractionation regimens such as continuous hyperfractionated accelerated radiotherapy (CHART) offer higher 2-year survival. Palliative radiotherapy is useful for large volume local disease in alleviating local symptoms such as pain, dyspnoea, cough and haemoptysis.
3. Neoadjuvant *chemotherapy* is routinely offered to suitable patients before radical radiotherapy. Its value prior to surgery is unclear. The value of chemotherapy, either concurrently with radiotherapy or following definitive treatment, is unresolved.

What treatments are there for SCLC?
Surgery has almost no role. Micrometastatic spread is invariable at diagnosis. All patients are considered for multiagent chemotherapy. Response rates are excellent but short lived.

What are the main causes of an anterior mediastinal mass?
● Thymoma ● Thyroid enlargement ● Teratoma ● Lymphoma ● Lymph node spread from carcinoma.

CASE STUDY   2.3 COLLAPSE (ATELECTASIS)

Instruction: *This patient has been short of breath recently. Please examine her chest and discuss your findings.*

RECOGNITION

There is *tracheal deviation (to the affected side). Decreased chest expansion, dullness to percussion* and *decreased breath sounds occur on the affected side.*

INTERPRETATION

Look for/consider causes

- Previous pneumonectomy/lobectomy (*thoracotomy scar*)
- Carcinoma obstructing a bronchus (page 16)
- Extrinsic compression, by, for example, mediastinal lymph nodes (*SVCO* – page 9)
- Benign tumour
- Mucus plugs, e.g. asthma
- Foreign body
- Granuloma, e.g. TB, sarcoid

Obstruction may predispose to pneumonia or segmental bronchiectasis.

DISCUSSION

You would likely be asked questions similar to those in Case study 2.2.

CASE STUDY   2.4 BRONCHIECTASIS AND CYSTIC FIBROSIS

Instruction: *This young man has been troubled by recurrent chest infections. Please examine his respiratory system and discuss the possible causes.*

RECOGNITION

There is a *large volume* of *sputum* in the sputum pot beside the bed in this *underweight*, *dyspnoeic* and *cyanosed* patient with finger *clubbing*. Auscultation reveals *coarse, late inspiratory crackles* ± inspiratory clicks and wheeze (mucus obstructing distal airways).

INTERPRETATION

Confirm the diagnosis

This is difficult clinically, but the differential diagnosis of clubbing and crackles includes lung cancer (page 16) and cryptogenic fibrosing alveolitis (page 27). Tell the examiners that you would ask about sputum volumes, usually large in bronchiectasis.

Look for/consider causes

Tell the examiners that you would consider the following causes of bronchiectasis:

- Cystic fibrosis (CF)
- Postinfective (pneumonia, TB, measles, whooping cough)
- Allergic bronchopulmonary apergillosis (APBA)
- Hypogammaglobulinaemia

- Primary ciliary dyskinesia or Kartagener's syndrome (associated *situs inversus* with right sided heart sounds)
- Localised/segmental bronchiectasis may occur secondary to endobronchial obstruction.

Assess other systems

Tell the examiners that you would ask about chronic diarrhoea and diabetes (cystic fibrosis).

Evidence of decompensation

Look for signs of cor pulmonale (page 13).

DISCUSSION

What is meant by the term bronchiectasis?

Chronic infection of permanently dilated distal airways (often a self-perpetuating cycle).

What are the potential complications?

- Empyema/abscesses ● Cor pulmonale ● Secondary amyloidosis.

What investigations might prove helpful in diagnosing bronchiectasis?

- Chest X-ray (*tramline shadows* indicate thickened bronchial walls; ring shadows and fluid levels may also be present)
- High resolution CT (HRCT) scanning.

Discuss the pathophysiology of cystic fibrosis (CF)

CF is autosomal recessive with a gene carriage rate of around 1 in 20 in Caucasians and a disease incidence of around 1 in 2000. Most CF is due to a mutation in chromosome 7 at position 508 where the codon for phenylalanine is deleted, although many other mutations in the same gene have been described. The result is that the cystic fibrosis transmembrane regulator (CFTR) protein is not produced in its normal form. CFTR normally permits chloride channel opening. Chloride channel opening at the luminal surface of airway epithelial cells normally permits chloride escape into the lumen. In CF, chloride fails to escape but this is associated with excess sodium influx into the cell. It is thought that this seduces water from the lumen, resulting in viscous secretions, although much remains unclear about CF pathophysiology. Certainly, the epithelial surfaces affected by CF have different actions in their native state (airways and intestinal epithelial surfaces are volume absorbing, sweat ducts salt absorbing and the pancreas volume secreting), causing diverse clinical sequelae.

How is CF diagnosed?

It often starts with clinical suspicion in a child with unknown carrier parents. Chronic productive cough, poorly responsive 'asthma', chronic sinusitis, nasal polyps, chronic diarrhoea or failure to gain weight/thrive may raise suspicion. A sweat sodium concentration > 60 mmol/L is indicative. Genetic testing is more reliable.

What are the main clinical features and complications of CF?

- Respiratory (thick sputum, chronic cough or wheeze, recurrent acute infection – pneumonia or bronchitis, chronic low grade infection with periodic relapses, bronchiectasis, chronic sinusitis, nasal polyps, allergic bronchopulmonary aspergillosis, pneumothoraces, cor pulmonale, clubbing, respiratory failure)
- Intestinal (ileal obstruction and rectal prolapse in infancy, intussusception, pancreatic failure and malabsorption – diabetes mellitus/steatorrhoea/osteoporosis, gallstones, biliary cirrhosis, chronic liver disease)
- Infertility (males are infertile due to failure of development or obstruction of the vas deferens and seminiferous tubules; females are subfertile due to altered cervical mucus and menstrual irregularity)
- Arthropathy.

A baby born with CF now might be expected to live past their fortieth birthday, such that diabetes, biliary cirrhosis and arthropathies are seen with greater frequency.

Discuss treatment options for CF

- Daily chest percussion and physiotherapy with postural drainage helps reduce respiratory exacerbations.
- Early institution of high dose, broad spectrum antibiotics, continued for a long duration (2–3 weeks is a usual minimum), is needed to minimise lung damage from infective exacerbations. Oral, intravenous and nebulised antibiotics are used, intravenous usually preferred for exacerbations in chronically infected patients. *Staphylococcus aureus* tends to affect infants, with *Haemophilus influenzae* and *Klebsiella pneumoniae* tending to appear through childhood, but eventually *Pseudomonas aeruginosa* colonisation occurs in nearly all patients. Chronic *S. aureus* and *P. aeruginosa* colonisation are almost impossible to eradicate. *Burkholderia (Pseudomonas) cepacia* infection may result in a rapid downhill course. An oral or intravenous fluoroquinolone, in combination with a nebulised antibiotic, is often used initially, but resistance and chronic carriage are typical and require combinations of intravenous antibiotics. CF nurses, administering intravenous antibiotics at home, enable many patients to remain out of hospital.
- Pancreatic enzyme replacement therapy helps to avoid malabsorption and its consequences.
- Bronchodilators may provide symptomatic relief.

- Dornase-alpha, administered as an aerosol spray, which inteferes with sputum neutrophil DNA, helps liquefy sputum and encourages expectoration. It reduces cough. Teenagers, in particular, report being able to go out more. The psychological and social consequences of CF are often overlooked, but these are paramount for patients. Teenagers find their illness interferes with friendships and school, adults find it difficult to work, and patients often have low self esteem.
- Immunisation (routine childhood and pneumococcal/influenza vaccination) is important.
- Lung transplantation is considered for patients with pulmonary function below 30% with chronically infected, purulent bronchiectasis, but the side effects of immunosuppression are significant. At least 70% of patients currently survive > 1 year following surgery and 50% > 5 years.
- ABPA (page 125) and TB (below) are more common in CF, requiring specialised management.
- Gene therapy is not yet practical.
- Palliative care specialists have a role in the management of advanced CF.

CASE STUDY 2.5 PREVIOUS TUBERCULOSIS (TB)

Instruction: *Examine this patient's chest and comment on your findings.*

RECOGNITION

You may still see the legacy of surgical treatments for TB. The broad aims were to render affected lung hypoxic (to kill the organism) and to close cavities. The results of these aims may include:

1. *Thoracotomy scarring* posteriorly/previous rib resections. There is *chest deformity*. The *trachea deviates to* the *same side*, where there is *decreased expansion* and *breath sounds* are *reduced*.
2. Scarring from iatrogenic pneumothoraces.
3. *Supraclavicular fossa/e scarring* indicating previous phrenic nerve crush procedures. Again, there may be *diminished chest expansion*.

INTERPRETATION

Confirm the diagnosis

Former TB may also be suggested by *apical flattening* and *upper lobe crackles* from fibrosis. Note:

1. Thoracoplasty was a common treatment for TB before days of antimicrobial therapy. This may be associated with a 'white out' of lung collapse on chest X-ray.
2. Pneumothoraces may leave calcified/thickened pleura visible on chest X-ray.

3. A raised hemidiaphragm may be seen on chest X-ray in patients who underwent a phrenic nerve crush procedure.

| DISCUSSION | |

What is happening to the prevalence of TB?

Mycobacterium tuberculosis is increasing in prevalence worldwide, infecting both previously healthy and immunosuppressed (notably HIV infected) individuals with increasingly multidrug resistant (MDR) strains.

What do you know about primary TB?

The tubercle bacillus is initially inhaled, giving rise to *primary pulmonary TB*, although it may occasionally infect the tonsils or ileocaecum. It multiplies at the primary infection site, usually subpleural, and this, together with regional caseating lymph nodes, is termed the *primary complex*. Clinically, this may:

- Remain asymptomatic
- Cause persistent cough
- Stimulate a significant cell medicated immune (CMI) response, producing fever, erythema nodosum or phlyctenular conjunctivitis
- Cause compression of a bronchus, leading to collapse.

Primary TB may be discovered as an incidental finding on chest X-ray or on tuberculin testing. 90% of primary TB heals, with calcification (*Ghon focus*), and spread is arrested by regional nodes.

What is meant by tuberculin sensitivity?

After 4–8 weeks of primary TB, sensitisation to the tuberculin protein has occurred, a CMI response.

What do you know about postprimary TB?

TB may progress, rather than heal. It usually progresses within an unhealed lesion within the first 12 months, but reactivation of older lesions or reinfection may occur at any time. Progression may occur locally, as *postprimary pulmonary TB*, or there may be *haematogenous* spread, and with both there may be systemic symptoms—anorexia, weight loss, night sweats and fever.

In postprimary pulmonary TB there is caseation (necrosis) within the centre of the lesion, leading to discharge of its contents and cavitation. The following problems may arise:

1. Discharge into a bronchus, with endobronchial symptoms (cough, sputum, haemoptysis).
2. Compression of a bronchus by lymph nodes leading to collapse of a lobe or segment (more commonly a problem with primary TB).

3. Spread via the lymphatics to the pleura or pericardium or direct discharge into these, giving rise to pleuritic pain, effusion, empyema or occasionally pneumothorax.
4. Aspergilloma formation within a cavitated lesion (usually an old healed cavity).

Haematogenous spread may give rise to *acute miliary TB*, or be insidious. Both forms are more common in immunosuppressed patients. Haematogenous spread may result in hepatosplenomegaly, renal TB, TB osteomyelitis, septic arthritis and meningitis.

How is TB diagnosed?

1. *Tuberculin skin tests* inject purified protein into the volar aspect of the forearm. In the *Mantoux* test (strength 1 : 1000 = 10 TU), induration > 10 mm at 72 hours is positive, implying immunity (usually from previous BCG vaccination, but if strongly positive, it may indicate active infection). The *Heaf* test is the screening test, which employs a circle of primed needles. False negative tests occur when the CMI response is impaired, as in HIV infection. This is called anergy.
2. Chest X-ray may show patchy upper lobe opacification, volume loss or cavitation. Other lobes can be involved.
3. Microbiological isolation of the bacillus is needed for diagnosis. Sputum is usually negative because acid fast bacilli in lesions tend not to communicate with bronchi. Morning gastric washings are sometimes helpful. Other options include pleural aspiration/biopsy, lymph node biopsy, bone marrow biopsy, bronchial lavage, morning urine specimens (renal TB) and cerebrospinal fluid examination.

CASE STUDY   **2.6 CRYPTOGENIC FIBROSING ALVEOLITIS (CFA) AND INTERSTITIAL LUNG DISEASE (ILD)**

Instruction: *This 55-year-old man has been increasingly short of breath on exertion. Please examine his hands and chest and discuss your findings.*

RECOGNITION

There is *finger clubbing*. There are *bilateral fine end-inspiratory ('Velcro') crackles at the lung bases*, which do not clear with coughing.
CFA usually occurs in patients 40–70 years old, is more common in males, and symptoms include slowly progressive dyspnoea and a dry, non-productive cough.

INTERPRETATION

Confirm the diagnosis

● CFA should be distinguished from other causes of basal lung

crackles, especially *left ventricular failure* (listen for a *third heart sound*).
- 50% of patients with CFA have finger clubbing. Other causes of clubbing, especially *bronchial carcinoma*, should be considered.

Look for/consider causes

CFA should also be distinguished from other causes of lung fibrosis.

- Note any obvious signs of *connective tissue disease* in the face or hands, especially *rheumatoid hands*, the *malar rash* of systemic lupus erythematosus (SLE) or the *skin changes* of scleroderma.
- Tell the examiners that you would take a detailed *drug* and *occupational* history (*pneumoconiosis*—asbestosis, silicosis; *hypersensitivity pneumonitis*—farmers, bird keepers).
- *Sarcoidosis* should always be considered, but fibrosis is not present in its more common triad of bilateral hilar lymphadenopathy, erythema nodosum and arthralgia.

Assess severity

Tell the examiners that you would like to know the results of pulmonary function tests (page 114), which would show a restrictive pattern.

Evidence of decompensation

In advanced CFA there may be *central cyanosis* and signs of *cor pulmonale* (page 13).

Look for/consider associated diseases

- Bronchial carcinoma develops in up to 15% of patients with CFA.
- Connective tissue diseases (rheumatoid arthritis, SLE, scleroderma, polymyositis) are more common in patients with CFA. You might ask about *Raynaud's phenomenon*.

DISCUSSION	

What do you know about the histopathology of CFA?

Also known as idiopathic pulmonary fibrosis (IPF), there is a spectrum from inflammatory/cellular alveolitis (*desquamative interstitial pneumonitis—DIP*) to more advanced inflammation with fibrosis (*usual interstitial pneumonitis—UIP*). UIP is much more common. The end stage is severe fibrosis with honeycomb scarring radiographically.

What investigations are useful in CFA?

Investigations in CFA are described in Box 2.4.

What is the overall prognosis in CFA?

Poor. The importance of tests supporting an inflammatory picture is that there is likely to be a better response to steroids and immunosuppression.

| Box 2.4 | Investigating Cryptogenic Fibrosing Alveolitis |

1. *Spirometry* shows a restrictive lung defect (RLD, page 114) with impaired gas transfer.
2. In early disease hypoxia may only be present following exertion.
3. *Autoantibodies* against rheumatoid factor (RF) or antinuclear antibodies (ANA) are positive in low titre in around one-third of patients.
4. The *chest X-ray* invariably shows diffuse interstitial shadowing in CFA, with or without honeycombing.
5. *CT scanning* is helpful in distinguishing CFA from other causes of diffuse parenchymal lung disease and in determining disease extent and activity. CFA is generally a disease of the periphery. A predominantly *ground glass* pattern on CT suggests more cellular, inflammatory disease *(with a greater likelihood of response to treatment)*, whereas a predominantly *reticular* pattern suggests fibrosis.
6. With *bronchoalveolar lavage* (BAL), lymphocytic fluid tends to be associated with inflammation, whereas neutrophilic fluid tends not to correlate with the histopathological abnormality.
7. *Open lung biopsy* (rather than transbronchial biopsy because disease is peripheral) may be indicated if patients are young, if no specific diagnosis can be made or if there are systemic symptoms or extrapulmonary signs.

What treatments are there for CFA?

- Steroids are widely used to treat CFA (often with azathioprine) and may improve symptoms and pulmonary function, although evidence for improved survival is limited. Treatment is generally reserved for patients with a ground glass appearance on CT scan (Box 2.4), or patients with symptoms or deterioration on pulmonary function testing. Cyclophosphamide or ciclosporin are sometimes used.
- Antifibrotic agents are still under evaluation (fibroblast proliferation appears to occur from the earliest stages of disease).
- Sudden deterioration may be due to superadded infection or pulmonary emboli, which should be looked for and treated.
- Cor pulmonale is treated with diuretics and oxygen.

What other causes of pulmonary fibrosis are there?

1. **Connective tissue disease:**
   - Rheumatoid arthritis/disease ● Systemic sclerosis ● SLE ● Polymyositis/dermatomyositis ● Mixed connective tissue disease ● Ankylosing spondylitis.
2. **Drugs** (over 100 have been implicated):
   - Chemotherapy agents (e.g. methotrexate, cyclophosphamide, busulfan, bleomycin) ● Amiodarone ● Sulfasalazine, gold ● Antibiotics (e.g. sulphonamides, nitrofurantoin).

3. *Radiotherapy.*
4. *Pneumoconioses (inorganic dust disease):*
   - Asbestosis ● Coal worker's pneumoconiosis ● Silicosis
   - Berylliosis.
5. *Hypersensitivity pneumonitis (organic dust disease)—also called extrinsic allergic alveolitis (EAA).*
6. *Sarcoidosis*
7. *Other:*
   - Cystic/nodular lung disease (Langerhans' cell histiocytosis, lymphangioleiomyomatosis, tuberous sclerosis) ● Lymphangitis carcinomatosis ● Cryptogenic organising pneumonia (COP)
   - Pulmonary vasculitis ● Pulmonary eosinophilia.

What are the effects of asbestos on the lung?

Patients with asbestos related disease may have a history of work in shipbuilding, lagging, building, docks, or factories engaged in the manufacture of asbestos products. Effects on the lung include:

Asbestosis

- Usually occurs > 20 years after exposure
- Generally proportional to intensity of exposure
- Characterised by exertional dyspnoea, dry cough, inspiratory crackles in lower zones
- Chest X-ray may show irregular opacities, and with more advanced disease honeycombing
- Pulmonary function tests (PFTs) reveal restrictive lung disease (page 113) with a reduced transfer factor and coefficient (pages 116–118)
- Lung cancer is increased synergistically with smoking, and the risk of mesothelioma is markedly increased
- Patients are eligible for industrial injury benefit.

Benign pleural disease

The following may occur:
- Plaques ● Diffuse pleural thickening ● Effusion ● Calcification.

These changes generally occur > 20 years after low intensity exposure and may affect not just the parietal pleura, but also the pericardium and mediastinum. Benign pleural disease is usually asymptomatic and detected on chest X-ray. Patients are usually ineligible for industrial injury benefit.

Mesothelioma

- Malignant pleural (and more rarely peritoneal) disease
- Usually latent period > 30 years
- Almost always caused by asbestos
- High risk asbestos is crocidolite (blue asbestos), followed by amosite (brown asbestos) then crysolite (white asbestos)

- Diagnosis is confirmed by pleural biopsy
- Patients are eligible for industrial injury benefit.

What do you know about coal worker's pneumoconiosis (CWP)?

This is related to total dust exposure. It is characterised by small rounded opacities (< 1.5 mm) on chest X-ray with or without focal emphysema. This is usually asymptomatic.

Progressive massive fibrosis (PMF) refers to the development of larger opacities (> 1 cm) on a background of simple CWP, usually in the upper zones and which may cavitate. PMF results in cough, sputum, dyspnoea and progressive respiratory failure.

In *Caplan's syndrome*, multiple rounded pulmonary nodules develop in patients with rheumatoid arthritis and CWP. There may be pleural effusions and calcification.

What do you know about silicosis?

This is caused by silicon dioxide, which is highly fibrogenic. Silicosis is discussed on pages 119–120.

What is hypersensitivity pneumonitis/extrinsic allergic alveolitis (EAA)?

This is a group of diseases triggered by hypersensitivity to inhaled antigens, usually the spores of microorganisms.

A vast array of types of EAA have been described, including farmer's lung (exposure to *Micropolyspora faeni*) and bird fancier's lung (exposure to avian proteins).

Some patients develop an early immune complex mediated *acute alveolitis* (type III hypersensitivity – page 203) within hours of exposure. There is dyspnoea, which may progress if the triggering agent is not removed, often with fever and myalgia. Other patients develop a delayed cell mediated *chronic alveolitis* (type IV hypersensitivity – page 203).

EAA tends to cause neutrophilia (not eosinophilia), especially acutely, and with time serum precipitins become detectable.

What is sarcoidosis?

Sarcoidosis is a multisystem granulomatous disease. Granulomata contain macrophages, lymphocytes, epithelioid cells and histiocytes, fused to form multinucleate giant cells. The cause is unknown.

1. **Acute sarcoidosis** (granulomatous 'jelly'). This commonly presents as a triad of: (i) bilateral hilar lymphadenopathy (BHL); (ii) erythema nodosum; (iii) arthralgia. This triad is benign, resolving over weeks, and tends to occur in Caucasians.
2. **Chronic sarcoidosis** (granulomatous 'shoe leather'). This commonly presents as pulmonary fibrosis or lupus pernio (page 436).

Any organ may be affected by sarcoidosis. Important complications include hypercalcaemia, seizures, bilateral facial nerve palsy, cardiac conduction defects, painless lymphadenopathy, splenomegaly, hepatic infiltration (liver disease is often asymptomatic but biopsy diagnostic) and anterior uveitis.

List some causes of upper zone lung fibrosis
- Pneumoconioses (except asbestosis) ● Extrinsic allergic alveolitis
- TB ● Allergic bronchopulmonary aspergillosis (ABPA)
- Ankylosing spondylitis.

List some causes of lower zone lung fibrosis
- Cryptogenic fibrosing alveolitis ● Asbestosis.

CASE STUDY | 2.7 PULMONARY VASCULAR DISEASE

Instruction: *This patient is thought to have pulmonary hypertension. Please examine her and report the signs you find.*

RECOGNITION

Look for the signs of *pulmonary hypertension* (Box 2.2).

INTERPRETATION

Look for/consider causes

Primary pulmonary hypertension tends to affect younger women. The pathophysiology is uncertain, but there is almost certainly an imbalance of vasoactive endothelial molecules promoting vasoconstriction.

Pulmonary hypertension is more commonly *secondary* to:

- Parenchymal lung disease or airway disease with hypoxia (*cor pulmonale*).
- Pulmonary emboli. Covert, recurrent pulmonary emboli are not unusual in the elderly (*history of stepwise breathlessness*).
- Left heart disease, such as mitral stenosis (Case study 5.1).

DISCUSSION

How might you diagnose pulmonary embolus (PE)?

Diagnostic steps are described in Box 2.5.

Pre-test clinical probability strongly modifies the positive and negative predictive value of any test and also applies to diagnosing deep venous thrombosis (Case study 8.18). A single negative ultrasound may be sufficient to exclude a DVT in a patient with a low clinical probability. D-dimer assays have also been used to help corroborate ultrasound results. Again, angiography is the gold standard.

Box 2.5	Diagnosing Pulmonary Embolus

1. The first step is an *index of suspicion. Predisposing factors* include immobilisation, age > 40 years, recent surgery or trauma, thrombophilia (page 470), previous venous thromboembolism (VTE), pregnancy/puerperium, obesity, oestrogens (oral contraceptives and hormone replacement therapy increase the relative risk but have a very low impact on absolute risk), malignancy, cardiovascular disease/heart failure and nephrotic syndrome (renal loss of antithrombin and other natural anticoagulants).

2. Suggestive *symptoms and signs* include dyspnoea, tachypnoea, pleuritic chest pain, pleural rub, haemoptysis and sinus tachycardia. Haemoptysis is rare. There may be signs of a deep venous thrombosis (Case study 8.18), including unilateral leg swelling/pitting oedema, tenderness and warmth.

3. *Investigations* can be especially difficult to interpret where there is pre-existing lung disease. Where there are significant chest X-ray changes from *pre-existing lung disease*, ventilation/perfusion (V/Q) scanning may be difficult to interpret and *spiral CT scanning* or *pulmonary angiography* (which remains the gold standard but is more invasive) may be more appropriate. Spiral CT is likely to miss the small percentage of patients with small, segmental pulmonary emboli. Some advocate the use of D-dimer testing prior to a gold standard test. The D-dimer test is sensitive for degradation products of thrombi, but not specific. Hence, if negative, some physicians feel this sufficient evidence to rule out thrombus.

4. In patients with previously *normal lungs, V/Q scanning* is more reliable, and the result is reported as low, intermediate or high probability. In general, an alternative diagnosis should be sought in patients with low probability (but PE is never 100% excluded), anticoagulation is needed for patients with high probability, and patients with an intermediate result may proceed to spiral CT scanning or angiography.

5. These recommendations apply to stable patients. Unstable patients, presenting with the syndrome of hypotension and elevated jugular venous pressure, may need urgent anticoagulation or thrombolysis if they have massive/submassive PE, but also urgent ECG/echocardiography to exclude right ventricular infarction, global dyskinesis from an extensive acute coronary syndrome or tamponade.

What is the treatment for venous thromboembolism (VTE)?

As a general rule, anticoagulation with unfractionated or low molecular weight heparin (LMWH) is indicated for patients with clinically suspected VTE. Warfarin is commenced in non-pregnant patients with confirmed VTE, aiming for an international normalised ratio (INR) in the range 2–3 following a first episode, and continued for at least 3 months, the overall duration depending upon the presence or absence of ongoing risk factors.

Should there be an overlap between warfarin introduction and heparin withdrawal?

Yes. Heparin should be continued for a few days after warfarin has been introduced. Warfarin inhibits hepatic synthesis of prothrombotic factors II, VII, IX and X, but also inhibits the production of the natural anticoagulant promoter protein C and its cofactor protein S. The half-life of proteins C and S is short, and thus in the first few days of warfarin therapy a state of procoagulation may be induced, especially in patients with underlying protein C or S deficiency.

CASE STUDY   2.8 PLEURAL EFFUSION AND PLEURAL DISEASE

Instruction: *Examine this patient's chest and discuss your findings.*

RECOGNITION

The *trachea* is *deviated to the opposite side* (if large pleural effusion). There is *stony dullness* to percussion. *Breath sounds* and *vocal resonance* are *reduced*.

INTERPRETATION

Confirm the diagnosis

The differential diagnosis of dullness at the lung base includes:

- *Consolidation* (*bronchial breath sounds and increased vocal resonance* because sound travels well through solid lung). Bronchial breathing may be absent if there is complete obstruction of a bronchus with collapse.
- *Collapse* (*absent breath sounds*, *trachea* may be *deviated to side of collapse*).
- Raised hemidiaphragm (due to *hepatomegaly*).
- Pleural thickening.

Look for/consider causes

Transudate (< 3 g/L protein)

- Cardiac failure (*raised JVP, sacral or pulmonary oedema, third heart sound*)

- Nephrotic syndrome (*generalised/facial/periorbital oedema*)
- Hepatic failure (*signs of chronic liver disease* – Box 3.1, page 41); note that in addition to hypoproteinaemia, right sided diaphragmatic lymphatic channels may open secondary to ascites and contribute to the effusion
- Hypothyroidism (*myxoedematous face*)
- Meig's syndrome, with benign ovarian fibroma
- Yellow nail syndrome (yellow nails and lymphatic hypoplasia).

Exudate (> 3 g/L protein)

- Bronchial carcinoma/mesothelioma (*cachexia, clubbing, tar staining*)
- Pneumonia (signs of *consolidation*)
- Tuberculosis
- Pulmonary embolus/infarction (*pleural rub, signs of DVT?*)
- Autoimmune/connective tissue disease, e.g. SLE (*malar rash*), rheumatoid arthritis (*rheumatoid hands*)
- Subphrenic abscess.

DISCUSSION

What investigations would you consider?

- Chest X-ray (AP and lateral). The earliest radiological sign is blunting of the costophrenic angle which may require the presence of at least 300 ml of fluid.
- Pleurocentesis.
- Pleural biopsy (essential).
- Ultrasound of abdomen (for hepatic cause) or chest ultrasound to confirm effusion and determine if loculated.
- CT chest/bronchoscopy/blood tests depending on likely cause.

Which tests on pleural fluid can help diagnostically?

Biochemistry

- Protein concentration pleural fluid : serum > 0.5 favours an exudate.
- Lactate dehydrogenase (LDH) pleural fluid : serum > 0.6 favours an exudate.

Microbiology

- Highly cellular fluid favours an exudate.

Cytology

- Neutrophil counts are high in a parapneumonic effusion.
- Lymphocyte counts are raised in malignancy, TB and autoimmune causes.
- Malignant cells may be present.
- The presence of blood may indicate malignancy, pulmonary infarction or TB.

What is a pleural rub?

> A superficial scratching/grating/creaking sound on deep inspiration (like the crackle of leaves underfoot on an autumn forest floor, or the crunching underfoot of freshly fallen snow!). A pleural rub sounds 'close to the stethoscope' and does not change with coughing. Common causes include pneumonia and pulmonary emboli.

What are the clinical signs of a pneumothorax?

> - Decreased chest movement on the affected side
> - Tracheal deviation to the contralateral side
> - Decreased breath sounds on the affected side
> - Increased vocal resonance on the affected side.

How might you classify pneumothoraces?

> - Small (rim of air around lung)
> - Moderate (lung collapses towards the heart border)
> - Complete (an airless lung, separated from the diaphragm).
>
> Any pneumothorax may be under tension (airflow through a 'one-way' valve into the pleural space can cause rapid cardiorespiratory compromise demanding immediate drainage).

List some causes of a pneumothorax

> - Spontaneous (especially tall, thin males)
> - Trauma
> - Asthma/COPD
> - Lung cancer
> - Pneumonia/TB
> - Cystic fibrosis
> - Mechanical ventilation
> - Marfan's syndrome
> - Catamenial (associated with menstruation)
> - Rare cystic/nodular lung diseases may cause spontaneous pneumothoraces—Langerhan's cell histiocytosis, lymphangioleiomyomatosis, tuberous sclerosis.

CASE STUDY   2.9 OBSTRUCTIVE SLEEP APNOEA (OSA)

Instruction: *This 54-year-old man was recently in a road traffic accident. He says that he doesn't recall what happened, but he thinks he must have 'blacked out' at the wheel. Your neurology and cardiology colleagues have investigated his loss of consciousness but have not found a cause. Please examine him and discuss your findings and management.*

RECOGNITION

> The patient is *overweight*. He may be *plethoric* or *cyanosed*. Tell the examiners that you would wish to know his body mass index (BMI – page 193).

INTERPRETATION

Confirm the diagnosis

Tell the examiners that you would ask about daytime somnolence, impaired concentration, irritability and mood disturbance. A history of snoring/apnoeas from a bed partner is helpful.

Look for/consider causes

- Hypothyroidism (*myxoedematous face*)
- Acromegaly (*facial features, large hands*)
- Craniofacial abnormalities.

Evidence of decompensation

Systemic hypertension and cor pulmonale may be associated with OSA. Ask to take the patient's *blood pressure* and consider whether or not the *signs of cor pulmonale* (page 13) are present.

DISCUSSION

What do you understand by the term OSA?

OSA refers to recurrent episodes of complete or partial airway obstruction during sleep. *Obstructive apnoea* is defined by cessation of airflow for > 10 seconds with continued respiratory effort. *Obstructive hypopnoea* refers to reduction, rather than cessation, of airflow. The consequences are impaired sleep quality and potential cardiovascular complications.

The most important symptom is daytime sleepiness (measured by Epworth score), although concentration problems and mood disturbances are common. Somnolence correlates with the amount of sleep fragmentation rather than nocturnal episodes of hypoxia; this is because apnoeic episodes are associated with arousal (demonstrated by electroencephalography) and impede entry into deeper phases of refreshing sleep.

The increased risk of road traffic accidents is significant. The risk of cardiovascular complications attributable to OSA has been difficult to quantify because obese patients already have a higher risk of hypertension and cardiovascular disease.

Partial collapse of the pharynx may also occur in the absence of apnoeic episodes, sufficient to disrupt sleep but not to trigger hypoxia.

What is the place of a sleep study?

Full polysomnography, which includes detailed recordings of electroencephalography (EEG) and electromyography (EMG), oximetry, oronasal airflow, respiratory effort and snoring, has been the gold standard. In practice more limited nocturnal recording is sufficient for diagnosis. Oximetery alone is insufficient because of the high false negative rate (in patients with partial obstruction but without hypoxia) and the high false positive rate (in patients with coexisting lung disease such as COPD).

Snoring per se is insufficient evidence for OSA and not an indication for a sleep study. An additional symptom, such as daytime somnolence, nocturnal choking or witnessed apnoeas, is an indication.

What management options are available for OSA?

General measures include weight reduction, smoking cessation and alcohol reduction. An ENT opinion may be sought if local nasopharyngeal pathology is thought to be a possible cause. Dental splints have been used to pull the jaw forward. Continuous positive airways pressure (CPAP) is the most effective therapy to date.

REFERENCES AND FURTHER READING

Armstrong P, Vincent JM. Staging non-small cell lung cancer. Clin Radiol 1993; 48(1):1–10.

British Thoracic Society Guidelines (Asthma, COPD, Community Acquired Pneumonia, Pulmonary Embolus). Online. Available: www.brit-thoracic.org.uk.

British Thoracic Society Recommendations. The diagnosis, assessment and treatment of diffuse parenchymal lung disease in adults. Thorax 1999; 54: (suppl 1).

Department of Health. Manual of lung cancer. Online. Avalable: www.doh.gov.uk/cancer/pdfs/lungmanual.pdf

Mountain CF. Revisions in the international system for staging lung cancer. Chest 1997; 111:1710–1717.

Scottish Intercollegiate Guidelines Network. Lower respiratory tract infection in adults. Edinburgh: SIGN 2002. Online. Available: www.sign.ac.uk.

3. ABDOMINAL SYSTEM

EXAMINATION: ABDOMINAL SYSTEM

Your patient should be lying comfortably supine, one pillow supporting the head, arms rested at the sides. The patient should be exposed from xiphisternum to pubic symphysis.

Inspection

1. Look at the skin for *jaundice, pallor* or *pigmentation* (haemochromatosis).
2. Look at the face, notably the sclera for *jaundice*, the eyelids for *xanthelasmata* (primary biliary cirrhosis) and the mouth for ulceration (Crohn's disease).
3. Look at the trunk for *gynaecomastia* and *spider naevi*.
4. Look at the hands for other *signs of chronic liver disease* (Box 3.1).
5. Look at the abdomen for *scars*, localised or generalised *swellings*, abnormal *pulsation* or *distended veins*. *Caput medusa* refers to veins radiating from the umbilicus and suggests portal hypertension.

Palpation

1. Ask if there is any pain or tenderness.
2. Palpate with your arm parallel to the patient's abdomen, kneeling at the bedside.
3. With the palmar aspect of the fingers of your right hand (fingers flexed gently at the metacarpophalangeal joints, finger pulps rather than tips making contact), palpate the nine regions—*right iliac fossa (RIF), hypogastrium, left iliac fossa (LIF), left flank, umbilical region, right flank, right hypochondrium, epigastrium, left hypochondrium*. Many candidates do not appreciate that gentle, superficial palpation often yields more information than deeper palpation. You should of course palpate more deeply for masses.
4. Note if the abdomen is generally soft, and note any *masses*, which you should attempt to describe with respect to *site, size, shape, surface, fixation or mobility to the skin or with respiration, tenderness and pulsatility*.
5. Examine specifically for liver, spleen or kidney enlargement (Fig. 3.1).

Liver

The normal liver may be palpable 2 cm below the costal margin, displacing downwards on deep inspiration to meet the finger pulps and radial border of your right hand. It *enlarges downwards*. Measure enlargement in centimetres from the costal margin.

Spleen

The spleen *enlarges towards the RIF*. It has a *medial notch*. An important discriminating feature of an enlarged spleen is that it is *not possible to feel its upper border*. Rolling your patient onto their right side may detect mild to moderate splenomegaly. Bimanual palpation of the spleen (Fig. 3.1) is preferred, although the purpose of the left hand is more that of steadying the patient than feeling the spleen, which is protected largely by the ribs posterolaterally.

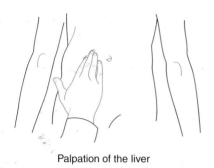

Palpation of the liver

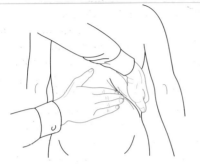

Palpation of the spleen

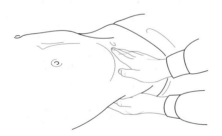

Palpation of the right kidney

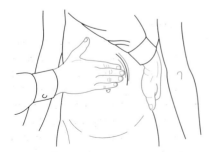

Palpation of the left kidney

Fig. 3.1 *Palpation for abdominal organomegaly*

Kidneys

Palpate for these bimanually and by ballottement. Ballottement refers to a 'flicking' movement in which the lower hand, in the renal angle, pushes the kidney towards the upper hand anteriorly. The kidneys are normally only palpable in thin subjects. They move with respiration and may appear resonant because of overlying bowel.

Other masses

Normal masses sometimes found include the normal liver edge, the kidneys, the aorta, the rectus abdominis, hard faeces, a distended bladder and small inguinal lymph nodes. Abnormal masses include carcinoma of colon/caecum (RIF), ovarian masses (RIF or LIF), carcinoma of the stomach or pancreas (epigastrium), lymphoma or secondary lymphadenopathy (hard, often bulky masses arising at any site) and abdominal aortic aneurysms, characterised by pulsatility.

Percussion

1. Percuss over the liver. The rib level of the upper border varies with the phase of respiration and the lower border is just below the costal margin.
2. Percuss over the spleen. The lower border is not palpable in normal circumstances.
3. Percuss for *shifting dullness* if you suspect *ascites* (generalised abdominal swelling):
(i) Firstly confirm ascites by percussing from the umbilicus (resonant unless ascites is massive and tense) to the flanks (stony dull).
(ii) Secondly ask the patient to roll onto their left side whilst marking (or keeping your finger over) the resonant–dull interface. Fluid from the right side further fills the left flank and the area of dullness extends towards the umbilicus.

4. In patients with large volume ascites, a *fluid thrill* may be elicited by tapping one flank and feeling transmission of the fluid wave to the other. An assistant's hand on the centre of the abdomen limits transmission of the wave through the abdominal wall.

Auscultation

Auscultate for bowel sounds, bruits (renal bruits are often heard over the epigastrium) and a venous hum (rare, but almost pathognomonic of portal hypertension).

Complete abdominal examination, not performed in PACES, includes examination of hernial orifices, genitalia and rectum.

REVISION: FAILURE OF LIVER FUNCTION

Many abdominal cases in PACES represent liver disease, and a brief revision of failure of liver function is useful for these cases.

Hepatocellular failure and hepatic decompensation

Histologically the liver is made up of hepatic lobules. Each lobule contains a *central hepatic vein*, a *peripheral portal 'triad'* comprising bile duct and branches of the portal vein and hepatic artery, and *hepatocytes* (liver cells) which run between the two.

Functionally, the liver is divided into *acini* which centre on the portal triad. The zone around the central vein sustains injury in venous congestion (as in right heart failure) whilst in hepatitis/cirrhosis damage starts at the portal triads and spreads outwards in 'ripples'.

The liver is integral to metabolising carbohydrate, fat and protein. Whilst liver enzymes are useful in assessing the cause of jaundice, serum *bilirubin*, serum *albumin* and a *prothrombin time* are a better reflection of synthetic liver function.

Most insults to the liver bring the threat of necrosis and liver failure. The end result of a wide range of causes of liver failure, from the causes of fulminant and acute liver failure to those of decompensated chronic liver disease and cirrhosis, can be similar—a series of functional changes which lead to the features in Box 3.1 (point C). Circulatory changes (hyperdynamic circulation, peripheral vasodilatation) and

---

Box 3.1 Signs of Chronic Liver Disease (CLD)

There are many signs of chronic liver disease and it can be difficult to classify them. One useful way is to consider *three categories of signs*:

A. General signs of chronic liver disease
These may include:

- *Jaundice*
- *Scratch marks* secondary to itch
- *Pallor/anaemia*
- *Cyanosis* (due to pulmonary venous shunts)
- *Purpura*
- *Spider naevi*

- *Gynaecomastia*
- *Paucity of body hair*
- *Testicular atrophy*
- *Muscle wasting*
- *Non-specific signs of chronic liver disease in the hands.* These may include, in addition to some of those signs above, *clubbing, leuconychia, koilonychia (chronic iron deficiency from blood loss), palmar erythema and a flapping tremor (asterixis)*
- *Hepatomegaly* (in cirrhosis the liver may be small or large and nodular due to regeneration. It may also be enlarged by acute inflammation)

B. Signs which suggest an underlying cause

Many of these are not signs of liver disease itself. They include:

- *Dupuytren's contracture, parotid hypertrophy* (alcohol)
- *Tattoos* or *'non-medical' needle track marks* (viral hepatitis)
- *Associated autoimmune disease e.g. hypothyroidism* (autoimmune hepatitis)
- *Xanthelasmata* (primary biliary cirrhosis)
- *Slate grey pigmentation* (haemochromatosis)
- *Kayser–Fleischer ring* (Wilson's disease)
- *Signs of obstructive airways disease* (alpha-1 antitrypsin deficiency)

C. General signs of hepatic decompensation

Hepatic decompensation can occur in both chronic and acute liver disease. The main signs are:

- *Jaundice* (Case study 3.1)
- Evidence of *hepatic encephalopathy* (e.g. asterixis, see below)
- *Ascites* (Case study 3.2)
- Evidence of *bleeding* (e.g. purpura, page 43)
- Evidence of *portal hypertension* (page 43). Portal hypertension is a major complication of cirrhosis (not necessarily decompensated), and signs of portal hypertension such as caput medusa and splenomegaly are not in themselves signs of hepatic decompensation. Variceal bleeding is the most important complication of portal hypertension, usually presenting with haematemesis and diagnosed endoscopically

a propensity to fever and sepsis are also problems in hepatocellular failure.

The extraordinary capacity for hepatic regeneration must be overcome if these changes are to occur. Jaundice, for example, is common in acute hepatitis because the speed of onset does not allow time for regeneration. Jaundice tends to occur in chronic liver disease either when hepatic reserve is exhausted or when an acute insult compromises an already limited regenerative capacity.

Jaundice

Jaundice is discussed in Case study 3.1.

Hepatic encephalopathy

The pathogenesis of hepatic encephalopathy is multifactorial:

1. Gut derived substances fail to be cleared because of hepatocellular failure and may be directly shunted to the brain through the portosystemic veins which open up when portal vein pressure is high (especially in CLD).
2. Impaired protein metabolism leads to build up of neuroactive toxins impairing neurotransmission.

That metabolic changes account for hepatic encephalopathy is supported by its tendency for reversibility. The clinical picture is complex and may include, in approximate order of onset, the features in Box 3.2.

Acute decompensation of liver disease may be induced by the following reversible factors:

- Gastrointestinal bleeding ● Drugs, especially sedatives ● Sepsis (including spontaneous bacterial peritonitis) ● Other catabolic states, such as surgery or trauma ● Transjugular intrahepatic portosystemic shunting (page 44) ● Fluid and electrolyte imbalance (vomiting, diuretics, large volume paracentesis) ● Constipation ● High protein intake.

Box 3.2   Clinical Features of Hepatic Encephalopathy

- Mild confusion
- Mood or behavioural change, especially flattening of affect
- Asterixis or 'flapping tremor' (metabolic myoclonus)
- Apraxia, notably constructional apraxia (inability to draw a five-pointed star) and impaired handwriting

- Dysarthria
- Drowsiness
- Hyperreflexia or hyporeflexia
- Coma and decerebrate posturing

Ascites

Ascites is discussed in Case study 3.2.

Bleeding

Bleeding is common in liver disease and has numerous causes:

- A prolonged prothrombin time (PT) consequent upon depletion of prothrombin and other coagulation factors (II,VII,IX,X) in impaired synthetic function.
- Thrombocytopenia due to splenomegaly and hypersplenism.
- Portal venous bleeding in portal hypertension.
- Gastritis and peptic ulceration associated with alcohol induced liver disease.

Portal hypertension

The portal vein enters the liver at the porta hepatis and sends a branch to each lobe. It receives blood from all veins draining the abdominal part of the gastrointestinal tract and is formed from the union of the superior mesenteric vein and the splenic vein. Normal portal flow rate is about 1–1.5 L/min with a pressure of 5–10 mmHg.

When portal flow is obstructed, either from within or outwith the liver, collateral circulation develops to carry blood into systemic veins (portosystemic shunting) Two problems then arise:

1. The liver's metabolic function is bypassed
2. Increasing pressure in collaterals (termed *varices*) causes bleeding.

Varices are commonly oesophageal, derived from the left gastric vein. There are multiple layers of veins in the oesophagus and varices usually develop in the deep intrinsic layer. Varices occur at other sites including the stomach, colon and rectum.

Hyperdynamic circulation accompanies portal hypertension and may in part develop to maintain portal flow as collaterals lower the pressure.

Causes of portal hypertension may be:

- *Prehepatic* (e.g. portal vein thrombosis, extrinsic compression)
- *Hepatic* (cirrhosis, acute hepatitis, congenital hepatic fibrosis)

Box 3.3   Clinical Consequences of Portal Hypertension

1. *Gastrointestinal bleeding*, often the first indication of varices
2. *Caput medusae*
3. *Venous hum*
4. *Splenomegaly* (but size correlates poorly with portal pressure)
5. *Secondary hypersplenism* (can cause peripheral blood cytopenias)

- *Posthepatic* (e.g. hepatic vein thrombosis/ Budd–Chiari syndrome, constrictive pericarditis).

Clinical consequences of portal hypertension are shown in Box 3.3.

Management of varices is discussed in Box 3.4.

Prognosis in hepatocellular failure

Prognosis in liver failure correlates with the severity of:

- Hyperbilirubinaemia (mmol/L) ● Encephalopathy ● Ascites ● Hypoalbuminaemia (g/L) ● Prothrombin time derangement.

Box 3.4   Management of Varices

1. *Resuscitation* includes urgent cross matching and initial restoration of circulating volume with colloid and 5% dextrose. Saline may aggravate ascites. Elderly patients or those with cardiac failure may need pulmonary artery wedge pressure monitoring. Fresh frozen plasma and vitamin K may be needed to correct coagulopathy. Platelet transfusion may be needed in thrombocytopenia.

2. *Octreotide*, a somatostatin analogue, reduces splanchnic flow and may be given as an intravenous infusion, aiding diagnostic and therapeutic endoscopy when there is active bleeding.

3. *Endoscopic sclerotherapy* involves injection of a sclerosant solution into a bleeding varix or its overlying mucosa. The former obliterates the varix lumen by thrombosis, the latter induces inflammation and fibrosis.

4. *Endoscopic band ligation* eradicates varices with fewer treatment sessions and complications than sclerotherapy.

5. *Balloon tamponade* may be life saving in patients with acute variceal bleeding either where sclerotherapy or banding is unavailable or where bleeding is too brisk to undertake the procedure.

6. *Transjugular intrahepatic portosystemic shunting (TIPS)* can be life saving for patients whose bleeding remains uncontrolled by endoscopic measures. The recurrence rate is up to 50% and the risk of encephalopathy up to 25%. Therefore its primary role is that of rescue or as a bridge to subsequent liver transplantation.

7. *Long-term secondary prophylaxis*, by repeated endoscopic treatment or with beta-blockers, reduces portal pressure and lowers the risk of subsequent bleeding. All patients without contraindications should be considered for beta-blockers, aiming to reduce portal pressure to < 12 mmHg.

8. All patients with cirrhosis should be screened by endoscopy, large varices meriting *primary prophylaxis* with beta-blockers.

CASE STUDY   3.1 JAUNDICE

Instruction: *Please look at this patient's skin and examine his/her abdomen. Discuss your findings.*

RECOGNITION

Jaundice is present. (Jaundice is most apparent in fluid/tissues with high protein concentration such as cerebrospinal/ocular fluid and elastic tissue—skin, sclera, blood vessel walls. Conjugated hyperbilirubinaemia tends to produce more intense jaundice because of its water solubility.)

INTERPRETATION

Look for/consider causes

Jaundice may be prehepatic, hepatic (hepatocellular) or posthepatic (cholestatic). The bilirubin pathway is discussed below.

Prehepatic

Look for *anaemia*.

Increased bilirubin load on hepatocytes, usually due to haemolysis, gives rise to anaemia, an elevated reticulocyte count, decreased haptoglobin levels and unconjugated hyperbilirubinaemia. Liver enzymes and synthetic liver function tests are otherwise normal.

Hepatocellular

Look for *signs of chronic liver disease* (Box 3.1).

Failure of the liver cell to take up, metabolise or excrete bilirubin may result from:

- Gilbert's syndrome and other enzymopathies (page 47)
- Acute hepatitis (alcohol, viral or drugs or toxins)
- Cirrhosis.

There is both unconjugated and conjugated hyperbilirubinaemia with deranged liver enzymes (transaminases tending to rise in greater proportion to alkaline phosphatase) and synthetic liver function tests. The enzyme rise may be very high in acute hepatitis on a background of a normal liver, but less in cirrhosis where fewer hepatocytes remain to be destroyed.

Cholestatic

Look for *cachexia*. Tell the examiners that you would ask about symptoms in relation to fatty meals and take a drug history.

Obstruction to bilirubin excretion may result from:

- Cholelithiasis ● Carcinoma of the pancreas or bile ducts
- Lymphadenopathy ● Drugs

There is conjugated hyperbilirubinaemia and a rise in alkaline phosphatase in greater proportion to a rise in transaminases.

Frequently an insult will cause a combination of hepatocellular failure and cholestasis (e.g. primary biliary cirrhosis) and the biochemical abnormalities in any of the above states may precede jaundice.

Evidence of decompensation

Look for signs of hepatic decompensation (Box 3.1, point C).

DISCUSSION

Give an overview of bilirubin metabolism

Bilirubin is the *end product of haem metabolism*, bound to haptoglobin in serum. Most bilirubin comes from the haemoglobin of destroyed red blood cells, but a small amount is from other haem proteins such as myoglobin.

Unconjugated bilirubin is bound to albumin, lipid soluble and transported to liver cell receptors before entering the liver cell. It is *conjugated* in the endoplasmic reticulum *by uridine diphosphate glucuronosyl transferase (UDPGT)*. Different forms of UDPGT exist but UDPGT$_1$ is predominant. Expression of the UDPGT gene sequence is

Fig. 3.2   *Bilirubin metabolic pathway (insert: conjugation process)*

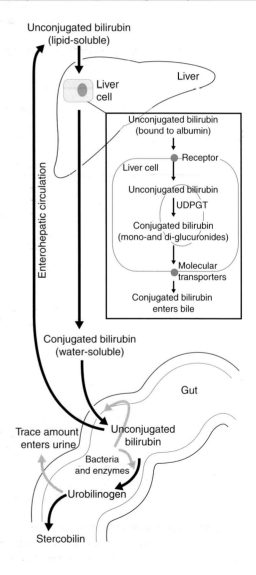

promoted by a 'promotor of transcription region' in a nearby exon containing the nucleotide sequence *TATAA*.

The conjugation process converts unconjugated bilirubin into conjugated *bilirubin mono- and diglucuronides*. These conjugated molecules are *transported out of the liver cell by molecular transporters* (Fig. 3.2).

Conjugated bilirubin glucuronides are water soluble and so poorly reabsorbed when they reach the intestine. Most are *hydrolysed back to unconjugated bilirubin* and *reduced to urobilinogen* by gut enzymes and subsequently converted to *stercobilin*. *Small amounts of remanufactured unconjugated bilirubin and urobilinogen are reabsorbed through the enterohepatic circulation. A trace of reabsorbed urobilinogen ends up in the urine.*

In what forms may hyperbilirubinaemia be detectable in the urine?

It follows from above that hyperbilirubinaemia may be detectable in the urine in various ways, outlined in Box 3.5.

Box 3.5	Hyperbilirubinaemia and the Urine

1. *Normally*, bilirubin is not present in the urine, except as traces of urobilinogen.
2. In *unconjugated hyperbilirubinaemia* or prehepatic jaundice (overuse of normal pathways), bilirubin is only detectable in the urine as increased levels of urobilinogen.
3. In *conjugated hyperbilirubinaemia* when outflow to the gut is obstructed, bilirubin enters the urine in its conjugated, water soluble form, giving rise to *dark urine*. The *stools are pale* because stercobilin is absent. Urobilinogen is absent from the urine.

What do you know about Gilbert's and Dubin–Johnson syndromes?

Gilbert's syndrome is a common, harmless, autosomal dominant defect of the TATAA sequence, giving rise to reduced levels of UDPTG. It results in mild, intermittent unconjugated hyperbilirubinaemia, occasionally with mild jaundice. Episodes may be precipitated by stress, fasting or intercurrent infection. It does not give rise to other abnormalities in liver function. Reassurance is all that is needed. *Crigler–Najjar syndrome* is a very rare and severe autosomal recessive defect in which UDPGT is absent.

Dubin–Johnson syndrome is a benign, autosomal recessive defect of molecular transporters responsible for transporting conjugated bilirubin out of liver cells. It gives rise to conjugated hyperbilirubinaemia and green-black liver pigmentation at autopsy.

How would you investigate cholestatic jaundice?

1. Investigation starts with ultrasound scanning to determine whether or not the bile ducts (BDs) are dilated. Dilated BDs

suggest extrahepatic cholestasis (EHC). Normal BDs suggest intrahepatic cholestasis (IHC).

2. Causes of EHC include gallstones, tumours, strictures and parasites. Causes of IHC include primary biliary cirrhosis, sclerosing cholangitis, sepsis and drugs. Endoscopic retrograde cholangiopancreatography (ERCP) or magnetic resonance cholangiopancreatography (MRCP) is an appropriate next step for EHC. Liver biopsy is more useful in IHC.

CASE STUDY 3.2 ASCITES

Instruction: *Examine this patient's abdomen and discuss your findings.*

RECOGNITION

There is *generalised swelling* (differential diagnosis fluid, fat, faeces, flatus, fetus) of the abdomen with *shifting dullness*. There may be a *fluid thrill* in tense ascites, and the umbilicus may be everted.

To palpate organs in the presence of ascites you must used a 'dipping' technique, pressing quickly, flexing at the wrist.

INTERPRETATION

Look for/consider causes

1. Chronic liver disease/cirrhosis: look for *signs of chronic liver disease* (Box 3.1, Fig. 3.3).
2. Malignancy (especially gastric, ovarian and liver metastases): look for *cachexia and lymphadenopathy*.
3. Right/biventricular failure: look for a *raised JVP* and *peripheral oedema*.
4. Nephrotic syndrome and other causes of hypoalbuminaemia. Tell the examiners you would check the *urinalysis*.
5. Rare causes include hypothyroidism, constrictive pericarditis, Meig's syndrome and serositis in familial Mediterranean fever.

Evidence of decompensation

Look for signs of hepatic decompensation (Box 3.1, point C).

DISCUSSION

What is the mechanism of ascites formation?

Over 75% of ascites is due to liver disease. The pathogenesis is uncertain but contributing factors include hypoalbuminaemia and portal hypertension. It is also likely that peripheral vasodilatation promotes sodium and water retention by stimulating the renin–angiotensin–aldosterone system.

What laboratory analysis would you request on ascitic fluid?

● Cell count and differential ● Protein, albumin and amylase concentration ● Cytology ● Gram stain and culture.

The macroscopic appearance of ascitic fluid is also important—straw coloured (most causes), turbid (pyogenic causes, TB), bloody (malignancy, TB), chylous (pancreatitis).

In chronic liver disease always consider *spontaneous bacterial peritonitis (SBP)*, diagnosed by paracentesis, microscopy and culture. Neutrophils are the predominant cells. Ascites may be minimal and detectable only by ultrasound.

What is the value of the serum : ascites albumin gradient?

Most causes of ascites are transudates (< 25 g/dL), malignancy and peritoneal TB being notable exceptions. Because diuresis affects the total ascitic protein concentration, the serum : ascites albumin gradient (SAG) is sometimes a preferred method of characterising ascites.

The SAG correlates directly with portal pressure. Patients with normal portal pressures have a gradient of < 1.1 g/dL. Conditions causing exudative ascites also tend to have a gradient < 1.1 g/dL, whereas ascites associated with heart failure, nephrotic syndrome or cirrhosis with portal hypertension usually has a gradient > 1.1 g/dL.

Is the chest X-ray ever abnormal as a consequence of ascites?

It may show a right pleural effusion because diaphragmatic channels open up and transmit fluid.

How would you treat ascites?

1. Identification and treatment of any underlying remediable cause of liver disease. Avoidance of alcohol is essential.
2. Salt restriction and diuretics, especially the aldosterone antagonist spironolactone, are central to treatment of ascites. The commonest reason for diuretic 'failure' is inadequate salt restriction. < 40–60 mmol (1–1.5 g) of salt daily is ideal but unpalatable and difficult to achieve; < 80 mmol daily is practical.
3. Therapeutic paracentesis may be necessary for tense ascites, and occasionally concurrent administration of albumin is indicated.

How might you detect the presence of a small volume of ascites?

One method is the 'tiger test' (author's term). The patient is asked to kneel down on all fours 'like a tiger', at which time percussion over the most dependent area—around the umbilicus—becomes dull. Not recommended in PACES.

| CASE STUDY | **3.3 CHRONIC LIVER DISEASE (CLD) AND CIRRHOSIS** |

Instruction: *Examine this patient's abdominal system. Discuss your findings and comment on possible causes.*

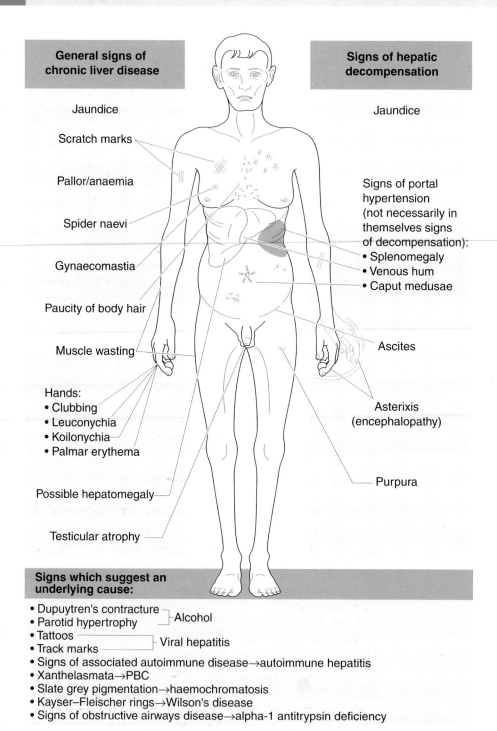

General signs of chronic liver disease

Jaundice

Scratch marks

Pallor/anaemia

Spider naevi

Gynaecomastia

Paucity of body hair

Muscle wasting

Hands:
- Clubbing
- Leuconychia
- Koilonychia
- Palmar erythema

Possible hepatomegaly

Testicular atrophy

Signs of hepatic decompensation

Jaundice

Signs of portal hypertension (not necessarily in themselves signs of decompensation):
- Splenomegaly
- Venous hum
- Caput medusae

Ascites

Asterixis (encephalopathy)

Purpura

Signs which suggest an underlying cause:

- Dupuytren's contracture ⎤
- Parotid hypertrophy   ⎦ Alcohol
- Tattoos ⎤
- Track marks ⎦ Viral hepatitis
- Signs of associated autoimmune disease→autoimmune hepatitis
- Xanthelasmata→PBC
- Slate grey pigmentation→haemochromatosis
- Kayser–Fleischer rings→Wilson's disease
- Signs of obstructive airways disease→alpha-1 antitrypsin deficiency

Fig. 3.3   *Possible signs in chronic liver disease*

RECOGNITION

Some *general signs of chronic liver disease* are present (Box 3.1, Fig. 3.3).

INTERPRETATION

Look for/consider causes

- Alcohol (*Dupuytren's contracture, parotid hypertrophy*)
- Viral hepatitis (*tattoos or 'non-medical' needle track marks*)
- Autoimmune hepatitis (associated autoimmune disease, e.g. thyroid)
- Primary biliary cirrhosis (*xanthelasmata*)
- Haemochromatosis (*slate grey pigmentation*)
- Wilson's disease (*Kayser–Fleischer rings*)
- Alpha-1 antitrypsin deficiency (*signs of obstructive airways disease*)
- Drugs.

Evidence of decompensation

Look for signs of hepatic decompensation (Box 3.1, point C).

DISCUSSION

What do you understand by the term cirrhosis?

Cirrhosis is a diffuse process of fibrosis and regenerative nodule formation. It is the end result of many insults to the liver, whose response has been:

- Initially, and perhaps recurrently, activation of an acute cell mediated proinflammatory immune response (pages 199–200).
- Chronic progression to fibrosis, mediated by fibrogenic cytokines, and repair.

The stages of cirrhosis (by no means always a sequence, but may be contemporaneous) are:

1. Liver cell necrosis
2. Inflammation
3. Fibrosis
4. Nodular regeneration.

Cirrhosis generally starts at the portal triads and progresses outwards in 'ripples', eventually abutting to form bridges of necrosis. Bridging necrosis progresses to fibrosis and the fibrous bands are termed septae. In advanced disease there will be more fibrosis and septae than regenerated liver. Regenerating liver grows between the septae, and the septae–regenerating junction is called the limiting plate. When there are tightly compacted septal bands with small islands of regeneration, this is termed micronodular cirrhosis. Macronodular cirrhosis involves larger islands of regeneration.

Which patients may be suitable for liver transplantation?

Where the benefits of transplantation outweigh the risks of surgery and will likely improve prognosis, indications for transplantation include:

- Fulminant hepatic failure ● Alcohol induced cirrhosis (if patient demonstrates ability to abstain) ● Hepatitis B or C virus induced cirrhosis (but frequently recurs) ● Primary biliary cirrhosis ● Hereditary haemochromatosis ● Wilson's disease ● Hepatocellular carcinoma (unifocal, small, no evidence of invasion) ● Cholangiocarcinoma.

Which areas are important in the history?

- Drug history ● Alcohol consumption ● Previous jaundice, transfusions or drug use (viral hepatitis) ● Medications, including complementary therapies ● Family history (hereditary haemochromatosis, Wilson's disease, alpha-1 antitrypsin deficiency) ● Occupational history ● Travel history ● Sexual history (viral hepatitis).

How do you distinguish caput medusae from inferior vena caval obstruction?

Caput medusae veins radiate from the umbilicus. Inferior vena caval obstruction (very rare) promotes venous flow upwards from the groin.

CASE STUDY   **3.4 ALCOHOL INDUCED CHRONIC LIVER DISEASE (CLD)**

Instruction: *Please examine this patient's abdominal system. You may briefly look for any other signs which you think may help you determine an underlying cause for his problem. Discuss your findings and the likely cause.*

RECOGNITION

Some *general signs of chronic liver disease* may be present (Box 3.1, Fig. 3.3).

INTERPRETATION

Confirm the diagnosis

Consider other causes of chronic liver disease (Box 3.1). In alcohol induced CLD, *Dupuytren's contractures* (not always due to alcohol) and *parotid enlargement* may be present. Other accompaniments to alcohol misuse include cerebellar signs *(past pointing, broad based gait)*, Wernicke's encephalopathy *(ophthalmoplegia)* and evidence of dilated cardiomyopathy *(displaced apex ± signs of heart failure)*. Tell the examiners that you would ask about alcohol consumption.

Evidence of decompensation

Look for signs of hepatic decompensation (Box 3.1, point C).

DISCUSSION

How would you classify alcohol induced liver damage?

- Fatty change, seen within days of ingestion on ultrasound.
- Alcohol induced hepatitis. The liver is swollen, smooth and tender.
- Cirrhosis, classically micronodular.

What abnormal laboratory indices may accompany alcohol misuse?

- Raised γ-glutamyl transferase (GGT), due to enzyme induction
- Raised aspartate aminotransferase (AAT) and transaminases
- Raised mean corpuscular volume (MCV), due to alteration in the red blood cell membrane lipid profile
- Thrombocytopenia (haematinic deficiency, hypersplenism)
- Low urea may occur due to nutritional deficiency.

CASE STUDY | **3.5 VIRAL HEPATITIS**

Instruction: *This 45-year-old man has a history of intravenous drug misuse. Please examine his abdominal system and discuss your findings.*

RECOGNITION

The *general signs of chronic liver disease* may be present (Box 3.1, Fig. 3.3).

INTERPRETATION

Confirm the diagnosis

Consider the other causes of chronic liver disease (Box 3.1).
Remember that two or more causes may coexist.

Look for/consider causes

Tell the examiners that you would ask about:

- Alcohol consumption ● Previous jaundice ● Previous transfusions ● Drug use ● Occupational history ● Travel history ● Sexual history.

Evidence of decompensation

Look for signs of hepatic decompensation (Box 3.1, point C).

DISCUSSION

Tell us about the stages of hepatitis B virus (HBV) infection

The virion comprises a surface envelope bearing the surface antigen (sAg) and a core containing the core antigen (cAg). A further antigen, eAg, arises from the same gene (C gene) as cAg. The C gene has two initiation codons, a precore and a core region. When translation is initiated at the precore region, the protein product is HBeAg, which has a signal peptide that facilitates its secretion into the serum. When translation is initiated at the core region, the protein product is HBcAg, which lacks a signal peptide, is not secreted and is not detectable in serum.

An intact immune system is vital to HBV clearance. The more vigorous the response (and florid the clinical condition), the greater

Box 3.6 Stages of HBV Infection

Stage 1: Incubation/active viral replication
This is usually asymptomatic, lasting a few weeks. HBsAg is positive, as are HBV DNA (indicating active viral replication), HBeAg and IgM antibody to HBcAg (anti-HBc IgM). Transaminases are normal.

Stage 2: Continued replication of virus and inflammatory response
HBeAg is still secreted by infected liver cells. But HBV DNA levels in serum fall as the number of infected cells declines due to direct cell lysis and the TH1 mediated (pages 199–200) proinflammatory response.

In patients with acute disease, stage 2 is the symptomatic stage of acute hepatitis with jaundice, lasting a few weeks. Transaminases are elevated. In patients with chronic disease, stage 2 may persist for years, leading to cirrhosis.

Seroconversion refers to loss of HBeAg and conversion to anti-HBe (antibodies to HBeAg) positivity. This may occur early after acute symptoms, signifying declining infectivity and resolving infection. But in chronic disease, the spontaneous seroconversion rate is only a small percentage of patients per year.

Stage 2 has a widely variable time course, from weeks to many years.

Stage 3: Post-seroconversion
Once an immune response eliminates or greatly diminishes the infected cell load, stage 3 begins. HBeAg is negative, and anti-HBe is positive. Transaminase levels are normal. HBV DNA may be detectable in some patients by polymerase chain reaction (PCR). Essentially, infection has cleared, but HBsAg remains positive because the sAg gene has been inserted into the host's genome.

Stage 4: Clearance
Most patients eventually become negative for HBsAg and develop anti-HBs antibodies. HBV DNA is undetectable by PCR and reactivation or reinfection is unlikely.

IgG antibodies to HBcAg (anti-HBc IgG), together with anti-HBe, are present in people with a past history of HBV infection, and persist lifelong. Anti-HBs antibodies are present after infection or vaccination.

the chance of clearance. Most offspring of affected mothers progress to chronic carriage, whereas only a small minority of adults are chronic carriers. The life cycle has four stages (Box 3.6).

Factors affecting evolution through these four stages include genetic predisposition, concurrent infection with other viruses, immune status and HBV mutant status.

What are the markers of high infectivity HBV carrier status?

● HBeAg positive ● HBsAg positive ● Negative/low titre anti-HBc IgM ● High titre anti-HBc IgG ● Anti-HBe negative ● HBV DNA detectable ● Raised transaminases ● Anti-HBs absent.

What are the markers of low infectivity HBV carrier status?

● HBeAg positive ● HBsAg positive ● Negative anti-HBc IgM ● Moderate titre anti-HBc IgG ● Anti-HBe positive ● HBV DNA absent ● Normal transaminases ● Anti-HBs absent.

What are the markers of past HBV infection?

Anti-HBs must be positive before complete recovery from HBV infection and immunity can be inferred. Anti-HBc IgG and anti-HBe remain positive. All other markers are negative.

What is HBV precore mutant disease?

A variant C gene fails to produce HBeAg capable of secretion into the serum but otherwise causes typical viral replicating disease. The negative HBeAg test is a misleading false negative and HBV DNA is necessary to detect the presence of disease activity. Precore mutant strains may develop late in the disease process and lead to reactivation of disease.

What do you know about HBV treatment?

The important complications of chronic HBV carriage are cirrhosis and hepatocellular carcinoma (HCC).

Treatment is considered for patients with active, replicating disease.

Patients positive for HBsAg but without abnormal liver biochemistry, no evidence of replicating disease and a normal ultrasound are generally at low risk of symptomatic liver disease or HCC. They require no further investigation but should be screened (screening frequency arguable, but at least annually) since reactivation may occur.

Patients with abnormal liver biochemistry, even without detectable HBV DNA, should proceed to liver biopsy; 5% of patients with isolated HBsAg carriage at presentation will have cirrhosis. Interferon-alpha is indicated for patients with abnormal liver histology. The optimal dose and duration of treatment is contentious.

The overall response rate (inhibition of viral replication) is around 40%, and successful treatment leads to sustained improvement in liver histology and may lower the risk of HCC. HBsAg usually remains positive despite treatment.

Interferon-alpha is more likely to benefit the following groups:
● Young ● Female ● Those with low HBV DNA titres ● Those with active inflammation (raised transaminases, histology).

The use of interferon-alpha is limited by side effects, notably flu-like symptoms, depression and fatigue, and occasionally haematological abnormalities.

What do you know about the epidemiology of the hepatitis C virus (HCV)?

HCV infection is a major public health concern. Globally, it is much more prevalent than HIV infection. The UK prevalence is unknown but estimated to be around 0.5%. Infection is usually silent, but associated with a high chronic carrier state (85%), eventual progression to cirrhosis in chronic carriers and a 1–4% annual risk of HCC in those with cirrhosis.

How is HCV transmitted?

HCV is a single-stranded RNA virus of various genotypes with differences in pathogenicity, treatment response and prognosis. The two most important routes of transmission are the sharing of needles or equipment by injecting drug users and transfusion of blood and blood products (now virtually eliminated in the UK since screening of donors in 1991). Other potential routes include sharing of toothbrushes and razors, tattooing, body piercing, electrolysis and acupuncture. Sexual transmission and maternal vertical transmission rates appear to be low.

Occupational risk in health care workers is significant, as HCV may be transmitted in many body fluids. The risk of transmission from an HCV needlestick injury is about 1 : 30.

How is HCV tested for?

The HCV antibody test is positive at 6 months after exposure but the RNA virus can be detected by the polymerase chain reaction (PCR).

How is HCV disease severity assessed?

Liver biopsy is the only satisfactory way to assess severity, since serum transaminases may fluctuate disproportionately to activity.

What do you know about HCV treatment?

Combination treatment enhances efficacy and reduces resistance. Optimal treatment combines subcutaneous interferon-alpha with oral ribavirin for 6 months in patients with non-genotype-1 HCV, and for 12 months in those with genotype-1 HCV. Sustained viral clearance— defined as PCR negativity at 6 months—is around 40%, but may be improved by more effective interferon formulations.

List some causes of viral hepatitis which do not lead to chronic liver disease

Hepatitis A virus, Ebstein–Barr virus, pravovirus, atypical pneumonia organisms.

CASE STUDY **3.6 AUTOIMMUNE HEPATITIS (AIH)**

Instruction: *Please examine this 45-year-old lady's abdominal system and comment on possible diagnoses.*

RECOGNITION

Some *general signs of chronic liver disease* may be present (Box 3.1, Fig. 3.3)

(AIH is a relatively uncommon diagnosis that mainly affects young women. The usual presentation is with fatigue, right upper quadrant pain, polymyalgia/arthralgia and abnormal liver function tests. Other autoimmune conditions are present in up to 20% of patients. AIH can produce transient jaundice or may be detected serendipitously as an isolated transaminase rise. It may remain subclinical and undetected until cirrhosis with hepatic decompensation.)

INTERPRETATION

Confirm the diagnosis

Consider the other causes of chronic liver disease (Box 3.1). Look for signs of other autoimmune diseases, especially *thyroid disease (face)* and *rheumatoid arthritis* and *scleroderma (hands)*.

Evidence of decompensation

Look for signs of hepatic decompensation (Box 3.1, point C).

DISCUSSION

What types of AIH do you know of?

1. Type 1 AIH, the classical 'lupoid' type, is seen especially in young women. It is responsible for around 80% of AIH, and is associated with HLA B8/DRw3, high circulating titres of antinuclear antibody (ANA) and polyclonal (but especially IgG) hypergammaglobulinaemia. Anti-smooth muscle antibodies (anti-SMA) directed at actin are frequently present although non-specific.

2. Type 2a AIH affects around 10% of patients, especially children. It is associated not with ANA but with anti-liver/kidney/microsomal (anti-LKM) antibodies. It is rapidly progressive without treatment. Type 2b AIH is associated with anti-LKM antibodies and hepatitis C infection.

3. Type 3 is similar to type 1 and rapidly progressive. ANA and anti-LKM antibodies are not present and there is no significant

hypergammaglobulinaemia, but antisoluble liver antigen (anti-SLA) antibodies, directed at cytokeratin, are present.

How would you investigate a patient with an isolated transaminase rise?

AIH illustrates the importance of investigating patients with 'incidental' raised transaminase levels in whom no clear diagnosis is apparent. Biochemical and serological tests for causes of CLD (HBV/HCV serology, ANA/anti-SMA, antimitochondrial antibodies, iron studies, occasionally copper studies) are important, as is a liver ultrasound, but liver biopsy is often needed to secure the diagnosis.

What is the treatment for AIH?

Immunosuppression with steroids and azathioprine produces lasting remission and an excellent prognosis.

CASE STUDY | **3.7 PRIMARY BILIARY CIRRHOSIS (PBC)**

Instruction: *Examine this lady's skin and abdomen. Discuss your findings.*

RECOGNITION

There may be prominent *scratch marks* (due to itch), *xanthelasmata* and multiple *xanthomatous deposits* (Case study 5.16). There is sometimes *finger clubbing*. There may or may not be other *signs of chronic liver disease* (Box 3.1, Fig. 3.3).

PBC predominantly affects middle-aged women. Intense itch may be a prominent, early feature of PBC, which may later present as cholestatic jaundice. PBC may first present as variceal bleeding, illustrating the importance of pre-emptive investigation of patients with isolated alkaline phosphatase elevation.

↑ALK Phos.

INTERPRETATION

Confirm the diagnosis

Consider the other causes of chronic liver disease (Box 3.1). Primary biliary cirrhosis is also more common in women. Look for *xanthelasmata*.

Evidence of decompensation

In addition to hepatic decompensation (Box 3.1, point C), steatorrhoea and malabsorption may lead to osteomalacia with bone pain. Tell the examiners that you would ask about this.

Look for/consider associated diseases

These include rheumatoid arthritis, Sjögren's syndrome and thyroid disease.

RA
Sjögrens
Thyroid.

DISCUSSION

What diagnostic tests are there for PBC?

Antimitochondrial antibodies (AMA) are invariably positive, especially the M$_2$ subtype, and the AMA profile present can give prognostic information. IgM is commonly increased. Liver biopsy may show increased copper deposition with destruction of interlobar ducts, small duct proliferation, fibrosis and cirrhosis.

What is the treatment for PBC?

Ursodeoxycholic acid may slow disease progression. PBC is one of the more common indications for liver transplantation.

What is primary sclerosing cholangitis (PSC)?

Do not confuse PBC with PSC, the latter is characterised by chronic fibrosis of intra- and extra-hepatic ducts and is associated with other autoimmune diseases. 70% of PSC occurs in the presence of ulcerative colitis. Secondary sclerosing cholangitis follows numerous insults including bacterial cholangitis and graft versus host disease.

CASE STUDY   3.8   HEREDITARY HAEMOCHROMATOSIS (HHC)

Instruction: *Examine this patient's skin and abdomen and proceed as you think is most appropriate.*

RECOGNITION

There may be *slate greyish pigmentation*. There is *firm, smooth hepatomegaly ± splenomegaly*. There may be *general signs of chronic liver disease* (Box 3.1, Fig. 3.3).

INTERPRETATION

Confirm the diagnosis

Consider the other causes of chronic liver disease (Box 3.1). The pigmentation in HHC is characteristic and affects most patients. Generally, the disease presents in middle age, women tending to be diagnosed later than men because of the protection afforded by menstruation. Tell the examiners that a liver biopsy is diagnostic. Genetic testing is also used (below).

Assess other systems

The clinical manifestations of HHC result from iron deposition in major organs, notably the skin, pancreas, heart, liver and anterior pituitary. Arthralgia may be an early symptom.

Tell the examiners that you would wish to determine the presence or absence of:

- *Arthropathy* or *arthritis*, including pseudogout of wrists, hips and knees
- Diabetes mellitus (*glycosuria*)
- Cardiomyopathy (*signs of heart failure*)
- Pituitary failure (Case study 11.5).

Evidence of decompensation

- Signs of hepatic decompensation (Box 3.1, point C).
- Hepatocellular carcinoma is the commonest cause of death, the relative risk some 200-fold times that of the normal population. Tell the examiners that an ultrasound scan is important.
- Glycosuria.
- Signs of heart failure.
- Hypopituitarism.

DISCUSSION

What do you know about the genetic basis of HHC?

Haemochromatosis is an autosomal recessive disorder of excessive absorption of dietary iron leading to deposition in several organs and organ failure. The genetic defect responsible for 90% of cases in the UK is homozygosity for a single base mutation (cytosine to tyrosine, C282Y) in the HFE gene, closely associated with HLA A3 on the short arm of chromosome 6.

How is HHC diagnosed?

Early symptoms are non-specific and may include fatigue, arthralgia, impotence and loss of libido, amenorrhoea and increased skin pigmentation. Diabetes mellitus, cardiomyopathy, arrhythmias, cirrhosis and anterior pituitary failure ensue if HHC is not detected.

Diagnosis may be suggested by a high transferrin saturation, and confirmed by liver biopsy (excessive iron storage) or genetic testing.

What is the treatment for HHC?

Regular venesection is needed, at least initially, and early treatment improves outcome, an argument in favour of screening.

What are the factors in favour of HHC screening?

Patients do not usually develop symptoms until they are over 40 years of age, by which time iron deposition in affected organs may have caused irreversible tissue damage and incipient organ failure. Treatment in early disease can restore normal life expectancy.

And against?

Although HHC is detectable at a presymptomatic stage, and treatable, it does not fulfil all of the criteria for screening. It is relatively uncommon (although many would argue that its incidence justifies screening), and the optimal test is contentious. Transferrin saturation only detects expressed disease.

Based on the above, who would you screen?

Ideally, the general population, but this has not been practical to date. A suitable compromise is to screen anyone in whom symptoms or signs suggest the possibility of HHC, relatives of patients with HHC and anyone with unexplained abnormal liver biochemistry (especially if diabetic).

CASE STUDY	3.9 WILSON'S DISEASE

Instruction: *This patient has a family history of his disease. Please examine his abdominal system, then look briefly at his eyes before discussing your findings.*

RECOGNITION

Some *general signs of chronic liver disease* may be present (Box 3.1, Fig. 3.3).

Wilson's disease is very uncommon, but might just appear in PACES. The clue from the instruction is to look at the eyes for *Kayser–Fleischer rings* (KFRs, Fig. 3.4).

INTERPRETATION

Confirm the diagnosis

Consider the other causes of chronic liver disease (Box 3.1).

KFRs are rusty brown deposits of copper within Descemet's membrane of the cornea and are pathognomonic of Wilson's disease. They start at 6 and 12 o'clock, are not always present, and sometimes only detectable with a slit-lamp.

Fig. 3.4   *Kayser–Fleischer ring.*
Reproduced with permission from Haslett et al. (2002) Davidson's Principles and Practice of Medicine, 19th edn. Churchill Livingstone, Edinburgh.

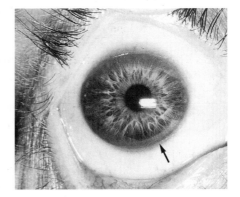

Assess other systems

Other features of Wilson's disease include neuropsychiatric sequalae due to basal ganglia deposition (often *choreiform movements*), and less commonly *sunflower cataracts* and Fanconi's syndrome due to copper infiltration disrupting renal tubular exchange (*glycosuria*).

Evidence of decompensation

Look for signs of hepatic decompensation (Box 3.1, point C).

DISCUSSION

What is the underlying abnormality in Wilson's disease?

Hepatocytes are unable to excrete copper into bile due to a mutation in a copper transporting ATPase. Different mutations run in different families. They are autosomal recessively determined, on chromosome 13.

What biochemical abnormalities would you expect?

- Low serum caeruloplasmin (copper carrying protein)
- Serum copper may be high, low or normal
- High urinary copper excretion.

Liver biopsy may be diagnostic.

What treatments are available?

Penicillamine may be effective.

Asymptomatic siblings should be screened.

CASE STUDY 3.10 HEPATOMEGALY

Instruction: *Please examine this patient's abdomen and discuss your findings.*

RECOGNITION

There is *hepatomegaly*, the *liver enlarged to (cm) below the costal margin*. The spleen is not enlarged.

INTERPRETATION

Look for/consider causes

1. **Cirrhosis**. Look for *signs of chronic liver disease* (Box 3.1, Fig. 3.3).
2. **Malignancy**. The liver is often *hard*, with a 'knobbly' or *nodular edge*. Look for *cachexia*.
3. **Right heart failure**. The liver is *firm*, with a *smooth, tender edge*, and may be *pulsatile*. Liver tenderness suggests recent stretching of its capsule due to heart failure or acute hepatitis. Look for a *raised JVP* and *peripheral oedema*.

DISCUSSION

List some other causes of hepatomegaly

- Pyogenic liver abscess ● Amoebic liver abscess ● Hydatid disease.

From where might a pyogenic liver abscess arise?

- Subphrenic abscess ● Biliary sepsis ● Diverticulitis
- Appendicitis ● Crohn's disease ● Bacterial endocarditis.

What causes an amoebic abscess?

Entamoeba histolytica, transmitted by the faecal–oral route with ingestion of protozoal cysts. 10% of the world's population is chronically infected. Cyst walls degrade in the small bowel to release trophozoites which migrate to the large bowel and, if a pathogenic strain, cause colitis and invasive disease. Symptoms include RUQ pain and fever.

What is hydatid disease?

This is caused by the dog tapeworm, *Echinococcus granulosus*. The life cycle involves ingestion by the dog of hydatid cysts from sheep liver. The dog, the definitive host, harbours the adult tapeworm in its small bowel, from which eggs are passed into its faeces and reingested by sheep. Humans may be inadvertent intermediate hosts. Eggs hatch in the sheep small bowel into larvae which penetrate into the bloodstream, travel to the liver and form cysts.

CASE STUDY 3.11 HEPATOSPLENOMEGALY/SPLENOMEGALY

Instruction: *Please examine this patient's abdomen and discuss your findings.*

RECOGNITION

There is *hepatomegaly*, the *liver enlarged to (cm) below the right costal margin*. There is *splenomegaly*, the *spleen enlarged to (cm) below the left costal margin* towards the right iliac fossa.

INTERPRETATION

Look for/consider causes

- Cirrhosis with portal hypertension (congestive splenomegaly)
- Lymphoproliferative disorders (Case studies 3.12 and 3.13)
- Myeloproliferative disorders (Case study 3.14)
- Infection/infiltrative disorders (glandular fever, brucellosis, leptospirosis, sarcoid, amyloid, glycogen storage disorders)

DISCUSSION

What are the causes of isolated splenomegaly?

Similar to hepatosplenomegaly, but an important additional cause is infective endocarditis.

What are the causes of a very large spleen?

- Chronic myeloid leukaemia
- Myelofibrosis
- Visceral leishmaniasis.

CASE STUDY   **3.12 CHRONIC MYELOID LEUKAEMIA (CML)**

Instruction: *This 50-year-old man has an abnormal blood count. Please examine his abdomen and discuss your findings.*

RECOGNITION

The *spleen is markedly enlarged* (Fig. 3.5). *Lymphadenopathy* may be present. Signs of bone marrow failure (*anaemia, petechial rash, signs of sepsis*) may be present.

INTERPRETATION

Confirm the diagnosis

- Confirm splenomegaly. The spleen *enlarges towards the RIF*, has a *medial notch* and it is *not possible to feel its upper border*. The lower border of the spleen is felt with the finger pulps and radial border of your right hand. Like the liver, it is displaced downwards on deep inspiration, meeting your fingers. Measure any enlargement in centimetres from the costal margin.
- Tell the examiners that you would ask about weight loss, fever and night sweats.
- Look for a bone marrow aspiration/trephine dressing or bruising over the iliac crest.

Fig. 3.5   *Chronic myeloid leukaemia*

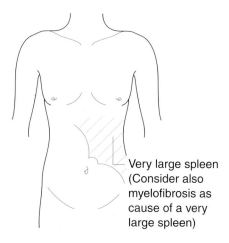

Very large spleen (Consider also myelofibrosis as cause of a very large spleen)

- Tell the examiners that you would request a peripheral blood film.

Evidence of decompensation

- Evidence of bone marrow failure (anaemia, infection, petechiae).

DISCUSSION

What is the underlying genetic abnormality in CML?

In most cases of CML there is a reciprocal translocation between chromosomes 9 and 22 to form the Philadelphia chromosome which contains the chimeric gene BCR/ABL. ABL, an oncogene encoding a tyrosine kinase, is translocated from chromosome 9 to a specific breakpoint cluster region BCR on chromosome 22. Chimeric BCR/ABL mRNA encodes a protein with aberrant tyrosine kinase activity which accelerates growth and differentiation of the myeloid line.

This cytogenetic defect arises as a somatic defect within a haematopoietic stem cell precusor from which the clone of leukaemic cells are born.

What is the difference between a somatic and a germline mutation?

Somatic mutation refers to mutation of genetic material within a particular cell and its clonal offspring. *Germline* mutation implies that every cell in the body carries the mutation. Somatic mutations underlie leukaemias and many malignancies.

How may CML be diagnosed?

↑WCC, splenomegaly.

CML is most common in middle-aged men.

It is characterised by a raised white cell count (WCC) and splenomegaly. It may be diagnosed incidentally from a blood film, or present with abdominal pain or swelling, lymphadenopathy, constitutional symptoms or bone marrow failure.

A markedly raised WCC of $50-500 \times 10^9$/L and thrombocytosis are typical. The complete spectrum of myeloid cell differentiation may be seen on the peripheral blood film and basophils are often prominent. Vitamin B_{12} levels may be high.

The Philadelphia chromosome may be identified by cytogentic or DNA based (Southern blot or PCR) studies. The small number of variant translocations may be identified by novel strategies including fluorescence in-situ hybridisation (FISH).

What is the natural history of CML?

An initial chronic phase of clonal myelopoiesis (> 5% blasts) progresses inevitably to an accelerated phase with new cytogenetic changes and finally to blast cell crisis.

How is CML treated?

Treatment should target the chronic phase, since normal stem cells are gradually replaced by Philadelphia positive stem cells as disease progresses. Potential cure has only been possible with bone marrow transplantation (BMT) from an HLA-identical donor. Tyrosine kinase inhibitors, which induce long-term remission, have an increasingly important role.

Modern cytogenetic testing allows detection of minimal residual disease following allogeneic BMT, early detection of relapse and assessment of cytogenetic responsiveness to treatment. Further, these techniques can be used to monitor the cytogentic changes which herald blast transformation.

What are haemopoetic stem cells (HSCs)?

HSCs have the capacity for self-renewal and are pluripotent. They live in the bone marrow where they divide and differentiate into populations of *progenitor cells* which are committed to each of the main marrow cell lines.

Briefly describe normal haemopoiesis

In the bone marrow developing cell differentiation is directed by *haemopoietic growth factors*. These include colony stimulating factors (CSFs) such as granulocyte-CSF (G-CSF), thrombopoietin (TPO) and erythropoietin (EPO) which are lineage specific.

Erythropoiesis

Proerythroblasts are large with dark blue cytoplasm and primitive nuclear material or chromatin. As they differentiate they become smaller, with increasing amounts of haemoglobin and a polychromatic cytoplasm, and their nuclear chromatin condenses. The nucleus is eventually extruded giving rise to a *reticulocyte*. Reticulocytes still contain RNA and are capable of haemoglobin synthesis, but spend only a few days in the bone marrow before travelling to the spleen where they lose RNA and become fully fledged erythrocytes or red blood cells (RBCs).

Leucopoiesis

Whilst the bone marrow is the primary site of granulocyte and lymphocyte formation, most circulating mature lymphocytes are produced after migration to peripheral secondary lymphoid tissue — lymph nodes, spleen, thymus and gastrointestinal associated lymphoid tissue. Lymphocytes normally comprise < 10% of bone marrow cells. Plasma cells are typically basophilic cells with a blue tinge and an eccentric nucleus.

Granulocytes (neutrophils, eosinophils, basophils) adopt a central role in inflammation. Large numbers of *neutrophils* are held in reserve in the bone marrow. Those that enter the circulation spend only hours within it before adhesion and migration into the tissues under the influence of chemokines (page 201). Of the circulating pool, about half are loosely adherent to the endothelium, a phenomenon called margination. *Monocytes* may survive for months or even years in tissues, functioning as phagocytes (circulating monocytes enter tissues within hours to days and become wandering macrophages) or as antigen presenting cells (APCs) (page 196).

How may bone marrow (BM) examination aid diagnosis in haematological disease?

Bone marrow aspirates yield films which may be examined for:

● Morphology of individual cells
● Proportions of different cells
● The presence of abnormal cells such as leukaemic, metastatic or infective cells, and organisms
● Iron status.

Bone marrow trephine biopsies provide cores of bone and marrow for histological assessment. They are useful for examining marrow architecture and cellularity and are the most reliable way of detecting marrow infiltrates.

List some causes of neutrophilia and neutopenia

Neutrophilia is common in bacterial infection. Steroids cause apparent neutrophilia by inducing demargination.

Neutropenia may be seen in viral infections, overwhelming sepsis, chemotherapy, myelodysplasia and in bone marrow infiltration—leukaemias, myeloma, lymphomas, myelofibrosis, secondary carcinoma.

All cytopenias may be classified as *increased peripheral destruction/utilisation* (there may be a compensatory bone marrow response as in sepsis, when the bone marrow response causes a *left shifted* peripheral blood film) or *deficient bone marrow production*.

What is meant by the term leucoerythroblastic change?

The presence of nucleated RBCs and white cell precursors in peripheral blood. It is seen in severe illness such as sepsis or trauma and in bone marrow infiltration.

How do acute leukaemias broadly differ from chronic leukaemias?

Acute leukaemias are characterised by their *rapid onset* and their *high proportion of undifferentiated blast cells* compared to chronic leukaemias. Aberrant myeloid or lymphoid precursors arise in the bone marrow after somatic mutation of a single cell and spill out into the blood. Blast cells on a peripheral blood film often provide initial evidence of suspected acute leukaemia.

Clinical features of acute leukaemias result from the consequences of bone marrow failure (neutropenia, thrombocytopenia, anaemia) and organ infiltration (lymph nodes, spleen, liver, meninges, testes (especially acute lymphoblastic leukaemia (ALL)), skin and gums (some acute myeloid leukaemias (AML)).

Chronic lymphocytic leukaemia (CLL) arises from mature lymphocyte precursors. CML is a stem cell disorder in which differentiation is possible. AML represents a more mature but arrested stage.

How is AML classified?

Morphologically

The French American British (FAB) classification (Table 3.1) has traditionally distinguished subtypes of AML based on peripheral blood and bone marrow morphology and cytochemistry stains.

Immunologically

Monoclonal antibodies to cell surface markers can now be used to phenotype leukaemic cells. Immunophenotyping may employ flow cytometry.

Cytogenetically

It is now evident that the most important prognostic indicator is the specific mutation within a leukaemic clone. Increasingly, cytogenetic methods are used to define specific subtypes of AML and guide treatment.

TABLE 3.1   FAB classification

Category	Features
M0	*Acute myeloblastic leukaemia with minimal differentiation* Least differentiated, with large, agranular myeloblasts
M1	*Acute myeloblastic leukaemia without maturation* Non-erythroid blasts comprise ≥ 90% of myeloid population
M2	*Acute myeloblastic leukaemia with maturation* Non erythroid blasts 30–89% but definite promyelocyte differentiation
M3	*Acute promyelocytic leukaemia* Mostly abnormal promyelocytes, containing granules of procoagulant material
M4	*Acute myelomonocytic leukaemia* (An eosinophilic subtype is recognised)
M5	*Acute monocytic leukaemia* 80% of non-erythroid cells are monoblasts, promonocytes or monocytes
M6	*Erythroleukaemia* Erythroid component of marrow comprises > 50% of all nucleated cells
M7	*Megakaryoblastic leukaemia*

Auer rods are aggregates of granules seen in M1, M2 and especially M3.

What is acute promyelocytic leukaemia (APML)?

APML is due to the fusion of the PML gene on chromosome 15 with the RARα gene on chromosome 17 to form a chimeric fusion protein which interferes with factors essential for differentiation of myeloid precursors. These cells contain procoagulant 'junk' material. Cell lysis can cause disseminated intravascular coagulation (DIC) but all-*trans* retinoic acid (ATRA) may be used to induce remission in the absence of chemotherapy without causing DIC. Postinduction chemotherapy is needed to maintain remission.

What are the treatment principles in AML?

Remission induction followed by postinduction treatment (consolidation is better than low dose maintenance therapy), bone marrow/HSC transplantation (below) and supportive therapy (blood products, broad spectrum antimicrobial therapy for febrile neutropenia, haemopoietic growth factors).

What are the principles of haemopoietic stem cell transplantation (HSCT)?

Bone marrow transplantation (BMT) or HSCT involves harvesting HSCs from donor marrow (posterior iliac crest) or peripheral blood ('peripheral blood SCT', the HSC content of blood being augmented by chemotherapy and G-CSF prior to harvest) and using these to repopulate and regenerate recipient marrow, thus rescuing the recipient from aplasia. BMT and HSCT rely on the fact that HSCs infused into the peripheral vein of a recipient 'home' to the marrow to re-establish haematopoiesis. Donors may be autologous (same patient) or allogeneic (HLA matched relative or unrelated donor). A specific concern in autologous transplantation is the potential for tumour cells to contaminate the graft, and numerous purging techniques have been employed in attempt to reduce rates of disease relapse. Transplantation (in conjunction with intensive supportive therapy until the infused HSCs are able to produce adequate numbers of red and white cells and platelets) allows the use of high dose chemotherapy in recipients, and is used in many myeloproliferative (CML, AML) and lymphoproliferative (CLL, lymphomas) disorders as well as non-malignant disorders such as aplasia. HSCT for solid tumours has not proven beneficial. Supportive therapy includes blood products, haematopoietic growth factors and broad spectrum antimicrobials for neutropenic sepsis. Of emerging interest is the therapeutic use of stem cells from other tissues to repair diseased or degenerating tissue. Stem cells may have the ability to transdifferentiate ('plasticity'), and it may be possible to redirect HSCs and stem cells from muscle, brain, skin, liver and other sites to differentiate into tissue different from that originally intended.

What is graft verses host disease (GVHD)?

In allogeneic transplants activation of donor lymphocytes may cause immune damage to the skin, gut and liver of the recipient (GVHD). However, a graft versus tumour effect may also occur, donor lymphocytes recognising and eliminating residual malignant cells in the recipient. This has led to interest in donor lymphocyte infusion for antimalignancy effects, notably in chronic myeloid leukaemia.

What are the myelodysplastic syndromes (MDS)?

These are clonal disorders of haemopoiesis characterised by progressive peripheral blood cytopenias. The marrow is hypercellular but exhibits defective maturation, and there are frequently morphological abnormalities in all three cell lines. There is usually dyserythropoieis with nuclear atypia and the presence of ringed sideroblasts.

These disorders predominantly occur in elderly people who may remain asymptomatic or present with bone marrow failure. There are typically no other reticuloendothelial signs.

Cytogenetic abnormalities are common and 10–40% of patients with MDS progress to AML. Therefore, they have also been termed 'preleukaemic' syndromes.

The FAB classification identifies five types of MDS:

● Refractory anaemia (RA) ● Refractory anaemia with ring sideroblasts (RARS) ● Refractory anaemia with excess blasts (RAEB) ● Refractory anaemia with excess blasts in transformation (RAEB-T) (the World Health Organization (WHO) classification categorises RAEB-T as secondary AML) ● Chronic myelomonocytic leukaemia (CMML).

CASE STUDY	3.13 POLYCYTHAEMIA RUBRA VERA (PRV)

Instruction: *This gentleman reports pruritus after a hot bath. Please examine his abdomen and report your findings.*

RECOGNITION	

There is moderate *splenomegaly*.

INTERPRETATION	

Confirm the diagnosis

PRV is predominantly a disease of the middle aged and elderly. There is often *facial plethora, suffusion of the conjunctivae and engorgement of retinal vessels.*

It may present with headaches, lethargy, dyspnoea, fluid retention, bleeding, weight loss, night sweats or pruritus (exacerbated by a hot bath). Tell the examiners that you would ask about these symptoms.

Evidence of decompensation

Tell the examiners that priapism and vascular occlusive events such as stroke are important complications.

DISCUSSION

What types of polycythaemia are there?

Polycythaemias are characterised by an increased haemoglobin concentration, packed cell volume and RBC count (Fig. 3.6). Polycythaemias may be categorised as:

1. PRV
2. Secondary polycythaemias (appropriately or inappropriately elevated erythropoietin (EPO) as in smokers and high altitude)
3. Apparent polycythaemia (without true elevation of the red cell mass, as in dehydration).

What are 'myeloproliferative' syndromes (MPS)

These are clonal disorders of haemopoietic lines in which there is increased sensitivity of marrow cells to normal regulatory factors, and a hypercellular marrow with overproduction of red cells, white cells or platelets. There is often overlap of erythropoietic, granulopoietic and megakaryocytic expansion, lending support to the notion of a clonal stem cell defect. Cells are morphologically normal, although the World Health Organization classification now recognises overlap with *myelodysplastic syndromes*.

The myeloproliferative disorders include:

● PRV ● CML ● Essential thrombocytosis (ET) ● Myelofibrosis (MF).

What happens to the neutrophil alkaline phosphatase (NAP) score in PRV?

Most of the myeloproliferative disorders give rise to a high NAP score, with the exception of CML, in which the NAP score is low.

How is PRV treated?

Treatments include venesection and hydroxyurea.

CASE STUDY   3.14   CHRONIC LYMPHOCYTIC LEUKAEMIA (CLL)

Instruction: *Please examine this 74-year-old patient's lymphoreticular system and discuss your findings.*

INTERPRETATION

There is widespread *lymphadenopathy* and moderate *hepatosplenomegaly/splenomegaly* (Fig. 3.7).

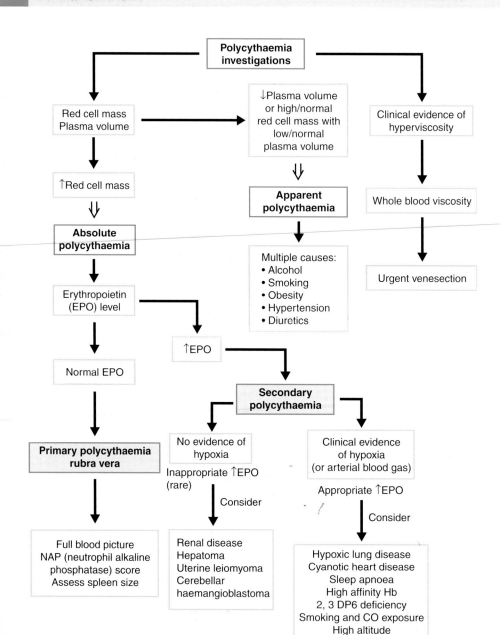

Fig. 3.6   *Scheme for assessing causes of polycythaemia*

| INTERPRETATION |

Confirm the diagnosis

- Lymph nodes are often markedly enlarged, painless and rubbery.
- Tell the examiners that you would request a peripheral blood film. This would demonstrate an excess of small, mature lymphocytes

Fig. 3.7 *Chronic lymphocytic leukaemia*

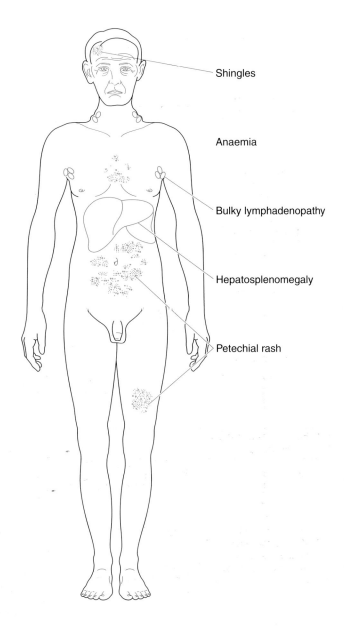

Shingles

Anaemia

Bulky lymphadenopathy

Hepatosplenomegaly

Petechial rash

with smear/smudge cells (broken in vitro by slide preparation). Immunophenotyping for the cluster designation (CD) surface marker profile of blood or bone marrow clonal cells is diagnostic.

Evidence of decompensation

The CLL clone invades the lymph nodes, liver, spleen and bone marrow (bone marrow failure causing sepsis, bruising/bleeding and anaemia). Look for *petechial haemorrhages* and *pallor*.

Tell the examiners that:

- T cell dysregulation also contributes to immune deficiency and recurrent infection. Further, the B cell leukaemic clone suppresses the normal B cell population and hence impairs the diversity of immune competence.
- Autoimmune haemolysis and thrombocytopenia are common.
- Transformation of lymph node tissue to Richter's large cell lymphoma is a rare but serious complication. Ebstein–Barr virus (EBV) related transformation is more common now because of immunosuppression induced by purine analogue treatment.

DISCUSSION

What is the underlying defect in CLL?

CLL is the most common leukaemia, and tends to occur in the elderly. A range of mutations is possible, arising in B lymphocyte precursors, with differing prognoses. One subgroup of CLL involves deletions in chromosome 13 associated with a mutated immunoglobulin heavy chain variable region, indicating postgerminal cell origin.

When should CLL be treated?

Treatment is for symptomatic disease, aiming to decrease tumour cell load, since CLL is not curable. The long natural history means that many patients remain asymptomatic and die from an unrelated problem.

What is the differential diagnosis of generalised lymphadenopathy?

- Lymphoproliferative disorders ● Infections such as EBV, cytomegalovirus (CMV), toxoplasmosis, HIV, TB, brucellosis.

What other lymphoproliferative disorders do you know of?

- Acute lymphoblastic leukaemia ● Non-Hodgkin's lymphoma (NHL) ● Hodgkin's disease ● Myeloma and paraproteinaemias.

What do you know about lymphoma classification?

NHL embraces a range of diseases traditionally classified by cell origin, which does not carry prognostic information. As with AML, reclassification will utilise cytogenetic methods. Clinically, NHL may be low, intermediate or high grade and prognosis broadly relates to age, stage and extent of extranodal involvement, markers of tumour load (such as lactate dehydrogenase (LDH) levels) and performance status. Diagnosis is usually from biopsy of an affected node or extranodal site.

The presence of the Reed Sternberg cell is pathognomonic of *Hodgkin's disease*, a disease with bimodal age distribution and classified histologically as lymphocyte predominant (a separate subtype more related to NHL), mixed cellularity, nodular sclerosing or lymphocyte deplete. Hodgkin's disease presents typically with peripheral (especially cervical) and mediastinal lymph node enlargement.

3.15   ADULT POLYCYSTIC KIDNEY DISEASE (APCKD)

Instruction: *Please examine this patient's abdomen and discuss your diagnosis.*

RECOGNITION

The *kidneys are palpable* (confirmed by bimanual palpation and ballottement, but often large enough to cause loin distension). The *liver may also be enlarged with an irregular surface*, also affected by polycystic disease. There may be a transplanted kidney in the right or left iliac fossa. Bulky polycystic kidneys are usually excised at transplantation.

INTERPRETATION

Confirm the diagnosis

If there are bilateral flank masses the diagnosis is very likely. Ensure that you can 'get above' the masses. This may be difficult on the right if the liver is also polycystic.

Assess other systems

Tell the examiners that you would like to:

- Take the blood pressure
- Ask about a family history
- Ask about haematuria.

Evidence of decompensation

Look for evidence of current or previous renal failure:

- A haemodialysis arteriovenous fistula in one or both forearms
- Scarring at internal jugular or subclavian haemodialysis catheter sites or even a catheter in situ
- Renal transplantation (Case study 3.18).

DISCUSSION

What is the natural history of APCKD?

Adult polycystic kidney disease is a common autosomal dominant disease (mutations in one of several proteins, including polycystin-1 and polycystin-2) presenting in the fourth or fifth decades, usually with one or more of:

- Haematuria ● Hypertension ● Renal failure ● Large kidneys/loin pain ● Urinary sepsis.

Hepatic, pancreatic and ovarian cysts are common and usually asymptomatic. Approximately one-third of patients develop renal failure, one-third hypertension without renal failure, and one-third remain asymptomatic through life.

What other complications can occur in APCKD?

- Loin pain from bleeding into cysts/infected cysts
- Mitral valve prolapse
- Anaemia of chronic renal failure
- Some patients develop polycythaemia (increased erythropoietin activity)
- Cerebral aneurysms and subarachnoid haemorrhage.

List some other causes of renal cysts

- Simple cysts, which are extremely common and benign
- Medullary cystic disease, which causes chronic renal failure
- Acquired cystic disease, which may be found in any scarred kidney
- Von Hippel–Lindau syndrome.

| CASE STUDY | 3.16   NEPHROTIC SYNDROME |

Instruction: This 40-year-old gentleman has developed oedema and an elevated creatinine. Please examine him and ask him some questions.

RECOGNITION

There is *fluid overload* as evidenced by *sacral and peripheral oedema*. There may be *periorbital or facial oedema*. There may be *leuconychia*.

INTERPRETATION

Confirm the diagnosis

Tell the examiners that you would like to perform urinalysis to check for proteinuria.
Nephrotic syndrome comprises:

- Heavy albuminuria (> 3 g/day) because the glomerular filter is *more leaky* than usual
- Hypoalbuminaemia
- Oedema
- Dyslipidaemia.

Look for/consider causes

The two common primary causes of nephrotic syndrome are *minimal change disease* and *membranous nephropathy*. Minimal change disease is usually primary but occasionally associated with Hodgkin's disease. Membranous nephropathy is usually primary but secondary causes include non-Hodgkin's lymphoma, carcinoma, melanoma, gold, penicillamine, diabetes, systemic lupus erythematosus, amyloid, malaria, hepatitis B virus infection, syphilis and HIV infection. Tell the examiners that you would take a history for these.

Evidence of decompensation

Tell the examiners that you would ask about infection and venous thromboembolism (Box 3.7).

DISCUSSION

What are the clinical responses to glomerular disease?

Clinical manifestations of glomerular disease are given in Box 3.7.

Which factors tend to be associated with a poorer prognosis in glomerular disease?

● Male sex ● Hypertension ● Heavy proteinuria ● Renal failure ● Heavy interstitial inflammation.

What are the histopathological responses to glomerular disease?

The glomerulus is a filter transferring material from capillary to nephron tubule across an endothelium, basement membrane and epithelial cell layer (the latter with podocytes to enhance transfer surface area). The epithelium is surrounded by mesangial cells. The glomerulus has a limited histopathological response to a huge array of insults. It is useful to classify glomerulonephritis (GN) histopathologically, but clinicopathological correlation is pivotal to diagnosis (Table 3.2).

CASE STUDY   3.17   RENAL FAILURE

Instruction: *This 45-year-old man has renal failure. Please ask him about uraemic symptoms and assess his fluid status.*

RECOGNITION

Uraemic symptoms are listed in Box 3.8.
Assessment of fluid status is described in Box 3.9.

INTERPRETATION

Look for/consider causes

Tell the examiners that you would ask about common causes of renal failure:

● Glomerulonephritis (CRF or ARF) ● Diabetes (CRF) ● Drugs, especially NSAIDs (ARF or CRF) ● Renovascular disease (CRF) ● Hypertension (CRF) ● Adult polycystic kidney disease (CRF).

| Box 3.7 | Clinical Manifestations of Glomerular Disease |

Haematuria

Dipstick urinalysis (for the presence of an active sediment) and microscopy is one of the most simple, rewarding yet forgotten investigations in renal diagnosis. *Glomerular haematuria* arises from diseased glomeruli. Typically cells are irregular in size and shape (*dysmorphic*) and form *red cell casts*. (Non-glomerular haematuria arises distal to the glomerulus. Hyaline casts are formed from Tamm Horsfall protein in fever or exercise and do not imply renal disease. Granular and white casts are found in many, notably pyogenic, conditions.)

Proteinuria

Persistent proteinuria usually implies renal disease. Glomerular proteinuria is usually > 500 mg/24 h and comprises mostly albumin. True orthostatic proteinuria (no proteinuria early morning, proteinuria with ambulation) and tubulointerstitial disease are usually associated with minor proteinuria.

Nephrotic syndrome

In nephrotic syndrome (notably *minimal change disease, membranous nephropathy, focal segmental glomerulosclerosis*), there is *heavy albuminuria* (> 3 g/day) because the glomerular *filter is damaged and more leaky than usual*. This leads to *hypoalbuminuria* and *oedema*.

The selective nature of the proteinuria tends to alter lipoprotein profiles causing *dyslipidaemia*, a *prothrombotic tendency* through loss of natural anticoagulant proteins and *mild immunosuppression* through loss of immunoglobulin subtypes.

Nephritic syndrome

In nephritic syndrome the glomerular *filter is damaged but inflammation renders it less leaky than normal*. Glomerular *haematuria, hypertension, oliguria* and *acute renal failure* are common.

Acute renal failure (ARF)

ARF is discussed in Case study 3.17.

Chronic renal failure (CRF)

CRF is discussed in Case study 3.17.

Hypertension

Blood pressure control is often the most significant factor determining the rate of progression of CRF.

TABLE 3.2   Histopathological types of glomerulonephritis and clinical correlation

Histopathological type	Clinical response	Light microscopy (LM), immunofluorescence (IF), electron microscopy (EM)	Treatment and prognosis
Non proliferative			
Minimal change disease	Selective proteinuria Nephrotic syndrome Mostly children, decreasing incidence with age	LM: Normal EM: Effacement of podocytes	Good response to steroids, but may relapse
Membranous nephropathy	Non-selective proteinuria Nephrotic syndrome Increasing incidence with age	LM: Deposition of immune deposits on basement membrane ± thickening and sclerosis	Good prognosis but associations include Hodgkin's disease Prognosis without treatment—30% improve, 30% static, 40% worsen May respond to steroids/immunosuppression Secondary causes include NHL, carcinoma, gold, penicillamine, diabetes, SLE, amyloid, malaria, hepatitis B and HIV infection
Focal and segmental glomerulosclerosis (FSGS) *May progress from minimal change disease*	Mostly young adults Proteinuria of variable selectivity Nephrotic syndrome	*Focal (unlike diffuse)* implies that not all glomeruli are involved *Segmental* implies that only part of each glomerulus involved	May be steroid responsive If unresponsive tend to progress to CRF Most require renal transplantation
Proliferative			
Diffuse mesangial GN *Also known as IgA nephropathy (IgAN)*	The most common GN, causing any of recurrent macroscopic haematuria (often precipitated by 'synpharyngitic'—concurrent—upper respiratory tract infection), asymptomatic microscopic haematuria, proteinuria, nephritic syndrome, nephrotic syndrome, ARF, CRF, hypertension	LM: Mesangial proliferation IF: Immune deposits, often IgA EM: Mesangial dense deposits	No satisfactory treatment Strict blood pressure control Prognosis of symptomatic IgAN variable, but high asymptomatic prevalence

TABLE 3.2   (Cont'd)

Histopathological type	Clinical response	Light microscopy (LM), immunofluorescence (IF), electron microscopy (EM)	Treatment and prognosis
Diffuse exudative and proliferative endocapillary GN *Also known as postinfectious/ poststreptococcal GN(PIGN)*	Mostly young Often triggered by infection Latent period of 7–10 days between infection and immune complex damage giving rise to nephritic syndrome	LM: Proliferation of endocapillary cells (endothelial and mesangial) IF: 'Starry sky' of immune deposits around capillary loops (especially C3 complement) EM: Subepithelial humps	No specific treatment other than of any identified infection Good prognosis
Diffuse proliferative GN with crescents *Also known as crescenteric GN*	Any age group, often older adults Rapidly progressive GN Oligoanuric ARF Often renal manifestation of systemic vasculitis	Accumulation of cells in Bowman's space to form crescents and often focal necrosis	Prognosis poor without rapid treatment but good with early treatment (steroids, cyclophosphamide ± plasma exchange)
Focal and segmental proliferative GN (FSGN)	Nephritic syndrome/ARF	*Focal (unlike diffuse)* implies that not all glomeruli are involved *Segmental* implies that only part of each glomerulus involved	May be associated with a systemic disease such as SLE Prognosis good, especially if treating a systemic disease
Membranoproliferative (also confusingly called mesangiocapillary) GN	Type 1 is idiopathic. Type 2 is associated with complement abnormalities and alternative pathway activation (C3 nephritic factor) Haematuria, proteinuria, nephrotic syndrome and/or renal failure	Type 2 EM: dense deposits	Poor overall prognosis for renal function

Non-proliferative disease tends to give rise to leaky glomeruli and nephrotic syndrome. Proliferative disease tends to give rise to inflammed glomeruli and nephritic syndrome.

Box 3.8	Uraemic Symptoms

- Anorexia, nausea and vomiting
- Cramps and restless legs
- Peripheral neuropathy symptoms (Case study 6.29) and sexual dysfunction
- Cognitive disturbance and drowsiness
- Hiccups
- Itch
- Pericarditis symptoms
- Myoclonus

Box 3.9	Assessment of Fluid Status

- Blood pressure measurement
- JVP assessment
- Examination for oedema (peripheral, sacral or pulmonary)
- Daily weight (1 L = 1 kg) and fluid balance charts

Frequently patients present with small 'burnt out' fibrotic kidneys, the cause not established.

Evidence of decompensation

Look for evidence of renal replacement by haemodialysis, peritoneal dialysis or renal transplantation (Case study 3.18).

DISCUSSION	

What do you understand by the term renal failure?

Renal failure (RF) refers to acute (ARF) or chronic (CRF) loss of renal function. Isotope measurement of the glomerular filtration rate (GFR) is the 'gold standard' for determining renal function, and reveals impairment before a serum creatinine rise. *CRF is defined as kidney damage or GFR < 60 ml/min for ≥ 3 months.* The kidneys have enormous reserve. Mildly elevated creatinine may imply that 75% of functioning renal tissue is lost and in CRF referral to a nephrologist is generally recommended before serum creatinine reaches 150–180 µmol/L.

Serum creatinine alone is a poor indicator of the degree of renal failure because it is influenced by muscle mass, age, sex, weight, diet and drugs. An elderly patient with a small body mass index and creatinine of 300 may develop uraemic symptoms whilst a young muscular patient with a creatinine of 1000 might not. Because measuring GFR is cumbersome, creatinine clearance is often used as a correlate of GFR, commonly estimated by the Cockroft–Gault formula:

$$\text{Cr clearance} = \frac{(140 - \text{age})\ (\text{weight in kg})}{\text{serum Cr (µmol/L)} \times 0.81} \times \frac{(0.85 \text{ if female}) \text{ ml/}}{\text{min}/1.73 \text{ m}^2}$$

What are the causes of renal failure?

Combinations of causes are common. Causes may be considered as prerenal, renal and postrenal.

Prerenal causes of renal failure

The kidney is underperfused when there is low blood pressure or shock. Causes include:
- Cardiogenic/left ventricular failure ● Sepsis ● Hypovolaemia.

Renal causes of renal failure

The kidney comprises three main groups of tissue: glomeruli, tubules and interstitial substance, and blood vessels.

Disease in any of these structures can cause renal failure. Revision of clinically important renal physiology may be helpful at this point (Box 3.10).

1. **Glomerular disease**. This is discussed in Case study 3.16.
2. **Tubulointerstitial disease.** There are many causes of diffuse tubulointerstitial damage which can give rise to renal failure, including drugs, hypoxia/acute tubular necrosis, autoimmune and cystic diseases. The commonest cause is interstitial nephritis secondary to drugs such as NSAIDs. Patients present with renal failure and have a normal urine sediment. Molecular advances have also revealed many genetic conditions attributable to a specific defective tubule transport mechanism. Many of these in isolation do not give rise to renal failure. Examples of these are given in Box 3.10.
3. **Vascular disease and the kidney.**
   (i) *Renovascular disease* is a leading cause of CRF. Given the prevalence of coronary artery and cerebrovascular disease it is no surprise that the renal arteries and microvascular tree are susceptible to the traditional cardiovascular risk factors. Diabetes mellitus and hypertension are the two most common causes of CRF and end stage renal disease (ESRD). Further, accelerated cardiovascular disease (mortality in patients with ESRD 10–20x normal) is a major problem in CRF.

   Macrovascular renal artery disease (renal artery stenosis) is usually atherosclerotic, and because the juxtaglomerular apparatus perceives low volume it stimulates hyperreninaemic hyperaldosteronism (page 253). *Fibromuscular dysplasia* is a rare cause of distal, 'sausage string' renal artery stenosis seen especially in younger females. Some patients present with 'flash floods' of dramatic pulmonary oedema. Clinical assessment may detect a renal artery bruit (commonly at the epigastrium) and investigations include Doppler ultrasound, captopril renography or

Box 3.10   **Clinically Important Renal Physiology**

Two sequential fundamental processes underlie kidney function:

1. Glomerular filtration

The glomerulus is a filter producing a cell- and protein-free ultrafiltrate of plasma which enters the tubule.

GFR is determined by the driving force of hydrostatic pressure from the heart and counteractive forces including Bowman's space hydrostatic pressure, oncotic pressures, filter permeability and surface area. GFR is greatly reduced in inflammatory glomerular disease.

Normal GFR is around 125 ml/min or over 150 L of ultrafiltrate daily, most of which is reabsorbed by the tubules. Filtration is tightly autoregulated.

2. Tubular transport

The renal *clearance* of a substance is an overview of its net handling. Clearance = urine concentration × urine flow rate/plasma concentration (ml/min).

(i) Proximal tubule

H^+-sodium exchange occurs proximally, providing luminal H^+ for reclaiming filtered bicarbonate (Fig. 3.8 and page 93). Two-thirds of sodium is reabsorbed in the proximal tubule. Regulation of sodium is the prime determinant of extracellular fluid volume.

Glucose, amino acids and phosphate are reabsorbed completely from the proximal tubule via a carrier protein. *Glycosuria* may result when the 'renal threshold' for reabsorption (plasma glucose 10 mmol/L) is exceeded, as in diabetes mellitus, or in an autosomal recessively determined defect in the sodium–glucose transporter. Various *aminoacidurias* may result from defective amino acid transporters. In *cystinuria* there is excess secretion of cystine, ornithine, arginine and lysine (COAL), causing high urinary cystine levels and calculi. The *renal tubular acidoses* are discussed on pages 94–95.

(ii) Thick ascending loop of Henle (TAL)

A sodium-potassium ATPase in the basal membrane maintains a baseline low intracellular sodium concentration but this encourages sodium influx from the lumen, and this is coupled with one potassium and two chloride ions in a unique 'triple cotransporter' (sodium, potassium, chloride) carrier molecule.

Loop diuretics bind to the chloride site of this carrier molecule and inhibit triple cotransport and water transport. A potassium channel normally redirects some intracellular potassium back into the lumen but loop diuretics inhibit this too and encourage a gradient for calcium and magnesium to efflux into the lumen. Traditional thinking was that diuretic induced hyponatraemia prompted aldosterone action (point iv) and that resultant loss of H^+ caused alkalosis. However, loop diuretics seem to also enhance local bicarbonate uptake as the H^+-sodium pump operates faster to compensate for the diuretic action. Therefore, *loop diuretics cause a hyponatraemic, hypokalaemic, hypomagnesaemic, hypocalcaemic, hypercalciuric (predisposing to calculi) metabolic alkalosis. Bartter's syndrome* is a genetic defect of the triple cotransporter. It is a *genetic loop diuretic!*

(iii) Early distal tubule
Fluid entering the distal tubule is hypo-osmotic. Here an apical sodium chloride cotransporter promotes sodium reabsorption and calcium efflux into the lumen. *Thiazide diuretics* block the cotransporter and cause *similar biochemical changes to loop diuretics, except that they may cause hypercalcaemia. Gitelman's syndrome* is a genetic defect of the cotransporter. It is a *genetic thiazide!*

(iv) Terminal distal tubule and collecting duct
Aldosterone stimulates absorption of sodium ions (via a H^+-sodium pump), exchanging them for potassium or hydrogen ions. Some *potassium sparing diuretics* inhibit aldosterone. Potassium transport is regulated mostly by aldosterone, released from the adrenal gland, triggered by rising potassium levels. Aldosterone disorders are discussed on page 254.

The final common regulator of volume is *antidiuretic hormone (ADH)*, which acts on water channel proteins in the collecting ducts called aquaporins to enhance their permeability. A defective aquaporin (aquaporin-2) causing end organ resistance to ADH gives rise to *nephrogenic diabetes insipidus (NDI)*, discussed on page 553.

magnetic resonance angiography. Where hyperaldosteronism is refractory to medical therapy, angioplasty, stents, artery bypass or nephrectomy may be necessary.

Microvascular renovascular disease may be atherosclerotic or embolic. Thrombolysis, anticoagulants or invasive procedures which shear endothelial plaques occasionally trigger embolic showers which scatter through the renovascular system. Episodes of cholesterol emboli may be associated with eosinophilia.

Renal infarction is underdiagnosed. It may be asymptomatic or induce loin pain with or without haematuria. A high lactate dehydrogenase (LDH) is a strong clue.

(ii) Whilst renal failure itself may promote hypertension, chronic inadequately controlled *hypertension* causes *nephrosclerosis*

Fig. 3.8 *Renal buffering*

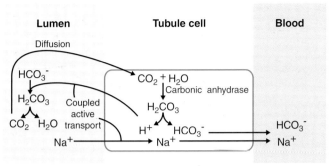

(a) Bicarbonate reabsorption (proximal tubules)

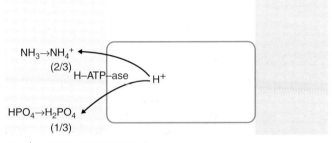

(b) H$^+$ excretion (distal tubules)

which may prompt CRF or accelerate progression of pre-existing renal disease. Hypertension is discussed in Case study 5.17.

(iii) The kidney may be involved in numerous *systemic vasculitides* (Box 3.11). These multisystem disorders are associated with deposition of immunoglobulin in vessel walls and vessel inflammation.

Wegener's granulomatosis is accompanied by granulomata, typically in the lungs and upper airways, and frequently presents with nasal stuffiness, nasal ulceration, sinusitis or otitis media. The major organs threatened are the lungs, with pulmonary haemorrhage, and the kidneys, with crescentic glomerulonephritis and its clinical correlate—rapidly progressive renal failure. Other manifestations include episcleritis, sight threatening 'meltdown' keratitis and uveitis. *MPA* presents similarly to WG. These conditions are sometimes placed under the wider umbrella of *pulmonary–renal syndromes. SLE* can also cause a wide array of histopathological insults in the kidney and lung.

Antineutrophil cytoplasmic antibodies (ANCAs) are directed against neutrophil granules and detected by indirect immunofluorescence. *Anticytoplasmic (cANCAs)* are seen to be directed against proteinase

Box 3.11	Types of Vasculitis

Large vessel
- Takayasu's arteritis ● Giant cell arteritis

Medium vessel
- Polyarteritis nodosa ● Kawasaki's disease

Small vessel
Granulomatous
- Wegener's granulomatosis (WG) ● Churg–Strauss syndrome (CSS)

Non-granulomatous
- Microscopic polyarteritis (MPA) ● Vasculitis associated with connective tissue disorders, e.g. RA, SLE ● Leucocytoclastic vasculitis (non-systemic, with polymorph infiltrate in skin vessel walls, often drug induced) ● Henoch–Schönlein purpura (page 464) ● Infective endocarditis (Case study 5.9) ● Cryoglobulinaemia (page 202)

3 (PR3) on enzyme-linked immunosorbent assay (ELISA) testing. They are predominant in patients with WG. *Antiperinuclear (pANCAs)* are seen to be directed against myeloperoxidase (MPO) on ELISA testing. They are most common in MPA. There is no conclusive evidence that ANCAs are pathogenic but the strength of association with disease activity is such that ANCA titres may monitor disease activity and indicate risk of relapse.

Treatment of the systemic vasculitides with renal involvement requires urgent, specialist institution of immunosuppression.

Postrenal causes of renal failure

Obstructive (urological) causes include prostatic hypertrophy, chronic calculus disease, transitional cell carcinoma of the bladder obstructing the ureters, ovarian and other pelvic masses obstructing the ureters, and urethral strictures.

What is Goodpasture' syndrome?

Goodpasture's syndrome is another pulmonary-renal syndrome which may cause renal failure, although it is not a vasculitis. Pathogenic antiglomerular basement membrane (GBM) antibodies target pulmonary and renal type IV collagen.

What is Alport's syndrome?

Alport's syndrome is a genetically mediated disease due to absence of the α-5 chain of type IV collagen. It is characterised by sensorineural deafness and glomerulonephritis and frequently causes end stage renal failure. Since donor kidneys contain the α-5 chain,

Alport's recipients may establish an immune response against it. This is called anti-GBM disease and can lead to graft failure.

How may renal failure be staged?

Staging (adapted from the National Kidney Foundation guidelines for CRF) on the basis of GFR in ml/min/1.73 m^2 (a surrogate creatinine clearance) is given in Box 3.12.

Box 3.12   Stages of Chronic Renal Failure

1. Normal or increased GFR (people at increased risk or with incipient renal damage): GFR > 90
2. Early renal failure: GFR 60–89
3. Moderate renal failure: GFR 30–59
4. Several renal failure (pre end stage renal disease): GFR 15–29
5. End stage renal disease (ESRD): GFR < 15

What are the effects of renal failure?

Assessment of the effects of renal failure and need for urgent treatment usually involves an assessment of three areas (Box 3.13).

Box 3.13   Three Areas to Assess in Renal Failure

1. Uraemic symptoms
2. Fluid status
3. Metabolic/biochemical status

Uraemic symptoms

Uraemic symptoms are listed in Box 3.8. Patients are usually asymptomatic until approaching end stage renal disease.

The syndrome of uraemia is complex and results from retention of multiple substances, many not yet established. The role of urea as a direct contributor to the uraemic syndrome is uncertain.

Fluid status

Early CRF may cause nocturia, due to the body's attempt to remove excess toxins, tubular dysfunction and sometimes polyuria. Later, CRF progresses to oliguria (a late sign) and oligoanuria. ARF usually causes oligoanuria. It is important to try to decide whether a patient is fluid overloaded, fluid depleted or normovolaemic. The presence of any oedema suggests that a patient is at least a few litres overloaded. Assessment of fluid status is given in Box 3.9.

Metabolic/biochemical status

'Renal blood tests' and their abnormalities are given in Box 3.14.

| Box 3.14 | Blood tests in Renal Failure |

- *Potassium* (hyperkalaemia occurs in severe renal failure)
- *Bicarbonate* (a low bicarbonate with a high anion gap metabolic acidosis occurs in severe renal failure)
- *Urea* and *creatinine* (proportionately elevated*)
- *Phosphate*** (hyperphosphataemia due to phosphate retention tends to occur in moderate to severe CRF; however, precipitation of calcium phosphate in renal tissue due to an increased calcium phosphate product may begin early)
- *Calcium*** (hypocalcaemia due to decreased production of active vitamin D_3 (pages 509–510) with decreased calcium absorption occurs in moderate CRF)
- *Parathyroid hormone* (PTH)** levels start to increase in early renal failure to compensate for hypocalcaemia (*secondary hyperparathyroidism*). If the parathyroid glands are persistently stimulated, over years, *tertiary hyperparathyroidism* can result. Whilst secondary hyperparathyroidism is due to appropriately reversible hyperplasia, aiming to correct hypocalcaemia, tertiary hyperparathyroidism is state of 'overshoot' with irreversible, autonomous secretion of PTH leading to hypercalcaemia. The mechanisms of renal bone disease (renal bone dystrophy) are complex but include hyperparathyroidism.
- *Haemoglobin*** (normochromic normocytic anaemia begins in moderate CRF when the GFR is 30–35% below normal, primarily caused by failure of erythropoietin (EPO) synthesis)
- *Lipids* (dyslipidaemia may be evident in early renal failure and contributes to cardiovascular risk)

*A rise in urea disproportionately higher than a rise in creatinine may be caused by dehydration, diuretics, gastrointestinal bleeding, high protein intake, catabolic states such as stress, starvation and steroids, or tetracyclines. A disproportionate creatinine rise occurs in rhabdomyolysis, in which myoglobin released from damaged muscle in severe crush injury, peripheral ischaemia or infarction 'clogs' renal tubules. There is usually other evidence of cell lysis such as raised potassium, phosphate and creatine kinase.
**Usually in CRF

Renal failure also causes platelet dysfunction, which may respond to synthetic ADH (DDAVP/desmopressin).

What investigations are important in renal failure?

Established renal failure

In established renal failure, investigations aim to determine *cause*,

TABLE 3.3   Urine protein quantification

Normal albumin excretion	< 30 mg/24 hours
Microalbuminuria	30–300 mg/24 h (20–200 mcg/min) *or* a spot urine albumin/ceatinine ratio of 2.5–25 mg/μmol in males or 3.5–35 mg/μmol in females
Macroalbuminuria	> 300 mg/24 h (> 200 mcg/min) – equivalent to urine dipstix ≥ 'one plus' protein

determine if *acute* or *chronic*, assess *severity* and monitor *progress*. They may include:

- Urine sediment analysis (Box 3.7)
- Urine protein quantification (Table 3.3)
- 'Renal blood tests' (Box 3.14)
- Autoimmune screen (ANA – page 475, double stranded DNA, ANCA – page 85, complement components)
- Paraprotein screen (immunoglobulin levels, serum electrophoresis, urine for Bence Jones proteins)
- Anti-GBM antibodies (if suspicion) and cryoglobulins (if suspicion)
- Creatine kinase (if rhabdomyolyis likely)
- Ultrasound to determine kidney size (usually normal in ARF and small in CRF but may be large in diabetes, amyloidosis, renal vein thrombosis, hydronephrosis), the presence or absence of hydronephrosis (obstruction) and Doppler flow (signals may be lost in renal artery stenosis)
- HBV/HCV/HIV status if renal replacement therapy is likely
- Chest X-ray
- ECG (LVH commonly accompanies moderate CRF).

Early detection of renal damage

Renal disease is often progressive once GFR falls below 25% of normal. The haemodynamic changes (including angiotensin II activity) which sustain renal function initially in surviving nephrons are ultimately detrimental. Patients at high risk (age, diabetes, hypertension, family history, renal transplant) should be evaluated for markers of kidney damage (albuminuria, abnormal urine sediment, elevated serum creatinine).

How may prerenal failure (PRF) be distinguished from established acute tubular necrosis (ATN) or oliguric acute renal failure?

In PRF, the tubules can reabsorb and thus concentrate urine. In ATN, the tubules are damaged and 'everything leaks out' (Table 3.4). However, PRF often leads to ATN and results become indeterminate.

What are the treatment principles in renal failure?

1. *Treatment of reversible causes*

Potentially reversible causes should be identified and treated.

TABLE 3.4   Features that distinguish PRF from ATN

	PRF	ATN
Urine osmolality	Increased (> 500 mosm/kg)	Decreased (< 350 mosm/kg)
Urine sodium	Low (< 20 mmol/L)	Normal/high (> 40 mmol/L)
Urine concentration	Normal	Dilute

These include pre-renal causes (page 82), toxins (nephrotoxic drugs, radiocontrast), uncontrolled hypertension and obstruction. Chronic obstruction exerts abnormal pressure on tubules and impairs tubular function. Significant diuresis may follow relief of obstruction, requiring large volume fluid replacement. A common mistake is to assume that obstruction cannot be present with a good urine output – but obstruction may be unilateral or there may be a battle between antegrade and retrograde flow before the battle is lost.

2. *Limiting progression*

Factors which cause progressive decline in renal function after the onset of kidney damage include:

● Persistent activity of underlying cause
● Hypertension
● Poor glycaemic control
● Persistent proteinuria, which is the single best predictor of progression of renal disease
● Dyslipidaemia
● Smoking
● High phosphate or protein diet
● Hyperphosphataemia
● Anaemia (which leads to a high cardiac output state, pressure/volume overload, left ventricular hypertrophy and systolic dysfunction).

Treatment objectives in renal failure are given in Box 3.15.

Briefly outline the body's fluid distribution

The volume of total body water is approximately 45 L. One-third of this is extracellular fluid (ECF) comprising plasma (3.5 L) and interstitial or tissue fluid (8.5 L) and two-thirds is intracellular fluid (ICF). The predominant ion composition of fluids is given in Table 3.5.

Fluid flow between plasma and interstitium depends on the balance between outward pressures (capillary hydrostatic pressure, tissue oncotic pressure) and inward pressures (interstitial fluid pressure, plasma oncotic pressure). *Oedema* results when interstitial fluid increases due to a pressure gradient or excess capillary permeability.

| Box 3.15 | Treatment Objectives in Renal Failure |

ARF

The main objectives with ARF are to *determine and institute treatment of the underlying cause*. Acute haemodialysis via a temporary central venous catheter (e.g. internal jugular vein) may be indicated if there is symptomatic uraemia, serositis (pericarditis ± pericardial rub, pleuritis), fluid overload with pulmonary oedema, hyperkalaemia or severe acidosis (bicarbonate < 12 mmol/L). Early diuresis prompted by high dose diuretics can sometimes obviate the need for dialysis.

CRF

The main objectives with CRF are to *correct the cause* where possible, *slow the rate of progression*, institute *therapeutic adjuncts* and *plan for renal replacement therapy* when ESRD seems inevitable.

Important strategies to *slow progression* include:

- Meticulous blood pressure control (< 130/85 mmHg in all patients with renal disease and < 125/75 mmHg in patients with proteinuric renal disease). This is the most important intervention to slow progression.
- Meticulous glycaemic control. Refer to Case study 4.18 for specific management of diabetic nephropathy.
- Reducing proteinuria with ACEIs or angiotensin II receptor blockers (ARBs). These agents slow progression in both diabetic and non-diabetic kidney disease. They reduce the effects of angiotensin II on renal haemodynamics and may have glomerular permselectivity effects, thus providing renoprotection independent of their beneficial effect on blood pressure lowering.
- Correction of dyslipidaemia (statins).
- Smoking cessation.

Other *therapeutic adjuncts* in CRF include:
- Modest dietary phosphate restriction and phosphate binders to limit phosphate absorption. Adequate nutrition is essential in CRF and the role of dietary protein restriction remains controversial.
- Calcitriol (1-hydroxy vitamin D which is further hydroxylated to 1,25 hydroxy vitamin D in the liver) may correct hypocalcaemia and 'switch off' PTH stimulation.
- Recombinant human erythropoietin (EPO) to maintain haemoglobin (Hb) at a level at which patients are unimpeded in daily activities but below that which may result in excessive

thrombotic risk. The National Kidney Foundation recommends evaluation of anaemia if Hb is < 11 g/dL and consideration of EPO to maintain HB > 11 g/dL.

● Strict attention to fluid balance, using loop diuretics if necessary. Large doses, e.g. furosemide (frusemide) 500 mg to 1 g, may be needed to treat oedema in severe renal failure.

● Bicarbonate in severe metabolic acidosis.

TABLE 3.5   Predominant ion composition of fluids

	ECF	ICF
Cations	Sodium	Potassium Magnesium
Anions	Bicarbonate Chloride	Phosphate Proteins Organic acids

Osmolality (osm) refers to the number of particles (osmoles) dissolved in 1 kg of solution (osmolarity refers to 1 L rather than 1 kg). The main determinant of ECF osm is sodium and ICF osm potassium. Normal plasma osm = 280–295 mosmol/kg. Normal urine osm = 300–1400 mosmol/kg.

Antidiuretic hormone (ADH) is the great evolutionary stress hormone—when sabre tooth tigers rewarded their hunger by biting off the limbs of our ancestors, ADH retained fluid and made platelets sticky. ADH deficiency (diabetes insipidus) and SIADH are discussed on page 553.

What are the causes of hyponatraemia?

Hyponatraemia may be spurious or true. Spurious (laboratory assay) hyponatraemia occurs when protein (paraproteinaemias), lipid (hyperlipidaemias) or glucose (diabetic ketoacidosis) is high and plasma is hypertonic or isotonic. True hyponatraemia occurs in four settings:

1. Psychogenic polydipsia.
2. Unavoidable sodium loss—gastrointestinal loss, renal loss (renal failure is frequently associated with dysregulated sodium balance)/diuretics.
3. Appropriate ADH excess when the body perceives volume depletion—cardiac failure, cirrhosis or nephrotic syndrome.
4. Syndrome of inappropriate ADH excess (SIADH), in which plasma osm (< 260 mosmol/kg) and sodium are low and urine osm and sodium are high.

The body hates cell swelling, which causes seizures and ultimately death. ADH levels are therefore normally low. Relative ADH excess plays a role in most causes of hyponatraemia because the body sees sodium as the instigator of cell swelling and water as the innocently seduced bystander. Hypernatraemia is therefore rare. Rapid correction of hyponatraemia may cause central pontine myelinosis.

How is acid–base balance regulated by the kidney?

Acids are hydrogen ion (H^+) donors and bases are H^+ acceptors. The main source of H^+ is by oxidation of carbon compounds ($CO_2 + H_2O \leftrightarrow HCO_3^- + H^+$). *Buffers* minimise changes in pH either by binding H^+ or by dissociating to release H^+. Buffer systems include:
1. ICF (50%) and plasma bicarbonate, phosphate and protein buffers
2. The red cell
3. The kidney (Fig. 3.8).

What acid–base balance disturbances do you know of? (Table 3.6)

TABLE 3.6   Types of acid–base disturbance

Principal disturbance	Primary change	Secondary compensation
Metabolic acidosis	↓ HCO_3	↓ P_{CO_2}
Metabolic alkalosis	↑ HCO_3	↑ P_{CO_2}
Respiratory acidosis	↑ P_{CO_2}	↑ HCO_3
Respiratory alkalosis	↓ P_{CO_2}	↓ HCO_3

What are the causes of metabolic acidosis?

Anion gap = plasma (sodium + potassium) – (chloride + bicarbonate)

| 146 | 4 | 110 | 24 |

The normal value is 16 ± 2 mmol/L. The 'gap' comprises unmeasured anions such as albumin, phosphate and sulphate.

Increased anion gap metabolic acidosis

This is usually due to addition of endogenous or exogenous organic acid. A mnemonic for remembering its causes is KUSMALE—think of Kussmaul breathing in diabetic ketoacidosis (DKA)—in Table 3.7.

TABLE 3.7   Causes of increased anion gap metabolic acidosis

	Anions	Features
Ketoacidosis	Ketotic pathway	DKA
Uraemia	Organic acids	Renal failure
Salicylate poisoning	Salicylic acid	Also respiratory alkalosis
Methanol poisoning	Formic acid	Visual disturbance
Alcohol/starvation	Ketotic pathway	
Lactic acidosis	Lactic acid	Ischaemia/infarction/sepsis
Ethylene glycol	Glycolate/oxalate	Oxalate crystals/renal failure

Normal anion gap metabolic acidosis

This is usually due to loss of bicarbonate. Compensatory chloride retention maintains a normal gap and hence this is sometimes described as *hyperchloraemic (and often hypokalaemic) metabolic acidosis.*

Causes include:

- Diarrhoea (loss of bicarbonate)
- Ureterosigmoidostomy (loss of bicarbonate)
- Renal tubular acidosis (RTA) (loss of bicarbonate in proximal RTA, impaired H^+ excretion in distal RTA)
- Ammonium chloride
- Acetazolamide.

Metabolic alkalosis is due to loss of H^+ or addition of bicarbonate. Gastrointestinal H^+ losses include vomiting and intestinal secretions. Renal losses include diuretics, hyperaldosteronism, Cushing's syndrome and liquorice ingestion. *Respiratory acidosis* is caused by hypoventilation. *Respiratory alkalosis* is caused by hyperventilation, e.g. anxiety, salicylate overdose, hypoxia, fever, thyrotoxicosis.

What do you know about renal tubular acidosis (RTA)?

Various abnormalities of tubule mechanisms give rise to the normal anion gap hyperchloraemic metabolic acidosis of the various types of RTA. Type 1 RTA and type 2 RTA cause hypokalaemia; type 4 RTA causes hyperkalaemia. Renal function is usually normal.

Type 1 (distal) RTA

Because of a defective H^+ ATPase in the distal tubule, the tubule cannot excrete H^+ or reabsorb sodium. This stimulates aldosterone (Box 3.10), causing hypokalaemia. Bicarbonate buffering decreases serum bicarbonate levels and bone buffering leads to release of calcium. Causes include autoimmune diseases such as SLE, hypergammaglobulinaemia, nephrocalcinosis (primary hyperparathyroidism, vitamin D excess, medullary sponge kidney), tubulointerstitial damage from drugs such as NSAIDs and tubule pressure damage in obstructive uropathy. Patients may present with hypokalaemic complications, renal calculi or bone pain (late). Diagnosis is by serum biochemistry and confirmed by alkaline urine, which fails to acidify to pH < 5.2 following an ammonium chloride acid load.

Type 2 (proximal) RTA

The H^+-sodium pump in the proximal tubule (Box 3.10) operates but only slowly, so that bicarbonate recovery is slow. Causes include paraproteinaemias (amyloid), cystinosis and Wilson's disease, which may also induce wider proximal tubule damage resulting in *Fanconi's syndrome* (failure to reabsorb glucose, phosphate and organic amino acids). Diagnosis is by serum biochemistry and detection of alkaline urine (bicarbonaturia). The urine can acidify because there is slowing rather than complete inhibition of normal function.

Type 4 RTA (associated aldosterone deficiency or resistance)

Aldosterone deficiency may be primary (Addison's disease) or secondary (to hyporeninaemia). *Aldosterone resistance* may be congenital (pseudohypoaldosteronism) or acquired (SLE, amyloid, obstructive uropathy, amiloride). Aldosterone disorders are discussed on page 254.

How is serum potassium concentration regulated?

Acute changes in potassium concentration are usually the result of redistribution between the ECF and ICF. Alkalosis, catecholamines and insulin tend to redistribute potassium into cells. The hypokalaemic and hyperkalaemic periodic paralyses are due to redistribution abnormalities.

Chronic regulation of potassium concentration is undertaken by the kidney, in the distal tubule.

Potassium disorders may be evaluated with four questions:

1. Is redistribution likely?
2. Is the kidney involved in the pathogenesis (measure urinary potassium)?
3. If the kidney is involved, what is the role of aldosterone?
4. Is there tubular dysfunction?

What are the causes of hypokalaemia?

1. Redistribution.
2. Total body potassium depletion:
   (i) Decreased intake, e.g. anorexia
   (ii) Increased loss (gastrointestinal loss—urine $K^+ < 20$ mmol/day; renal loss—urine $K^+ > 20$ mmol/day).
3. Aldosterone excess (hypertensive)
   (i) Primary or secondary hyperaldosteronism (page 254)
   (ii) Pseudohyperaldosteronism/Liddle's syndrome (page 254).
   Aldosterone excess (normotensive)
   (i) Acidotic: Types 1 and 2 RTA
   (ii) Alkalotic: diuretics, Bartter's syndrome (Box 3.10).
4. Pseudohyperaldosteronism/Liddle's syndrome (page 254).

What are the causes of hyperkalaemia?

1. Redistribution or spurious (haemolysed sample)
2. Total body potassium excess (increased intake or renal retention in renal failure)
3. Aldosterone deficiency (page 255)
4. Aldosterone resistance (page 255), potassium sparing diuretics, angiotensin-converting enzyme inhibitors (ACEIs), ciclosporin.

How would you treat hyperkalaemia?

- Ideal treatment is to promote diuresis, but if oligoanuria persists then dialysis may be needed.
- Emergency measures include calcium gluconate (cardioprotective), and insulin with dextrose (redistribution) and beta-2 agonists (redistribution).
- Low potassium diets and resonium may control potassium levels in CRF.

CASE STUDY   3.18 END STAGE RENAL DISEASE (ESRD) AND RENAL TRANSPLANTATION

Instruction: *Please examine this patient's abdomen and discuss your findings.*

RECOGNITION

There is a *palpable renal transplant in the right/left iliac fossa* with an overlying *scar*. There may be *arteriovenous fistulae* at the forearms and *internal jugular/subclavian scarring* from dialysis catheters or *scarring from peritoneal dialysis catheters* (Fig. 3.9).

INTERPRETATION

Look for/consider causes

- Insulin injection sites on the abdomen
- Bilateral flank masses or nephrectomy scar on same side of transplant or laparotomy scar (APCKD)
- Hearing aids (Alport's syndrome, Wegener's granulomatosis).

Assess other systems

- Tell the examiners that you would ask about uraemic symptoms, assess blood pressure and fluid status and wish to see the renal blood results (Case study 3.17)
- Cushingoid appearance (prednisolone)
- Gum hypertrophy/hirsutism (ciclosporin)
- Skin tumours (immunosuppression)
- Parathyroidectomy scar
- Signs of previous (or current if transplant failed) dialysis infection.

DISCUSSION

What types of renal transplant are there?

Donor transplants may be cadaveric or live.

List some complications of renal transplantation

- Rejection
- Immunosuppression

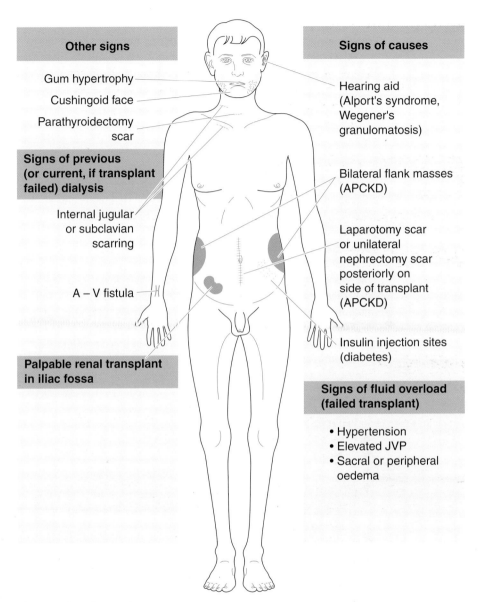

Other signs

Gum hypertrophy

Cushingoid face

Parathyroidectomy
scar

**Signs of previous
(or current, if transplant
failed) dialysis**

Internal jugular
or subclavian
scarring

A – V fistula

**Palpable renal transplant
in iliac fossa**

Signs of causes

Hearing aid
(Alport's syndrome,
Wegener's
granulomatosis)

Bilateral flank masses
(APCKD)

Laparotomy scar
or unilateral
nephrectomy scar
posteriorly on
side of transplant
(APCKD)

Insulin injection sites
(diabetes)

**Signs of fluid overload
(failed transplant)**

• Hypertension
• Elevated JVP
• Sacral or peripheral
  oedema

Fig. 3.9   *Renal transplant*

● Surgical—renal artery stenosis, ureteric stenosis, ureteric leak,
  infection, neoplasia.

Since transplant immunosuppressant drugs tend to inhibit interleukin
2 (IL-2) signalling, which is essential for T lymphocyte proliferation,
the profile of organisms tends to be that of depressed cell mediated
immunity (pages 199–200, 206).

What do you know about transplant rejection?

Following organ transplantation, a recipient's immune system tends to reject donor tissue, unless the donor tissue is genetically identical.

1. *Hyperacute rejection* may occur within minutes or hours and is due to preformed antibodies.
2. *Acute rejection* in the first few days is due to cytotoxic (CD8) mediated immunity.
3. *Late rejection* is due to antibody production against the graft and complement activation.

In both acute and late rejection, the initial reaction is between the T cell receptors of the recipient and the foreign HLA molecules of donor tissue bearing foreign peptides. This leads to a cascade of intracellular and extracellular events central to which is the production of IL-2 (pages 195–200).

Recipient/donor matching to reduce rejection involves HLA typing, blood grouping and lymphocytotoxic crossmatching. Renal transplantation is highly immunogenic (unlike cornea, bone and artery grafts), so that immunosuppressive drugs are mandatory for graft survival.

The final common denominator of many immunosuppressive drugs is inhibition of IL-2, a powerful inducer of T and B cell proliferation. Ciclosporin and tacrolimus (FK506) inhibit calcineurin, an intracellular molecule integral to IL-2 elaboration. Steroids inhibit nuclear regulatory proteins. Azathioprine inhibits lymphocyte DNA synthesis.

Which diseases recur in a transplanted kidney?

- Focal and segmental glomerulosclerosis (FSGS)
- Oxalosis
- Diabetes (but reasonable prognosis for graft survival)
- IgA nephropathy (IgAN)
- Haemolytic uraemic syndrome (HUS)/thrombotic thrombocytopenic purpura (TTP)
- Anti-GBM disease rarely recurs but linear staining for IgG is found in around 50% of biopsies.

What other forms of renal replacement are there for ESRD?

- Haemodialysis ● Peritoneal dialysis.

What are the forms of vascular access?

- Temporary double-lumen catheter inserted into the internal jugular or subclavian vein (the femoral vein is acceptable in an emergency but suboptimal)
- Permanent arteriovenous fistula (AVF) or gortex graft. An AVF is an anastomosis created surgically between an artery and vein, commonly at the forearm, which dilates over a number of weeks to become suitable for twin-needled dialysis access. By convention, the 'out' line is termed the 'A' line and the 'in' line the 'V' line. The

needles point in opposite directions to minimise mixing of outgoing and incoming blood and hence the dialysing of freshly dialysed incoming blood.

Discuss the principles of haemodialysis (Fig. 3.10)

From the point of vascular access, blood leaves the body and runs to a pump and thence to the dialyser ('artificial kidney'). The pump is designed not to crush blood cells. In the dialyser, blood enters thousands of semipermeable microtubules, not dissimilar to the diameter of a capillary. Between these microtubules and running in the opposite direction is *dialysis fluid*, against which the blood is dialysed. Dialysis fluid contains concentrations of substances such that an osmotic or ionic gradient is set up from blood to dialysis fluid. Since most patients with CRF are acidotic, dialysis fluid is alkaline and contains bicarbonate, thus allowing correction of acidosis in the blood. However, it is desirable to avoid large ionic shifts. Equally, dialysis fluid contains a low concentration of potassium (1–2 mmol/L) in order to draw potassium from the blood and usually a low concentration of calcium. Sodium and glucose concentrations are usually normal. Dialysed blood returns to the body via a separate lumen. The *dialysate* is discarded.

The transmembrane pressure gradient from blood to dialysis fluid is proportional to the rate and force of the pump. Adjusting the pump settings determines the amount of fluid removed at dialysis. The net amount of fluid removed is called the *ultrafiltrate*. Sometimes, patients are fluid overloaded but metabolically stable. In such cases, pure ultrafiltration, rather than dialysis, is indicated.

Fig. 3.10   *Principles of haemodialysis*

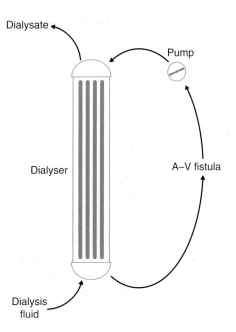

Measurement of dialysis adequacy is contentious.

Adjunctive treatments for dialysis patients are generally those outlined in Box 3.15.

What complications of haemodialysis may occur?

Complications include access problems, sepsis, haemodynamic instability and β_2-microglobulin accumulation. β_2-microglobulin is a non-dialysed molecule which forms amyloid deposits over many years in musculoskeletal tissues.

REFERENCES AND FURTHER READING

LIVER DISEASE

Krige JEJ, Beckingham IJ. Portal hypertension – 1: varices/portal hypertension – 2: ascites, encephalopathy and other conditions (ABC of diseases of liver, pancreas and biliary system). Br Med J 2001; 322: 348–351/416–418.

Sherlock S, Dooley J. Diseases of the liver and biliary system, 11th edn. Oxford: Blackwell Science; 2002.

Thomas HC. Hepatitis B and D liver infections. Medicine 1999; 27: 34–36.

HAEMATOLOGY

British Society for Haematology. Publishes British Committee for Standards in Haematology (BCSH) guidelines. Online. Available: www.bcshguidelines.com

Hoffbrand AV, Pettit JE. Color atlas of clinical hematology. London: Mosby-Wolfe; 1994.

Jandl JH. Blood. Textbook of hematology, 2nd edn. Boston: Little, Brown; 1996.

Johnson PWM, Orchard K. Bone marrow transplants. Br Med J 2002; 325: 348–349.

Provan AB, Weatherall DJ. Red cells II: acquired anaemias and polycythaemia. Lancet 2000; 355: 1260–1268.

Stewart AK, Schuh AC. White cells 2: impact of understanding the molecular basis of haematological malignant disorders on clinical practice. Lancet 2000; 355: 1447–1453.

Stock W, Hoffman R. White blood cells I: non-malignant disorders. Lancet 2000; 355: 1351–1357.

RENAL DISEASE

National Kidney Foundation. Publishes Kidney Disease Outcome Quality Initiative (K/DOQ) guidelines including clinical practice guidelines for chronic kidney disease: evaluation, classification and stratification. Am J Kidney Dis 2002; 39(suppl 1): S1–266

Parmar MS. Chronic renal disease. Br Med J 2002; 325: 85–90.

Scott DG, Watts RA. Classification and epidemiology of systemic vasculitis. Br J Rheumatol 1995; 33: 897–899.

Whitworth JA, Lawrence JR. Textbook of renal disease, 2nd edn. Edinburgh: Churchill Livingstone; 1994.

HISTORY TAKING SKILLS

4. History Taking Skills

History taking skills

Traditional history taking model

The traditional model of history taking (Box 4.1) has served doctors and patients for many years and is an essential foundation for effective history taking.

The traditional history taking model correctly emphasises the value of a careful social history (Box 4.2).

The traditional history taking model does not, however, ensure that history taking is effective. Effective history taking is more than asking a checklist of questions, noting responses and formulating a diagnosis at the end.

Effective history taking

In PACES you have 15 minutes to elicit a history, witnessed by examiners who will be examining your *history taking skills*. This is a short time in which to take a medical history and can only be achieved by sharply tailored history taking.

If you think 15 minutes is a short time, consider that general practitioners regularly take histories in less than 10 minutes. For GPs, sharp *communication and consulting skills* are paramount in rapidly eliciting problems. Problems are not elicited through a rapid-fire checklist of questions without giving the patient room to speak, but through a *tailored* history. *In PACES, feeling*

Box 4.1   Traditional History Taking Model

Introduction and preamble
- Introduction from doctor
- Patient's name, age, address and general practitioner

Nature of presenting complaint or complaints
- Identifying the *main symptoms*—what is wrong and why the patient is in hospital.

History of presenting complaint or complaints
1. Eliciting positive *symptoms* and expanding on these:
   Considering possible *causes* for each symptom

Considering possible *risk factors* and *complications* if a diagnosis is likely
2. Excluding other symptoms (negative) through a *systems review*
3. Enquiring about *management* to date
4. Formulating an *active problem list* from the above

Past medical history
- Eliciting an ongoing problem list and inactive problem list

Drug history
- Drugs past and present

Allergy history

Family history

Social history

Box 4.2   Social History

A social history might explore details of:

Personal and home life
- Marital status and health of spouse or partner
- Other family members and relevant medical problems
- Involvement of social support services
- Description of home, e.g. flat with lift, house with stairs
- Interior modifications such as bathroom rails

Work life
- Current and past occupation/s
- Effects of work on symptoms
- Effects of symptoms on work
- Degree of work satisfaction
- Income adequacy (income verses expenditure)

Asking directly about financial affairs can be an insensitive invasion of privacy and a list of questions about a patient's pension arrangement, mortgage, debts and bills is inappropriate without cues from the patient that they are relevant to the presentation. However, financial stress is a major part of modern life and history taking skills can be sensitively employed to elicit relevant details.

Leisure activities
- Support from friends
- Interests and hobbies, including the effects of illness on the quality of these
- Alcohol intake, cigarette smoking and recreational drug use

Quality of life
- Major effects of illness viewed by patient
- Coping strategies of patient
- Daily effects on life—bathing, dressing, shopping, cooking and sleep are common starting points

---

pressured because you are short of time and trying to extract the 'facts' at all costs from your patient is less important than demonstrating your skills as a communicator and showing concern for your patient.

Patients often report things in what seems a chaotic order, dodging from one area of the history to another. Candidates often prefer patients to quickly and simply answer questions rather than volunteer extra information. However, the extra information often contains important elements of the real problem. You should therefore infuse *history taking skills* into the traditional model to rapidly elicit the right facts.

History taking skills

History taking is a way of guiding what patients say. The best way to understand how history taking skills can guide patients is to understand what patients are thinking.

What patients think

A PACES case study is shown in Box 4.3.

Having taken such a history, you should of course consider the possibility of a deep venous thrombosis (DVT). DVT is the most serious of the differential diagnoses, although intuitively you may have some doubts; the duration of symptoms is long and the flight 2 months ago is likely irrelevant. Hypothesis testing (pursuing possibilities in turn until they are either excluded or warrant further testing) may also bring a popliteal cyst and non-specific muscle strain into the differential diagnosis.

You may also wonder whether as a nurse she might be particularly worried about a DVT. She will have seen DVTs on the surgical wards and know them to be

Box 4.3　　PACES Case Study

You have taken a history from a 52-year-old woman admitted with a painful left calf and mild swelling in the region of the popliteal fossa. You discover that she has had worsening pain for 3 weeks, exacerbated when going up and down stairs, and that sometimes it is so painful it reduces her to tears. She has had to stop work. You discover that she is a nurse on a surgical ward, married, with two children. She has no significant past medical history but 2 months ago was on a long haul flight, returning from a visit to her sister in Australia. You have been told that examination confirms mild swelling in the popliteal fossa and calf tenderness but that examination is otherwise unremarkable.

dangerous. She may also be aware of the risks of air travel, unaware that 2 months is a long time to 'harbour' a thrombosis.

She is probably very apprehensive. Being a patient in hospital—as a health care professional to a greater or lesser extent—is being in an alien environment amidst other unwell or dying fellow human beings. Many patients have strong preconceptions about doctors and hospitals learned from relatives, friends or the media—doctors seem not to tell patients very much, and what they do tell can be difficult to understand; doctors make mistakes, sometimes with fatal outcomes.

This patient may have already decided that she has a blood clot in her leg until proven otherwise. She may know that blood clots can travel to the lung and prove fatal. Much convincing to the contrary may be needed if her grandmother died from a blood clot (albeit after a fractured hip). She may have seen patients on warfarin, a dangerous drug to be taken for life. She may be scared that she has a serious condition requiring dangerous treatment.

These sorts of thoughts going through a patient's mind may be summarised as their *beliefs, concerns and expectations about what their symptoms might represent.*

This patient may **believe** she has a blood clot, be **concerned** about *why* it has happened and *what* needs to be done about it and **expect** the worst if nothing is done.

A 30-year-old athlete with similar symptoms may believe them to represent a strained muscle, have very few concerns and expect them to go away.

Patients don't present just with symptoms, but with thoughts about their symptoms. Some patients volunteer their thoughts. When patients do not volunteer their thoughts, asking is much better than making assumptions. A simple question can often yield useful information:

D: *What have you been told before/so far about this?*

D: *What thoughts have gone through your mind about this?*

D: *Are you worried about anything in particular?*

Without asking such a question, you may not discover (as the candidate at this station failed to discover) that the PACES patient was worried that she might have multiple sclerosis (MS). Her sister in Australia presented 2 years earlier with a painful left leg, which was later been diagnosed as MS. She in fact **believed** that she had MS and that it had happened because it ran in her family, was **concerned** about needing a lumbar puncture, and **expected** to become wheelchair bound as her sister had.

D = doctor; P = patient

Establishing patients' thoughts about their symptoms is as important in PACES as it is in practice, and can prevent you from taking the wrong direction. Without establishing these thoughts, you are working purely on assumption. Assume nothing!

Failing to elicit a patient's thoughts can mean that doctor and patient are looking at the same problem from a different angle or even two different problems. Discovering these thoughts and any hidden agenda is important. For all sorts of reasons patients don't always report their concerns, and a simple question can sometimes confirm things:

D: *Your asthma has obviously been troubling you a lot recently. How do you feel we could best help you? By trying to improve the sleepless nights, or something else?*

Six important skills to ensure that you successfully pass the History Taking Skills station are outlined in more detail below. They are:

1. Listening skills
2. Eliciting skills
3. Identifying beliefs, concerns and expectations
4. Responding to cues
5. Exploring the context
6. Summarising.

Listening Skills

Introduction

Always introduce yourself first of all and seek permission to take a history.

D: *Good morning, I'm Dr -. It's Mrs -, isn't it? Would it be alright if I asked you some questions?*

Ideally, you should sit comfortably at the same level as your patient, allowing good eye contact. These simple beginnings encourage the likelihood of good rapport.

Listening

From the start, your 'awareness antennae' should be alert to all visual and verbal information presented to you. As with examining patients at the bedside and starting with inspection, good history taking candidates are alert to how patients look, talk and behave. Your patient may be relaxed or anxious, waiting for questions, or may have already started talking. They may pre-empt your opening question with:

P: *I don't know where to start.*
P: *I don't like hospitals.*
P: *I don't know what I'm going to do about my breathing.*

The important thing is not to rush in with questions, suppressing information that may provide a valuable insight into what your patient is thinking.

Useful opening questions might be:

D: *What seems to be the problem?*
D: *Your GP says you have had a painful leg. Could you tell me about that?*
D: *Could you tell me why you have come into hospital?*

The response might be:

P: *It's my heart, doctor.*
P: *I just don't seem to have any energy any more.*

Again, it is very important to continue listening. Many candidates respond immediately with questions, for example by asking about cardiac symptoms or by assuming the problem to be tiredness and asking about thyroid symptoms. Remember that *asking a direct question usually only gives you the answer to that question!* Careful listening for a minute or two, encouraging your patient to elaborate, will help you form a much more accurate assessment of what the problem is likely to be about:

P: *I just don't seem to have any energy any more ... It all started last October when I began to get short of breath ... I'd never been in hospital in my life before that...now I seem to be here every few weeks. I first noticed it when I was out walking my dog. He's always full of energy but I was beginning to find that I couldn't keep up with him any more. I went to see my own doctor because you hear about people suddenly dropping down with heart attacks at my age, don't you? I mean, I'd had a few pains in my chest as well. He said that the heart tracing was okay but thought I should have an X-ray —that was when he sent me into hospital.*

Your thoughts may now be quite different. Heart failure? Angina? Pulmonary emboli? Chronic obstructive pulmonary disease? Fibrosing alveolitis? The point is that listening, allowing your patient time to tell you what has been happening in their own words, will give you a clearer idea about the direction you need to take.

Active versus passive listening

Use active rather than passive listening throughout the history. Active listening is more than just listening. It is *showing that you are interested in what your patient is saying.* Active listening skills include:

● An attentive manner (it helps to sit forward—do not slouch!—and make eye contact).

● Not interrupting patients (at least, not immediately).

● Encouraging noises, posture and gestures, or the skilful use of silence.

● Reflecting back answers to create follow-up questions—*What do you mean by dizzy?*

Open and closed questions

Open questions are particularly important if you are to avoid jumping to conclusions. They are essential early on:

D: *Can you describe the pain in more detail?*
D: *Can you tell me a little more about that incident?*
D: *And what has been happening since then?*
D: *So you're worried about what this pain says about your health?*
D: *Have you noticed if the pain is brought on by anything in particular?*
D: *May I ask some general questions about your health?*
D: *What has been the result of all of this?*

Closed questions may be used to clarify what a patient has said or to obtain pieces of factual information that have not been volunteered:

D: *Have you coughed any blood?*

As a general rule, save closed questions until your patient has had the chance to tell their story. A relevant systems enquiry is, of course, an appropriate series of closed questions.

Eliciting skills

Some patients need little encouragement to talk, and it is important to guide their account towards what you see as most clinically relevant. Some patients are reserved and reticent, and need encouragement. Important eliciting skills include:

Active listening

Active listening is one of the most important eliciting skills.

Appropriate use of open and closed questions

As well as asking open and closed questions, remember that some questions may seem irrelevant to patients and it is important to explain why you are asking them. This may be especially important for sensitive issues:

D: *Some of my patients with emphysema get quite depressed. I often ask patients with emphysema if they have been feeling depressed.*

Encouragement

There are many ways of encouraging a patient to continue their account. The simplest yet very effective methods are silence with encouraging facial gestures (smiling and showing concern), nodding, saying *Mmn* or *Yes* and *echoing* what is said:

P: *I have this headache sometimes.*
D: *Headache?*
P: *Not all the time, but I get it a lot.*
D: *Which part of your head gets sore?*
P: *This bit. It comes and goes. I wondered if it was serious.*
D: *What do you mean by serious?*
P: *Well you hear about headaches.*
D: *What have you heard?*

Speaking the patient's language and 'matching'

Most important is to *speak clearly and simply*, in a way that you feel your patient will understand, and to avoid technical terms which might not be understood. It can sometimes help to 'match' your patient's verbal and non-verbal behaviour.

Patients often speak in visual or auditory terms or in concepts. They might say:

P: *I don't see a way out.*
P: *It sounds like bad news to me.*
P: *It's all a bit much.*

Sometimes harnessing the patient's language in this way can enhance rapport and you may find yourself doing it naturally:

D: *I see what you mean but whilst it may look that way...*
D: *It sounds bad and not what you wanted to hear but...*

D: *I can imagine what you must be going through.*

Sometimes, in subtle ways, it is possible to match body language as well as speech.

Matching is a two-way process. Speaking loudly and clearly will often encourage your patient to do the same.

'Questions in disguise'

'Questions in disguise' (questions that are not actually questions!) can be very useful for eliciting information:

Statements can be used as questions:

D: *It sound as though that incident alarmed you.*

Conjecture can be used as a question:

D: *I was wondering whether...*
D: *Sometimes people with headaches worry that it might be something serious...*
D: *Sometimes when women have pain like this they worry they might be pregnant...*

Shared experiences or examples can be used as questions:

D: *I had a patient recently who went through a similar...*

Legitimising

Legitimising a patient's feelings can also help them to talk openly:

D: *This is clearly worrying you a great deal.*
D: *You have a lot to cope with; I think most people would feel the same way.*

Summarising periodically

Summarising periodically, as well as at the end of the interview (page 110), can be useful.

Identifying beliefs, concerns and expectations

The concept of doctor and patient centredness is discussed on pages 365–367. Overt doctor centredness (pure fact gathering) and overt patient centredness (purely addressing the patient's perspective) are extremes of a spectrum. History taking naturally undulates within the spectrum, generally starting with *patient centred open questions*:

D: *Your GP says you have had a painful leg. Would you be able to tell me more about that?*

P: *Well, yes, I noticed it a week or two ago, but didn't do anything about it.*

D: *Why not?*

P: *I hoped it would go away. I hoped it wasn't anything serious.*

D: *And what has happened since then?*

Patient centred history taking aims to identify a patient's beliefs, concerns and expectations. The following questions are examples of this *patient centred* approach:

D: *I expect you've been thinking about this for a while. Are you worried about anything in particular?*

D: *I was wondering what thoughts you'd had yourself about this?*

D: *What were your own thoughts about this problem?*

D: *Have you had any thoughts yourself about what may be causing this?*

D: *What did you think might be causing it?*

D: *Were you worried it might be due to something in particular?*

D: *Some people might have thought it might be due to blood pressure. Did that worry you at all?*

D: *When you hear the word ..., what does that mean to you?*

D: *Tell me what you have heard about ...*

D: *What types have you heard of?*

D: *You mentioned a family history of stroke. Is that what really worries you at the moment?*

D: *What part of this bothers you most—is it what the surgeon said or what your wife might think or something else?*

D: *What exactly is it about the operation that worries you most?*

Patient centredness taken too far can render history taking just as ineffective as pure doctor centredness. History taking should certainly involve guiding a patient back on track if their account starts to wander into areas you feel will not yield more useful information. It is perfectly acceptable to say something like:

D: *That is obviously important to you and perhaps we could return to it later, but didn't you say that the main problem you were having was...*

Responding to cues

A cue is hard to define, but usually recognisable when presented to you. *A cue could be defined as a signpost to an area in the history that you might otherwise ignore but which may be very important to the patient.*

Cues are very common. They are often not consciously presented by patients, but offer an insight into undeclared concerns. Examples of verbal cues include:

P: *I hoped it wasn't anything serious.*

P: *I don't get paid when I don't work.*

P: *It's my chest again.*

P: *I just seem to be losing it.*

P: *Of course it could just be stress.*

P: *Of course it could be my heart.*

P: *I'm not worried ... after all a lot of those TV programmes just show the worst cases.*

P: *It doesn't help that my sisters aren't here.*

P: *I hope this won't mean lots of tests. I've got a lot on my plate at the moment.*

There may also be cues in the pace, pitch, volume, rhythm or modulation of speech and there may be cues in censored speech—in what is not said. Patients frequently hesitate or appear to omit information which we intuitively feel should be included:

P: *It's no better (what's no better?)*

P: *Something will have to be done (what will have to be done?)*

P: *I'm worried (about what?)*

P: *I feel worse (worse than what or when?)*
P: *I'm suffering (from what?)*
P: *I feel a failure (why?)*

Sometimes, patients use generalisations to express their concerns:

P: *I don't like hospitals.*
P: *No one understands.*
P: *I always get headaches.*
P: *It never seems to get any better.*

Cues may be non-verbal. A patient may look sad or anxious and it might be appropriate to respond:

D: *You look worried about that.*

You will not detect all cues and do not need to act on all cues that you detect. But examiners will certainly notice if you ignore what seems to be an important cue.

Not all cues need an immediate response. Sometimes storing a piece of information and returning to it later is effective:

D: *You mentioned earlier that you hadn't wanted to come into hospital. Was there anything worrying you in particular about hospital?*

Exploring the context

Frequently, through patient centred history taking, important details of a patient's social history (Box 4.2) will have emerged. These details may act as catalysts for further questioning. If not, the questions in Box 4.2 should help you remember important areas to explore. Opening questions could be:

D: *How is this affecting you at work?*
D: *How are you coping at home with this?*

The principle is that it is as important to understand the person who has the disease as it is to understand the disease itself.

Summarising

Always give your patient a chance to add information or ask questions before concluding. You might ask:

D: *Is there anything you would like to ask?*
D: *Is there anything else you feel I should know?*
D: *Is there anything important to you which you feel I have left out?*

It is good practice to confirm shared understanding:

D: *May I take a moment to summarise what you've told me so I can check that I've understood everything that is important to you.*

PACES examiners expect you to have agreed a summary and plan of action with your patient and given opportunity for questions. A precise plan of action may not be possible without the benefit of examination findings, but it may be possible to say the following:

D: *From what we have discussed, it is possible that your symptoms could be due to (problem). I think we should consider the following test/s (explain briefly) to help confirm this.*

You should ask if your patient has any questions.

Finish by thanking your patient.

HISTORY TAKING CASES

At the History Taking Skills station the examiners are observing skills as much as knowledge. The remainder of this chapter summarises the knowledge base for history taking cases you could encounter in PACES.

In the discussion about your case, the examiners will usually start by asking you to state the problem/s elicited. They may then ask you a questions such as *Which aspects of this patient's social history do you consider particularly important?* or they may ask clinically orientated questions about management of the problem. Often they will ask you a variety of types of question.

4.1 SHORTNESS OF BREATH AND COUGH

Instruction: *Please take a history from this patient. You are not expected to examine her/him.*

Patient A

This 30-year-old lady has had episodes of cough and 'tightness' in the chest for the last 3 months. She uses antihistamines for hayfever, which has been particularly bad this year. She has never smoked and works as a primary schoolteacher.

Patient B

This 69-year-old has smoked 20 cigarettes a day since he was a young man. He has noticed that over the past 6 months he has become progressively short of breath whilst out walking his dog. He acknowledges that he has a 'smoker's cough' and says that 'coughs and colds always seem to go to his chest.' His symptoms have not been helped by ipratropium and salbutamol inhalers from his GP.

Patient C

This 74-year-old lady with chronic obstructive pulmonary disease (COPD) diagnosed 8 years ago has been finding it increasingly difficult to put on her shoes because of swollen feet. Her GP has tried 40 mg of furosemide (frusemide) daily which has not helped. He thought he heard a heart murmur.

Patient D

This 64-year-old newsagent has had at least one exacerbation of COPD per year over the last few years requiring oral prednisolone and antibiotics. He is taking salbutamol and fluticasone inhalers. On this occasion his GP has arranged admission to hospital because of unresolving crackles in the right upper lobe.

Patient E

This 54-year-old man has been losing weight. He is an ex smoker, and for the last 4 months had been coughing up increasing amounts of sputum.

Patient F

This 44-year-old roadbuilder has been getting increasingly short of breath on exertion over the past year. He has a 'dry' cough. His GP notes that he is a non-smoker, has no history of atopic symptoms and has found 'nothing untoward' on examination.

Patient G

This 32-year-old woman has been getting short of breath on exertion. Her husband thinks her necks veins are unusually pulsating.

Patient H

This 70-year-old lady has been progressively short of breath on exertion over the last 2 years. She has no significant past medical history, has never smoked and has noticed that she gets occasional pains in her chest, at which time it hurts mostly 'when she breathes'.

Case Box 4.1	Shortness of Breath/Cough History Taking Points

Shortness of breath is a diagnostic challenge encompassing respiratory and cardiovascular disease as well as anaemia, hyperventilation and overall lack of fitness. A careful history, corroborated by examination, pulmonary function tests, full blood count, ECG and chest X-ray can diagnose the vast majority of patients with shortness of breath. Important history areas to cover include:

Dyspnoea details
- Acute or chronic/progressive
- Onset sudden or insidious
- Episodic, stepwise or continuous
- At rest or on exertion
- Triggers (e.g. exercise, cold, smoking, allergens, occupational exposure) and relieving factors

Associated respiratory symptoms
- Cough—productive (sputum characteristics and volume) or non-productive
- Haemoptysis (consider bronchial carcinoma, pneumonia, pulmonary tuberculosis (TB), bronchiectasis, pulmonary embolus, pulmonary vasculitis)
- Wheeze
- Symptoms suggesting a cardiac cause—exertional chest pain, syncope, orthopnoea, paroxysmal nocturnal dyspnoea, ankle swelling (may be cor pulmonale)
- Alarm symptoms (e.g. weight loss, anorexia, haemoptysis, hoarseness)

Relevant past medical history
- Respiratory disease, e.g. TB, recurrent pneumonia
- Coronary heart disease risk factors—family history, smoking, hypertension, lipid profile if known, diabetes
- Atopy (personal or family history)—asthma, eczema, hayfever/allergic rhinitis

Drug history
- Especially sedatives, NSAIDs (wheeze), angiotensin converting enzyme (ACE) inhibitors (cough)

Social history

- Smoking history (including passive smoking and pipe smoking)—starting/stopping/quantity/pack years (page 14)
- Occupational history. Ask specifically about asbestos exposure. Remember that all previous occupations are important, not just the current one
- Travel history (atypical pneumonia, TB)
- Pets (cats—commonly trigger asthma; birds—atypical pneumonia, extrinsic allergic alveolitis (EAA))
- Effect of symptoms on daily activities—e.g. a patient with COPD who lives alone and who cannot walk to the shops may need considerable social support
- Effect of daily activities on symptoms

Since pulmonary function testing is an integral part of the assessment of patients with respiratory disease, a brief revision of it follows:

Lung volumes (Fig. 4.1)

The three important lung volumes in assessing disease are:

1. *Total lung capacity TLC*: the total volume of air in the lungs at full inspiration.
2. *Vital capacity (VC)*: the volume of air exhaled from full inspiration to full expiration.
3. *Residual volume (RV)*: the volume always left in the lung after breathing out the vital capacity.

Dynamic volumes (volumes which change!)

The above are *static* volumes; what we measure mostly in practice are *dynamic* volumes (because patients are breathing!):

Fig. 4.1   *Useful lung volumes*

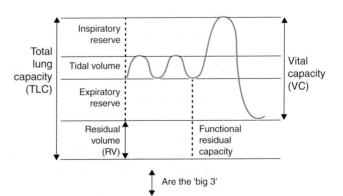

TABLE 4.1   Differences between OLD and RLD

	OLD	RLD
Examples	COPD Asthma	Interstitial lung disease Pulmonary vascular disease
Static volumes	There is air trapping or hyperinflation; therefore TLC may be increased (RV is increased because airways close early)	The lungs are small and fibrotic; therefore TLC is decreased (RV is decreased because alveoli are obliterated)
Dynamic volumes	FEV_1 markedly decreased FVC normal or decreased FEV_1/FVC decreased	FEV1 decreased FVC decreased FEV_1/FVC normal or > 80%
Flow rates	Expiratory flow rates decreased	Expiratory flow rates normal
Transfer factor (page 116)	Usually decreased in COPD, preserved in asthma	Normal or decreased

- *Forced vital capacity (FVC)*: This is the volume of air expired when your patient breathes out as hard and long as they can (as though trying to blow out all of the candles on a birthday cake!)
- *Forced expiratory volume over 1 second (FEV_1)*: This is the amount of air expired over the first second of FVC.

The normal *FEV_1/FVC* ratio is around 80%.

Spirometry can measure the FEV_1/FVC ratio and determine which of two major groups of lung disease we are dealing with, *obstructive* or *restrictive.*

Obstructive lung disease (OLD) and restrictive lung disease (RLD)

In OLD, FEV_1 is markedly reduced, and FVC normal or reduced, but giving a ratio less than predicted.

In RLD, FEV_1 and FVC are both reduced giving a normal or above normal ratio compared to predicted (Table 4.1).

Concept of flow rates

It is possible to plot the rate of airflow (e.g. the rate of expiratory airflow during a FVC manoeuvre) against lung volume (which changes as a person breathes out).

It may seem from Figure 4.2 that the expiratory flow rate in RLD is decreased. But if we correct this for the decreased lung volume seen in RLD, then the expiratory flow rate is actually normal or even increased. This is because the fibrotic lung provides more traction than normal on the airways, keeping them open.

In OLD, expiratory flow rates are decreased. Although the lungs are hyperinflated, inflammation, oedema and mucus in the smaller

Fig. 4.2 *Expiratory flow rate plotted against lung volume-normal, OLD, RLD*

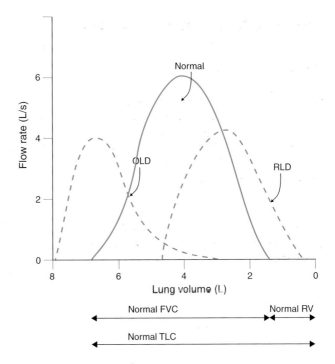

airways causes these small airways to close earlier than usual. This is despite the normal traction from the lung parenchyma which attempts to keep them open.

Concepts of compliance and elastic recoil

Compliance is essentially a measure of the 'give' of the lung when expanding, and *elastic recoil* a measure of the lung's ability to shrink to its original size again, like a deflating balloon. *OLD* lungs are very compliant, but have too little elastic recoil because there is too much airspace and not enough parenchyma. *RLD* lungs are not very compliant (they are too stiff) and have too much recoil, if anything.

Concept of flow rate variation

You can see from Figure 4.2 that flow rates in normal and diseased lungs vary according to lung volume. For example, in normal lungs the maximum flow rate, about 6 litres per second, occurs when about 4 litres of air are left in the lungs. This is sometimes called the *peak expiratory flow rate* (*PEFR*), and can be measured with a simple peak flow machine on the ward which measures flow in the first 10 milliseconds of expiration.

Sometimes, rather than plotting flow rate against volume, flow rate is plotted against percentage vital capacity. This is essentially doing the same thing, so don't be worried by it. It simply plots flow rate through the various stages of exhaling the vital capacity. For example,

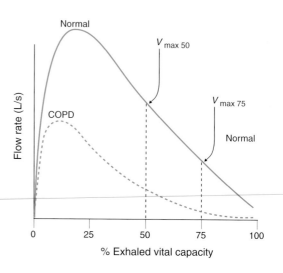

Fig. 4.3   *Flow rate variation in normal lung and in COPD*

when 75% of the vital capacity has been exhaled, the flow rate is called V_{max75}, or forced expiratory flow $(FEF)_{75}$.

Note from Figure 4.3 that flow rate is low in OLD at all stages of exhaling the vital capacity (i.e. at all lung volumes). Note how for OLD the curve is scooped out. This is one of the earliest signs of small airway damage (area between V_{max50} and V_{max75} often affected first) and is seen in young smokers before clinical features of disease.

Flow volume loops

Complex mathematics has been applied to produce the shapes of the above expiratory flow curves for normal and diseased lungs. Fortunately, physicians don't need to understand the maths, but merely recognise the shapes of certain curves and what they might imply. Curves have been created not just for expiration, but also for inspiration. Therefore as well as flow–volume curves, flow–volume loops (Fig. 4.4) which track the full inspiration–expiration cycle can be plotted, and these too have characteristic shapes. In OLD, for example, inspiratory flow rates are reduced, but not as dramatically as expiratory flow rates.

Transfer factor

Transfer factor (TLCO) measures the total transfer of carbon monoxide across the lung. It is a measure of total alveolar–capillary exchange. TLCO is also known as diffusing capacity (DLCO), and is best regarded as a measure of gas exchange or effective ventilation/perfusion (V/Q) matching.

KCO, or transfer coefficient, corrects TLCO for lung volume. For example, a TLCO of half the predicted value may occur after a pneumonectomy, but the KCO will be normal.

Fig. 4.4   *Flow-volume loops (maximal):*
(a) normally; (b) disease

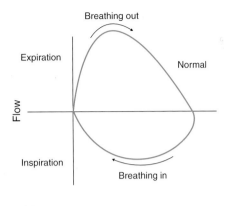

(a)

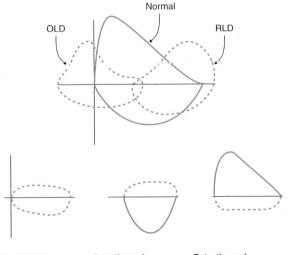

Fixed upper	Intrathoracic	Extrathoracic
airway obstruction	**variable obstruction**	**variable obstruction**
e.g. goitre	e.g. tracheomalacia	e.g. bilateral vocal cord
tracheal stenosis	(can't breathe out)	palsy (can't breathe in)

(b)

Decreased TLCO and KCO

This occurs in:

- COPD ● Interstitial lung disease ● Pulmonary vascular disease (pulmonary emboli, pulmonary hypertension, pulmonary oedema)
- Right to left shunts ● Anaemia.

In emphysema, TLCO is misleadingly elevated, because CO sits in the bullae. In fact, the obliterated alveoli cause markedly diminished gas exchange.

Increased TLCO and KCO

CO has a high affinity for blood cells, and so transfer is *apparently* increased in pulmonary haemorrhage, e.g. pulmonary vasculitis. It is also increased in polycythaemia and left to right shunts and exercise.

Decreased TLCO and normal KCO

This is due to extrapulmonary restriction functional volume loss, e.g. chest wall/neuromuscular disease) or volume loss post-peumonectomy.

What would be your approach to the management of?

Patient A

She probably has adult onset asthma. The history should explore any triggers. Has she, for example, recently taken up a new form of exercise? Has she moved in with a smoker? Has she come into contact with any new materials at work? Has she bought a pet? Has she moved house and come into increased contact with house dust mites? She should be asked about diurnal variation of cough (often worse at night), wheeze and shortness of breath. A family history of atopy is often elicited.

She should be asked to monitor her morning and evening peak flow on a peak flow chart, which may show more than 15% variability. A single normal peak flow measurement does not exclude asthma!

She should be managed according to the guidelines described in Case study 4.2. She should have a self-management plan, with long-term follow up by her general practitioner/practice nurse. An attempt to wean/withdraw her steroids should be made at the end of the hayfever season.

Asthma is discussed in Case study 4.2.

Patient B

This is a typical history from a patient with COPD.

Spirometry would confirm OLD with a markedly reduced FEV_1, reduced FVC and reduced FEV_1/FVC ratio. Reversibility of these baseline readings may be tested for with bronchodilators (salbutamol 5 mg by nebuliser) or a trial of oral steroids (30 mg prednisolone daily for 2 weeks). No significant reversibility (< 15%) is typical of COPD. COPD may be *mild* (FEV_1 60–80% predicted – cough, minimal breathlessness, no abnormal signs), *moderate* (FEV_1 40–59% predicted – breathlessness ± wheeze on minimal exertion, cough ± sputum, variable signs) or *severe* (FEV_1 < 40% predicted – breathlessness on any exertion or at rest, frequent cough and wheeze, hyperinflation, cyanosis and cor pulmonale in advanced cases). Inhaled short or long acting β_2 agonists and anticholinergics may help symptoms. The role of inhaled corticosteroids is unclear.

Stopping smoking, weight control and exercise are central to management but are not easy for patients. Patients should be aware that lung function inevitably declines if they continue to smoke and smoking cessation should be supported vigorously.

COPD is discussed in Case study 2.2.

Patient C

Possible diagnoses in this lady are biventricular failure or cor pulmonale. She should be asked about symptoms of heart failure and risk factors for coronary heart disease. A full respiratory history is mandatory, as her swollen ankles may be due to right heart failure consequent upon pulmonary disease.

Central to the development of cor pulmonale is pulmonary hypertension. Pulmonary hypertension sets up a cascade of back pressure events (Box 2.2).

Cor pulmonale is discussed on page 13.

Patient D

Pneumonia which fails to resolve in a smoker should always prompt investigation for the possibility of bronchial carcinoma. The history should specifically elicit any endobronchial symptoms (cough and haemoptysis) and constitutional symptoms such as weight loss or anorexia. Some patients with bronchial carcinoma present with hormonal related symptoms. Squamous cell carcinoma, for example, may cause hypercalcaemia. A small number of patients with an apical tumour may present with Horner's syndrome, brachial plexopathy or unilateral wasting of the small muscles of the hand.

An urgent chest X-ray is mandatory. Bronchoscopy and biopsy will be needed if a mass lesion is identified. It may also be needed to search for a tumour if the chest X-ray does not show a mass lesion or if appearances are difficult to interpret because of coexisiting infection or effusion. For some peripheral tumours open lung biopsy is more rewarding for histological sampling, and if pleural disease is suspected, pleural aspiration or biopsy is needed.

Lung cancer is discussed in Case study 2.2.

Patient E

Large volumes of sputum should always prompt consideration of bronchiectasis. In addition to the history points above, ask about possible causes, especially previous infection/pneumonia/TB.

Bronchiectasis is discussed in Case study 2.4.

Patient F

Pulmonary fibrosis should always be suspected in a patient with progressive exertional dyspnoea. Early on, it may be the only feature of disease, with examination and chest X-ray being unremarkable. A full history, examination and baseline investigations are important, as exertional dyspnoea also has cardiac causes including ischaemic heart disease, valvular heart disease and cardiomyopathy. Chest X-ray and spirometry are mandatory initial investigations in suspected pulmonary fibrosis.

Patient F's occupation is highly relevant and silicosis is by no means a disease of the past. Many occupations (e.g. stonemasons, roadbuilders) still involve exposure to quartz dust, highly concentrated in rock such as granite and sandstone.

Silicosis is caused by inhalation of crystalline silicon dioxide (quartz), which is highly fibrogenic. Particles are engulfed by macrophages and swept to hilar lymph nodes where inflammation, fibrosis and blockage to lymphatic drainage can occur. A similar process can occur in the lungs, provoking small fibrotic nodules.

Silicosis does not usually occur with brief exposure. Most patients have been exposed occupationally for years or decades. With high exposure, the small lung nodules can coalesce into large, destructive masses with surrounding bullae. Nodules continue to grow and merge, even after exposure has ceased, causing dyspnoea. Very high exposure occasionally causes an acute inflammatory destructive process with respiratory failure in the absence of nodules. The chest X-ray usually shows 'eggshell' hilar calcification and small (< 5 mm) diffuse nodular change.

The history, chest X-ray and workplace inspection by an occupational physician are usually sufficient for the diagnosis. Biopsy is seldom necessary, but mineral analysis can reveal fine quartz particles.

Patients with pneumoconioses are entitled to compensation and Industrial Injuries Benefit. An occupational physician or a medical inspector from the Health and Safety Executive should investigate the workplace to identify if other workers are at risk from enclosed surroundings, inadequate ventilation and so forth.

Interstitial lung disease is discussed in Case study 2.6.

Patient G

Primary pulmonary hypertension (PPH) is rare, and although there are alternative diagnoses, should be considered.

Pulmonary hypertension is discussed in Case study 2.7.

Patient H

Recurrent pulmonary emboli may present as stepwise exertional dyspnoea, especially in elderly patients.

Pulmonary embolus is discussed in Case study 2.7.

How would you define respiratory failure?

Type 1

- $Po_2 < 8$ kPa or 60 mmHg
- Pco_2 normal or decreased
- Causes include interstitial lung disease (in early disease hypoxic on exertion only), pulmonary vascular disease, asthma, COPD.

Type 2

- Pco_2 increased (> 6 kPa or 50 mmHg)
- Causes include hypoventilation, e.g. extrathoracic disease, COPD.

CASE STUDY	4.2 ASTHMA

Instruction: *Please read this letter from this patient's general practitioner and then conduct an appropriate consultation. You are not expected to examine the patient.*

> *Dear Doctor*
> *This 40-year-old asthmatic patient has developed worsening symptoms despite high dose inhaled steroid and long acting bronchodilators. She is generally otherwise well. I would be grateful for advice on her further management.*

What is asthma?

Asthma is characterised by airway inflammation (often failing to settle between attacks and now appreciated as a central problem in

---

Case Box 4.2   Asthma History Taking Points

The history should cover similar points to those in Case box 4.1.

A Royal College of Physicians document *Measuring Outcomes in Asthma* suggested that important questions to specifically ask asthma patients are:

In the last week/month:
1. Have you had any difficulty sleeping because of your asthma symptoms?
2. Have you had your usual asthma symptoms during the day?
3. Has your asthma interfered with your usual activities?

Many patients regard shortness of breath and wheeze as the main asthma symptoms. Difficulty sleeping because of cough or difficulty talking are not often volunteered and should be asked about.

In addition, try to determine:
- If there are any clear trigger factors. The most important allergens are the house dust mite (HDM), dog allergen, cat allergen, pollen and moulds. Respiratory infections, drugs (NSAIDs, beta-blockers), exercise, cigarette smoke, fumes, sprays and perfumes are other common triggers. Always ask about possible occupational triggers.
- The medications used to date and the current treatment step.
- If recurrent courses of oral steroids have been given (osteoporosis risk, Case study 4.16).
- Whether or not there have been previous hospital admissions and if so, which treatments were required. Ask specifically if artificial ventilation has ever been required.

asthma), giving rise to reversible airway narrowing, and airway hyperreactivity giving rise to the symptoms of cough, wheeze and dyspnoea.

What do you know about the pathophysiology of asthma?

Asthma and allergic diseases are increasing in prevalence in the Western world. Atopy refers to the predisposition to generate allergic antibodies (IgE) in response to environmental triggers.

Pages 195–200 describe how the immune system responds to foreign antigens by their being presented to naïve T helper lymphocytes (TH lymphocytes) which differentiate either to a TH1 response driving cell mediated inflammation or to a TH2 response driving B lymphocytes to switch to IgE production.

The optimal scenario is a well balanced ability to produce TH1 and TH2 responses. Allergy is increasingly regarded as a TH2 weighted imbalance. Atopic predisposition may start in early life, with impaired interferon gamma (IFNγ) production leading to impaired suppression of the TH2 activity involved in IgE mediated allergy. Studies have shown that normal neonates have a weakly TH2 biased immune response that is subsequently suppressed in early life. Exposure to bacteria in early life may increase IFNγ levels, lending weight to the 'hygiene' hypothesis which suggests that reduced exposure to bacteria together with antibiotics and modern infant diets result in the persistence of a dominant TH2 pathway.

Mycobacterial species are known to stimulate powerful IFNγ production and research has focused on bacterial vaccines to promote switching from TH2 to TH1 pathways.

What do you know about the British Thoracic Society (BTS) guidelines for the management of chronic asthma in adults?

Treatment is titrated in steps, starting with occasional use of *short acting beta-2 bronchodilators* (controlling 30% of all patients) followed by addition of *regular standard dose inhaled corticosteroids*, beclometasone or budesonide 100–400 mcg twice daily or fluticasone 50–200 mcg twice daily (controlling 50% of all patients). Options after this include the addition of an *inhaled long acting bronchodilator (LABD)* or *high dose inhaled corticosteroid*, beclometasone or budesonide 800–2000 mcg daily or fluticasone 400–1000 mcg daily (in divided doses) via a large volume spacer, or, less commonly, a *leukotriene receptor antagonist (LTRA)*. Evidence has suggested that a LABD is superior to doubling steroid doses. Theophylline may be used and there is interest in monoclonal anti-IgE antibodies in selected patients with an allergic trigger.

A combination of high dose inhaled steroids and an inhaled long acting beta-agonist may be required. The addition of regular steroid tablets to high dose inhaled steroids and an inhaled long acting beta-agonist may be needed in refractory cases.

Rescue courses of oral steroid may be needed at any step at any time. Oral or intravenous steroids used in asthma exacerbations reduce hospital admission and relapse rates.

Important adjuncts to drug therapy are identifying triggers (especially cigarette smoking), educating patients to manage their own asthma with individualised management plans, selection of appropriate inhaler devices, and regular monitoring with stepping up or down of treatment as required.

The ideal outcomes of treatment include minimal symptoms, minimal exacerbations, minimal need for relieving bronchodilators, unlimited normal activities and exercise, minimal side effects from medication and near normalisation in pulmonary function tests.

Do you know what effect guidelines have had on outcomes?

Since the introduction of guidelines, asthma mortality and admission rates have declined, but patients remain unable to predict their disease and its effects on daily life.

How would you explain to a patient how to use a metred dose inhaler (MDI)?

1. Shake the inhaler and remove the dust cap
2. Breathe out gently and fully
3. Place the mouthpiece between your teeth and seal your lips around it
4. Breathe in steadily, and at the moment you start breathing in ...
5. Press the inhaler to release the dose immediately after beginning to breathe in and keep breathing in to full inspiration (until your lungs are full)
6. Remove the inhaler from your mouth and hold your breath for 10 seconds or as long as is comfortable
7. If a second dose is needed, wait for 30–60 seconds.

How would you recognise and manage acute severe asthma (ASA) in adults?

Feature of ASA include:

- Peak expiratory flow (PEF) $\leq$ 50% of predicted or best
- Unable to complete sentences in one breath
- Tachypnoea with respiratory rate $\geq$ 25 breaths/min
- Heart rate > 110 beats/min.

Life threatening features include:

- PEF < 33% of predicted or best
- Silent chest, cyanosis or poor respiratory effort
- Bradycardia or hypotension
- Exhaustion, confusion or coma.

If oxygen saturations (Sao_2) are < 92% or there are any life threatening features, arterial blood gases are needed.

Immediate treatment includes 40–60% oxygen, nebulised beta-2 agonists and oral prednisolone or intravenous hydrocortisone. A chest X-ray is mandatory to exclude a pneumothorax. Life threatening features require nebulised ipratropium in addition to nebulised beta-2 agonists, and intravenous aminophylline or beta-2 agonists. Subsequent management includes repeated administration of the above treatments, with monitoring of PEF and Sao_2. Patients not improving should be discussed early with the intensive care team. Hypercapnia, persistent hypoxia or feeble respirations all imply progressive exhaustion, and are indications for assisted ventilation.

When would you consider it safe to discharge a patient from hospital after admission with acute severe asthma?

- Identification and modification of trigger factors achieved where possible
- Patient on discharge medication for at least 24 hours
- PEF > 75% of predicted or best and preferably PEF diurnal variability < 25%
- Patient on steroids in addition to bronchodilators
- Patent has individualised management plan, and, where possible, is able to self-monitor their PEF
- GP and specialist follow up arranged with good communication between all parties.

What might you consider when a patient has chronic asthma which is proving difficult to control?

- Persistence of triggers factors
- Poor compliance
- Poor technique/patient education
- Alternative diagnosis, e.g. heart failure, Churg–Strauss syndrome (the severity may be masked by steroid treatment).

What other pulmonary eosinophilic disorders do you know of?

- Allergic bronchopulmonary aspergillosis (ABPA).
- Churg–Strauss syndrome (allergic granulomatosis with angiitis) is an eosinophilic vasculitis associated with asthma, flitting pulmonary infiltrates, peripheral blood eosinophilia, peripheral neuropathy and renal failure. The cause is uncertain.
- Loeffler's syndrome, which refers to transient pulmonary infiltrates, often idiopathic but sometimes associated with parasitic infections or drugs (nitrofurantoin, sulfasalazine).
- Acute eosinophilic pneumonia, an idiopathic acute febrile illness with severe hypoxaemia, pulmonary infiltrates and no history of asthma.
- Chronic eosinophilic pneumonia, also idiopathic.
- Hypereosinophilic syndrome, an idiopathic disorder with a very high eosinophil count, weight loss, fever, night sweats,

hepatomegaly, lymphadenopathy, eosinophilic cardiomyopathy, renal failure and peripheral neuropathy.
● Tropical eosinophilia.

Many of these disorders are rare, possibly representing overlap of a group of heterogeneous disorders, and respond to steroids.

What is aspergillus and what diseases can it cause?
It is a ubiquitous fungus which can cause:

1. **Allergic bronchopulmonary aspergillosis (ABPA)**. This is an allergic mixed type I IgE and type III IgG/M hypersensitivity (pages 202–203) disease causing dyspnoea, wheeze, peripheral blood eosinophilia, positive skin testing, flitting X-ray shadows and upper zone fibrosis.

2. **An aspergilloma**. This is a fungus 'ball' which colonises a pre-existing lung cavity, e.g. post TB. It may cause life threatening haemoptysis. Serum precipitins are raised and skin testing is negative.

3. **Invasive aspergillosis**. This generally occurs in immunocompromised patients.

CASE STUDY **4.3 DYSPEPSIA AND GASTRO-OESOPHAGEAL REFLUX DISEASE (GORD)**

Instruction: Please take a history from this patient. You are not expected to examine her/him.

Patient A

This 28-year-old woman has symptoms of heartburn and regurgitation with a bitter taste in her mouth.

Patient B

This 40-year-old man has had episodic epigastric pain for 3 months, worse after meals.

Patient C

This 75-year-old lady has had 6 weeks of upper abdominal pain and nausea. She has been taking NSAIDs for a 'rheumatoid' condition'.

Patient D

This 36-year-old woman has a 3-month history of upper abdominal pain and nausea. She has a history of sinusitis, back pains, fibromyalgia and dysmenorrhoea.

Patient E

This 65-year-old man has a 4-month history of epigastric pain, anorexia and weight loss. His symptoms have improved with a proton pump inhibitor over the last 2 months.

| Case Box 4.3 | **Dyspepsia History Taking Points** |

Dyspepsia refers to a group of *symptoms arising from the upper gastrointestinal tract (UGIT),* including epigastric or upper abdominal discomfort, heartburn, nausea and bloating.

The *symptoms may indicate* gastro-oesophageal reflux (GORD), oesophagitis, gastritis, peptic ulcer disease or upper gastrointestinal malignancy. Heartburn is the primary symptom of GORD and some gastroenterologists restrict the term dyspepsia to epigastric discomfort, which excludes heartburn.

Important points to elicit are:
1. The nature of the symptoms
2. Whether the symptoms are of new onset, progressive, recurrent, episodic or persistent
3. Any precipitating or relieving factors, e.g. relationship to meals
4. Whether or not the symptoms have been investigated or treated before (has the patient heard of *Helicobacter pylori?*)
5. Age
6. The presence or absence of *alarm features (anaemia, loss of weight, anorexia, recent onset of progressive symptoms, melaena or haematemesis, dysphagia, abdominal mass)*
7. Medication history such as NSAIDs or corticosteroids
8. Past medical history such as chronic inflammatory conditions requiring recurrent course of corticosteroids (asthma, inflammatory bowel disease, connective tissue disorder)
9. Occupational history
10. 'Stress' and the psychosocial context
11. Alcohol and smoking history

Patient F

This 40-year-old man has a 5 year history of intermittent retrosternal chest discomfort and regurgitation of food. He has recently had difficulty swallowing liquids.

What do you know about GORD?

GORD is more common than peptic ulcer disease. It is potentially (although rarely) serious. It is associated with transient lower oesophageal sphincter (LOS) relaxation unrelated to swallowing. The LOS comprises oesophageal smooth muscle and diaphragmatic striated muscle, the latter incompetent in a hiatus hernia (which in itself does not diagnose GORD). GORD can lead to oesophagitis, Barrett's oesophagus (upward propagation of columnar epithelium, replacing squamous epithelium) and oesophageal adenocarcinoma. Most oesophageal carcinomas are squamous carcinomas.

The key to diagnosis is the history. A clear history of heartburn (a burning feeling rising from the stomach to the neck) is unlikely to be due to anything else and quality of life is affected in proportion to the frequency and severity of this, irrespective of the presence or severity of oesophagitis. Atypical symptoms include chronic cough and odonyphagia (painful swallowing).

Is there a role for endoscopy in patients with GORD?

Many gastroenterologists believe it to be of limited diagnostic role since most patients do not have endoscopically visible lesions. There is no consensus as to which patients merit endoscopy. Indications include alarm symptoms, exclusion of other causes (especially if symptoms are refractory to treatment) or assessment for GORD complications (Barrett's oesophagus, stricture, very rarely ulcer). Barrett's oesophagus confers an increased risk of oesophageal adenocarcinoma, but optimal practice for endoscopic detection and surveillance remains unclear. Free reflux on barium swallow is specific but poorly sensitive for GORD. The most accurate test is ambulatory oesophageal pH monitoring.

What treatments might you recommend for a patient with GORD?

1. Most people worldwide take antacids. Proton pump inhibitors (at high or standard dose) are more effective than histamine H_2 receptor antagonists and antacids. Prokinetic agents (e.g. metaclopramide) may help since many patients with reflux have delayed gastric emptying. The aim is to step down therapy to a regimen which is least costly yet which controls symptoms. Patients with GORD complications should remain on a PPI.
2. Avoidance of precipitating foods and drinks may help.
3. Smoking cessation and weight reduction are sound health measures, but may have little benefit on GORD.
4. *H. pylori* eradication does not heal oesophagitis or prevent symptom relapse.

What do you know about the physiology of gastric juice secretion?

Appoximately 3 litres of gastric juice is produced daily. *Parietal (oxyntic) cells* produce *hydrochloric acid* and *intrinsic factor*. *Chief (peptic) cells* secrete *pepsinogen*, a pepsin precursor. Stimulation of gastric secretion has three main inputs: neuronal (vagal), hormonal (gastrin) and histamine. Inhibitors of secretion are sympathetic nerve activity, low pH and small bowel enzymes.

Gastrin is produced from *G cells* in the *gastric antrum*. Its secretion is stimulated by food, distension, vagal input and low pH. It *promotes acid, intrinsic factor (page 133) and pepsin secretion* (the H_2 receptor being the final common pathway), gastric emptying, pancreatic bicarbonate release and secretin release.

What is Zollinger–Ellison syndrome?

Peptic ulcer disease resulting from a gastrin secreting adenoma, usually arising in the pancreas. It may be part of multiple endocrine neoplasia type 1 (MEN1) syndrome (page 561).

What do you know about *H. pylori* and its eradication?

A high proportion of the UK population suffer from dyspeptic symptoms and most do not have peptic ulceration. There is strong evidence that *H. pylori* has an important causative role in > 90% of duodenal ulcers (DUs), and also has a role in benign gastric ulcers (GUs) that are not attributable to NSAIDs. There is evidence for its causative role in gastric carcinoma and gastric lymphoma, and it may have a role in non-ulcer dyspepsia (NUD).

Eradication triple therapy is indicated for peptic ulcer and gastric lymphoma, and may be indicated for NUD.

What do you know about referral guidelines for endoscopy in patients with dyspepsia?

Most gastrointestinal units are receiving an increasing number of referrals for endoscopy. Various guidelines have attempted to rationalise increasing demand.

The *British Society of Gastroenterology guidelines* suggest, for first presentation of dyspepsia, that:

- Patient < 45 years (threshold may be raised to 55) without alarm symptoms should have *H. pylori* serology checked and receive antisecretory treatment. Patients testing positive, or patients testing negative in whom symptoms persist post treatment, should proceed to upper GI (UGI) endoscopy.
- Patients 45 (or 55) years or over or patients with alarm symptoms should be referred for UGI endoscopy.

The *European H. pylori study group (the Maastricht Consensus report)* differs in it management of patients < 45 years without alarm symptoms. These patients, it suggests, should be tested for *H. pylori* by serology or ^{13}C urea breath testing. If positive, these patients should receive a triple therapy eradication regimen, and if symptoms subsequently resolve, do not require further investigation. This has clearly favourable cost implications.

However, the few UGI malignancies that do occur in patients under 45 years of age are usually associated with *H. pylori*, lending support to the British guidelines. Although not stated in the guidelines, the Maastricht consensus clearly supports further investigation for patients with ongoing symptoms despite eradication therapy.

Different recommendations highlight that there are insufficient data to provide a more universal guideline and currently different gastroenterology units adopt different approaches.

Explain the urea breath test

Urea is hydrolysed by *H. pylori* urease to carbon dioxide and ammonia. Following ingestion of ^{13}C or ^{14}C labelled urea, ^{13}C or ^{14}C labelled carbon dioxide is detected in the breath of patients harbouring *H. pylori*.

How would you manage persistent symptoms after endoscopically proven peptic ulcer disease treated with eradication triple therapy?

Breath testing for *H. pylori* is appropriate for patients who have had an uncomplicated DU. If still infected an alternative eradication regimen may be used. If not infected an alternative diagnosis and further investigation may be appropriate.

H. pylori eradication should always be confirmed in cases where a peptic ulcer has bled, and all patients with a GU should be re-endoscoped to confirm healing, regardless of *H. pylori* status or symptoms, to exclude carcinoma.

How would you proceed in your management of:

Patient A

If the primary symptom is clearly heartburn, and there are no alarm symptoms, endoscopy is likely to be of limited value. It may be normal, even with severe symptoms. A barium swallow may show reflux or a hiatus hernia. Optimal treatment would be a proton pump inhibitor or an antacid. There is no strong evidence to support testing for and treating *H. pylori*.

Patient B

He has dyspeptic symptoms and is under 45 years of age. If there are no alarm symptoms, *H. pylori* testing is appropriate. If positive, eradication therapy is indicated, and some physicians would proceed to endoscopy whilst others would observe — if symptoms disappear, no further investigation is warranted; if symptoms persist or recur, endoscopy and repeat *H. pylori* testing (with a second line eradication therapy regimen if positive) are indicated.

Patient C

This lady may have NSAID induced peptic ulceration. Endoscopy is indicated if the NSAID cannot be stopped or if symptoms persist after stopping. NSAID induced ulcers usually heal with an H_2 receptor antagonist, misoprostol or a proton pump inhibitor. The least gastrotoxic NSAID should be used if treatment must continue, with concurrent administration of a 'gastroprotective' agent. The place of cyclo-oxygenase-2 (COX-2) inhibitors awaits long-term evaluation.

Patient D

The approach to this patient is along the same lines as patient B. Many patients with dyspeptic symptoms will have no ulceration at endoscopy, so called non-ulcer dyspepsia (NUD). Positive *H. pylori* testing can be managed by *H. pylori* eradication therapy. Most physicians or general practitioners would opt for a trial of eradication therapy first, and reserve endoscopy for persistent symptoms. However, the benefits of eradication therapy on NUD (an endoscopy diagnosis of exclusion) are unclear.

A number of patients with NUD also have features of a functional somatic syndrome, which may include irritable bowel syndrome, premenstrual syndrome, chronic pelvic pain, fibromyalgia, chronic (postviral) fatigue syndrome, atypical or non-cardiac chest pain, hyperventilation syndrome, temporomandibular joint dysfunction, atypical facial pain, globus syndrome and sensitivity to multiple chemicals. These 'somatisation' symptoms are more correctly assuming the term 'medically unexplained symptoms'.

Patient E

Alarm symptoms almost always warrant further investigation, usually by endoscopy. Investigation is difficult to justify in every case. Occasionally, for very elderly or unfit patients with other medical problems in whom overall prognosis is poor or in whom the risks of treatment would outweigh the benefits, further investigation may not be justified. The patient's informed choice, is, of course, important.

Patient F

Most patients with alarm symptoms would proceed initially to UGI endoscopy. Occasionally, benign strictures are discovered as the cause of anorexia and weight loss. Other non-malignant conditions such as oesophageal pouch or achalasia also cause dysphagia. Achalasia is best diagnosed by a barium swallow and manometry, the latter showing failure of relaxation of the lower oesophageal sphincter.

CASE STUDY	4.4 ABDOMINAL PAIN

Instruction: *This 50-year-old man has been admitted to your ward with acute abdominal pain. You suspect he should more correctly have been admitted under the surgical team. Please ask him some questions about his pain.*

Case Box 4.4	Abdominal Pain History Taking Points

There are two types of acute abdominal pain:
1. *Colicky* pain, which is gripping, often severe and comes in waves. It is due to abnormally strong peristalsis of a hollow viscus triggered either by obstruction (e.g. stone, tumour, hernia), or by irritation (e.g. gastroenteritis).
2. *Continuous* pain, present lying still and exacerbated by movement. It is due to inflammation, triggered by infection, ulceration, peritonitis or ischaemia.

These two types of pain may occur at one of *three main sites* in the abdomen because the brain receives *visceral pain* impulses from each of the three embryological components of the gut:
A. *Foregut* (stomach, proximal duodenum, gallbladder, biliary tree and pancreas) giving rise to *epigastric pain*.

B. *Midgut* (distal duodenum to two-thirds across the transverse colon) giving rise to *periumbilical pain.*
C. *Hindgut* (last third of transverse colon to rectum, and gynaecological areas of the pelvis, derived from the cloacal sac) giving rise to *suprapubic/pelvic pain.*

This knowledge of *types* and *sites* of pain can direct you towards common causes:
- *Colicky epigastric pain* is frequently due to biliary colic.
- *Continuous epigastric pain* is more likely to be due to peptic ulcer disease or pancreatitis.
- *Colicky periumbilical pain* in an elderly patient with weight loss and anaemia is right sided colonic cancer unless proven otherwise. In a young patient with episodic diarrhoea, constipation and bloating, without alarm symptoms, it may well represent irritable bowel syndrome.
- *Continuous periumbilical pain* may be due to peritonitis resulting from a perforated viscus, mesenteric ischaemia, or visceral peritoneal irritation in appendicitis.
- *Colicky suprapubic pain* with alteration in bowel habit may be due to colorectal cancer, inflammatory bowel disease or irritable bowel syndrome.
- *Continuous pelvic pain* in a young woman may be due to pelvic inflammatory disease, an ovarian cyst or ovarian torsion.

Visceral pain is often a vague, colicky midline pain, since it arises from visceral peritoneum in communicatation with a viscus. Continuous pain may be of visceral or parietal origin or both. *Parietal pain* tends to be more localised because the parietal peritoneum is innervated by spinal nerve roots which have specific sensory cortical representation. Hence, appendicitis, biliary colic and diverticulitis may all start as midline visceral pain but further localise to the RIF, right hypochondrium and LIF, respectively if the parietal peritoneum becomes inflamed.

Note that the kidneys and ureters (retroperitoneal structures) have parietal or spinal innervation from T8 to L1. Hence ureteric colic may be perceived as progressing from the loin (T8 dermatome) to the groin (L1 dermatome). Pain may also arise from structures outwith the abdominal cavity such as the abdominal wall or in a nerve root as in shingles.

The surgical team will care for this patient but would like to be persuaded by your account of the symptoms.

Report the typical symptoms of:

Biliary colic (intense, RUQ pain – with fever and tenderness indicating acute cholecystitis)

Pancreatitis (epigastric/central abdominal pain radiating to the back; pain could also be ruptured abdominal aortic aneurysm!)

Bowel obstruction (constipation, colicky abdominal pain, distension, vomiting)

Perforated viscus (progressive pain exacerbated by minimal movement, with rebound tenderness)

Mesenteric ischaemia/infarction (abdominal pain and rectal bleeding, usually on a background of cardiovascular risk factors)

Diverticulitis (LIF discomfort ± fever; history of constipation)

Ureteric colic (intense, intermittent pain from loin to groin, often with haematuria).

| CASE STUDY | **4.5 ALTERED BOWEL HABIT** |

Instruction: *Please read the letter from this patient's general practitioner and conduct an appropriate consultation. You are not expected to examine him.*

Dear Doctor

This 37-year-old man has complained of intermittent diarrhoea for 6 months. His stool culture is negative and his full blood picture, urea and electrolytes and liver function tests are normal. I would be grateful for your further assessment.

| Case Box 4.5 | **Altered Bowel Habit History Taking Points** |

Diarrhoea is difficult to define and definitions often refer to > 200 ml of stool per day or to increased stool frequency and decreased consistency. It may be *acute* or *chronic*, and predominantly a result of *small bowel disease* (often *large volume*, pale, with *steatorrhoea*) or *large bowel disease* (often *smaller volume* with *blood or mucus*).

  Small bowel causes of diarrhoea are sometimes classified as *secretory* (e.g. infectious causes, malabsorption), *osmotic* (e.g. osmotic laxatives) or due to *altered motility* (e.g. hyperthyroidism, autonomic neuropathy). Secretory symptoms tend to persist with fasting.

1. Try to determine if the symptoms suggest a predominantly small bowel or large bowel cause.
2. Ask about 'alarm symptoms' (anaemia, loss of weight — malabsorption itself will cause weight loss, anorexia, recent onset of progressive symptoms, melaena or haematemesis, dysphagia, abdominal mass).

If symptoms suggest small bowel disease
● Ask about any relevant past medical history—thyroid disease,
  diabetes, surgery (bacterial overgrowth in blind loops may
  increase deconjugation of bile salts, impairing micelle formation
  and causing steatorrheoa)
● Ask about alcohol intake (chronic pancreatitis, often presenting
  as relapsing steatorrhoea and back pain)
● Ask about medications, e.g. recent antibiotics
● Ask about foreign travel or unwell contacts (infectious causes)
● Consider the four commonest causes of malabsorption in the UK:
  (i)   Coeliac disease
  (ii) Cystic fibrosis (diagnosed in childhood)
  (iii) Postenteritis enteropathy
  (iv) Giardiasis.

Coeliac disease may cause diarrhoea and steatorrhoea with weight
loss and growth retardation. A wide spectrum of disease activity has
been recognised. Covert symptoms include malaise and recurrent
aphthous ulceration. It may cause hyposplenism. It may also present
as unexplained folate or iron deficiency anaemia (now the commonest
presentation). It is important to ask about itchy rashes (dermatitis
herpetiformis is rare, however) and bone pain (osteomalacia).

If symptoms suggest large bowel disease
Consider the above questions, and also consider the following
causes:
● Irritable bowel syndrome (IBS) characterised by episodes of
  constipation and diarrhoea with abdominal bloating in a younger
  adult without alarm symptoms
● Inflammatory bowel disease (ask about blood, mucus, pus, slime)
● Colorectal carcinoma, remembering to ask about a family history
● In older patients also consider diverticular disease and
  superior/inferior mesenteric ischaemia.

How would you investigate diarrhoea with a suspected small bowel cause?

● Full blood count for anaemia with iron, folate and B_{12} levels. The
  small bowel is the main site of absorption of nutrients. Iron is
  absorbed in the upper small bowel, folate in the duodenum and
  jejunem and B_{12}, bound to intrinsic factor, mainly in the terminal
  ileum.
● Inflammatory markers, e.g. erythrocyte sedimentation rate (ESR),
  C-reactive protein (CRP)
● Urea, electrolytes, liver function tests (especially albumin) and
  calcium
● Stool microscopy and culture for bacteria, ova, cysts and parasites

- A Schilling test, ^{14}C breath test for bacterial overgrowth (sometimes jejunal aspirates for bacterial quantification), xylose absorption test or 3 day faecal fat assay may be indicated to confirm malabsorption.
- Endoscopy and jejunal biopsy. Wireless capsule endoscopy is now possible for small bowel visualisation.

What do you know about infectious causes of diarrhoea?

1. *Acute secretory diarrhoea* is usually due to small bowel disease. In children this is often viral, and occasionally due to *Cryptosporidium*. In adults it is often due to *Escherichia coli*. Enterotoxigenic *E. coli* is a common cause (traveller's diarrhoea). Cholera is a very important cause worldwide. Food toxins also cause it.
2. *Acute bloody diarrhoea* implies invasive disease, usually colitis. The broad term for this presentation is 'dysentery'. The commonest causes in the UK are *Salmonella* spp. and *Campylobacter jejuni*. The enteric fevers *Salmonella typhi* and *Salmonella paratyphi* should be considered following travel to an area of risk. *Shigella sonnei*, enteroinvasive *E. coli*, *Clostridium difficile* (the main cause of pseudomembranous colitis), *Vibrio parahaemoylticus* (in salt water and shellfish) and *Yersinia enterocolitica* are others.
3. *Chronic secretory diarrhoea* is most commonly due to *Giardia lamblia* (giardiasis). Cryptosporidiosis, microsporidiosis and isosporiasis should be considered in immunosuppressed patients. Non-infectious causes, especially coeliac disease, must be considered.
4. *Chronic bloody diarrhoea* may be due to amoebic dysentery. The commonest non-infectious cause is inflammatory bowel disease.

What is coeliac disease?

Sensitivity to the gliadin component of gluten causing villous atrophy in genetically susceptible individuals. Tissue transglutaminase (TTG) may modify gliadin and act as an autoantigen. Coeliac disease has a wide range of presentations (Case study 4.5), is more common than previously recognised and confers an increased risk of malignancy, especially small bowel lymphoma.

How would you diagnose coeliac disease?

Endoscopy with jejunal biopsy for villous atrophy. Patients should be re-endoscoped after a period of gluten exclusion to confirm villous regeneration. Other causes of villous atrophy include Whipple's disease and small bowel lymphoma. Antiendomysial and anti-TTG antibodies are highly specific and nearly always positive. Antigliadin and antireticulin antibodies may be positive.

How would you treat coeliac disease?

A strict diet with complete exclusion of gluten-containing flour from wheat, rye, oats and barley is essential. Folate, iron and calcium supplements may be needed. Lifelong annual review should include assessment of symptoms, body mass index, haemoglobin, ferritin, folate, albumin, autoantibodies and osteoporosis risk (with bone densitometry for postmenopausal females and males aged over 55 years).

What are carcinoid tumours?

These are not uncommon incidental tumours, often found in appendix specimens. They arise from neuroendocrine cells and usually remain asymptomatic, their products metabolised by the liver. Rarely, they metastasise to the liver, whereupon they release serotonin into the systemic circulation. Its metabolite, 5-hydroxyindoleacetic acid (5-HIAA), is detectable by urinary assay. This is called carcinoid syndrome and may present with flushing, diarrhoea, bronchospasm and occasionally right sided heart valve dysfunction. Bronchial carcinoid tumours are less common, but may cause similar features, including left sided heart valve dysfunction. These tumours are generally very slow growing, but the syndrome has a poor overall prognosis.

CASE STUDY   4.6 INFLAMMATORY BOWEL DISEASE

Instruction: *Please read the letter from this patient's general practitioner and then conduct an appropriate consultation. You are not expected to examine her.*

> *Dear Doctor*
> *This 30-year-old lady has a 4-month history of bloody diarrhoea, passing at least six stools per day. There is associated mucus. She was previously well. I would be grateful for your further assessment and append her laboratory results. [FBC normal except for mild hypochromic microcytic anaemia, LFTs including albumin normal, ESR 45, stool microscopy and culture negative for bacteria, ova, cysts and parasites.]*

Case Box 4.6   Inflammatory Bowel Disease History Taking Points

This question is probably about inflammatory bowel disease (IBD). Crohn's disease (CD) and ulcerative colitis (UC) are idiopathic chronic relapsing and remitting disorders. They are increasing in prevalence and show a bimodal distribution with a major peak between 20 and 40 years and a lesser one between 60 and 80.

Questions should be similar to any case of altered bowel habit, but if there is a clear history of inflammatory symptoms (blood, mucus, pus or slime), then IBD is very likely. You would wish to exclude infectious causes (history and stool culture) and consider the possibility of colorectal cancer. Further investigation of this patient is mandatory. Sometimes, a non-specific diagnosis of 'colitis' will be made, but the underlying cause will likely be IBD.

Try to determine the subtype of IBD:

Acute severe UC

Usually total or subtotal colonic disease causing profuse diarrhoea (> 6 liquid stools/day), severe rectal bleeding (with mucus), abdominal pain, systemic disturbance (e.g. fever, tachycardia, anaemia, raised white cell count, raised ESR), anorexia and weight loss.

Moderately active UC

4–6 liquid stools/day, moderate rectal bleeding, some signs of systemic disturbance, or mild disease which fails to respond to treatment.

Mild UC

< 4 liquid stools/day, little or no rectal bleeding, no systemic disturbance.

Proctitis

Rectal bleeding, mucus discharge, tenesmus, constipation and sometimes pruritus ani.

Active ileocaecal disease

Pain, sometimes with a RIF mass, with or without diarrhoea and weight loss. The pain is constant if due to inflammation or abscess formation, and colicky with borborygmi and abdominal distension if due to small bowel obstruction.

Active Crohn's colitis

Symptoms are similar to active ulcerative colitis UC, but frank bleeding is less common.

Perianal Crohn's disease

There may be fissuring, fistulae or abscesses.

What causes IBD?

The cause is unknown. There is a 10-fold relative risk increase in first degree relatives. Environmental associations include non-smoking (UC), smoking (CD), enteric infection (UC), drugs (including NSAIDs, antibiotics and oral contraceptives) and stress.

What do you know about the pathology of IBD?

Crohn's disease is a chronic inflammatory disease with a TH1 mediated proinflammatory response (pages 199–200) at its core. It may affect the entire gastrointestinal tract from mouth to anus, especially the terminal ileum and anorectum. There may be skip lesions, with normal mucosa between affected areas. Inflammation is transmural, often with deep ulceration, fissuring and abscess formation. There may be non-caseating granulomas.

Ulcerative colitis is confined to the large bowel and almost always affects the rectum. Ulceration is usually superficial. Granulomas are not a feature.

What complications may arise from IBD?

Complications of Crohn's disease include fistulae (entero-enteral, entero-cutaneous, entero-vesical, entero-vaginal, perianal), a small increased risk of colorectal carcinoma, B_{12} deficiency, iron deficiency, abscess formation and systemic infection.

Complications of ulcerative colitis include toxic megacolon, an increased risk of colorectal carcinoma and iron deficiency. Fistulae are very rare.

Complications of drug treatments should also be considered, especially corticosteroid induced osteopenia/osteoporosis and bone marrow suppression from steroid sparing agents such as azathioprine.

What extraintestinal associations of IBD are you aware of?

● Enteropathic arthropathy, sacroiliitis ● Anterior uveitis ● Erythema nodosum ● Pyoderma gangrenosum ● Ureteric calculi (oxalate in CD, urate in UC) ● Gallstones (CD), sclerosing cholangitis, cholangiocarcinoma.

How would you manage IBD?

Management depends upon the diagnosis (Crohn's disease or ulcerative colitis), the site of disease, disease activity and the presence or absence of complications. Outpatient rigid sigmoidoscopy may be used to determine the type of inflammation, X-ray and colonoscopy to determine its extent.

There is no specific dietry advice in IBD. NSAIDs and antibiotics may provoke relapse and antidiarrhoeal (especially opioids), antispasmodic and anitcholinergic drugs may provoke colonic dilatation.

Ulcerative colitis

1. Acute severe ulcerative colitis requires intensive inpatient treatment with intravenous corticosteroids and, if no response, ciclosporin or proctocolectomy.
2. Mild to moderate attacks of ulcerative colitis may be managed with a systemic 5-amino salicylic acid (5-ASA) compound and/or twice daily 5-ASA or corticosteroid enemas. Oral corticosteroids in tapering doses may be needed for the first few weeks to induce remission. Azathioprine is used in steroid resistant or steroid dependent cases.
3. Proctitis may be managed with twice daily 5-ASA or steroid enemas.
4. The aim of treatment is to induce and then maintain remission. Maintenance with lifelong systemic 5-ASA significantly reduces the annual rate of relapse.
5. Colonoscopic colorectal carcinoma surveillance is needed, and usually begins no later than 10 years after diagnosis because the increased incidence of CRC starts at around this time frame.

Crohn's disease

1. Active ileocaecal inflammation usually responds to oral or intravenous corticosteroids with dosage tapering over a few weeks. Controlled, ileal release budesonide is an alternative to oral steroids. Azathioprine may be used to maintain remission in patients whose symptoms recur when steroids are reduced.
2. 5-ASA compounds are less beneficial in active disease than for ulcerative colitis. They probably confer no prophylactic benefit.
3. Smoking cessation aids maintenance of remission.
4. New therapeutic options also include anti-TNF-α (anti-tumour necrosis factor alpha) monoclonal antibodies, liquid formula diets, endoscopic stricture dilatation and laparoscopic surgery.

| CASE STUDY | 4.7 COLORECTAL CANCER AND SCREENING |

Instruction: *This 40-year-old lady's brother had a bowel tumour. She has no symptoms but wonders if she should be screened. Please ask her some questions.*

| Case Box 4.7 | Colorectal Cancer History Taking Points |

Colorectal cancer (CRC) screening is always topical and without clear guidelines. First degree relatives have a higher relative risk of CRC and often wonder if they should be tested.
The main issues here are:

1. To establish more details about the tumour in her brother. How did it present? Was it malignant? What treatment did he have? What was the outcome?
2. To establish if any other family members are known to be affected.
3. To establish any symptoms suggesting CRC in this lady. Right sided or proximal CRC tends to cause iron deficiency anaemia, abdominal pain or a mass. Left sided or distal CRC tends to cause altered bowel habit, per rectal bleeding and sometimes a mass or tenesmus.
4. To establish any other risk factors in this lady. Ask about inflammatory bowel disease. Diets low in fibre, fruit and vegetables and high in fat and red meat and alcohol are also thought to confer an increased risk.
5. To elicit her beliefs, concerns and expectations about her risk of CRC.

What do you know about the molecular basis and genetics of CRC risk?

More than 70% of CRCs develop from sporadic adenomatous polyps.
The commonest well defined hereditary syndromes are *familial adenomatous polyposis (FAP)* and *hereditary non-polyposis colon cancer (HNPCC)*/Lynch syndromes. Peutz–Jehgers syndrome is rare.

FAP is an autosomal dominant disorder in which there is a germline mutation in the tumour suppressor gene for adenomatous polyposis coli (APC) on chromosome 5. It accounts for < 1% of all CRC. Patients often have hundreds of pedunculated colonic polyps. Extracolonic manifestations may occur (previously referred to as Gardner's and Turcot's syndromes), including duodenal adenomas and cerebral and thyroid tumours.

In HNPCC there are germline mutations in DNA mismatch repair genes giving rise to pedunculated and flat polyps, predominantly in the proximal colon. The proportion of CRC attributable to HNPCC is unclear, but HNPCC likely accounts for a significantly higher proportion than FAP. Associations include endometrial, ovarian, gastric and other cancers.

Clusters of CRC also occur in some families without a recognisable syndrome, suggesting a genetic origin.

The immediate family members of a patient with CRC have a two- to three-fold relative risk of developing the disease.

Ulcerative colitis is unequivocally associated with increased CRC risk, high risk factors including disease > 10 years, extensive disease and the presence of primary sclerosing cholangitis.

Factors which may promote the adenoma to CRC sequence include APC gene mutations, k-ras mutations, deleted in colon cancer (DCC) mutations and p53 gene mutations.

Which factors determine a higher risk of malignant transformation within a polyp?

● Large size ● Sessile or flat ● Severe dysplasia or squamous metaplasia ● Villous rather than tubular architecture ● Multiplicity (e.g. FAP).

What do you know about CRC screening?

CRC is a major public health challenge. Outcome is directly related to histological staging and patients with Dukes' A lesions have a 5-year survival of > 83%. Early detection is imperative, and this includes prompt investigation of patients with symptoms, selective screening of high risk patients and population screening.

Patients at increased risk of CRC should be considered for surveillance. This group includes patients with a positive family history and patients with longstanding IBD. The lifetime risk of CRC is 1 : 50. This rises to 1 : 17 if one first degree relative is affected and > 1 : 10 if two or more first degree relatives are affected. Patients with a family history of HNPCC (suggested by three or more members affected by CRC or endometrial carcinoma) should be screened in early adult life. The timing of initial screening for patients with FAP or HNPCC is uncertain, and often determined by a family's risk pattern.

The arguments for a national screening programme are that CRC is common, with a known premalignant lesion (adenoma). As it takes a long time (years) for adenomas to undergo malignant change, intervention is likely to significantly reduce the morbidity and mortality burden of CRC.

The two problems faced by population screening are: *which patients to target* and *by which method. Faecal occult blood* testing is non-invasive, cheap and simple. It is relatively insensitive and non-specific, but has the potential to save many lives at an acceptable cost. *Flexible sigmoidoscopy* detects up to 80% of CRC as it examines the entire left colon and rectum. A strategy aimed at one-off testing of patients aged 55–65 for adenomas is under evaluation. *Colonsocopy* is the gold standard diagnostic test, but difficult to resource and inconvenient. Virtual colonoscopy using spiral CT or MRI scanning are non-invasive alternatives. Stool DNA analysis may have a future role.

CASE STUDY   4.8 CHEST PAIN AND CORONARY HEART DISEASE (CHD)

Instruction: *This 49-year-old gentleman has diabetes, smokes and has a family history of ischaemic heart disease. His blood pressure is 160/94. His TC : HDL ratio is > 6 mmol/L. He reports recent chest pain. Please take a history from him and discuss your proposed management.*

Case Box 4.8   Chest Pain History Taking Points

Elicit more details about the chest pain
- Site (ischaemic pain is poorly localised retrosternal discomfort, often described as tightness, pressure or burning)
- Character (ischaemic pain is 'heavy' or 'tight'; often patients deny the symptom of pain and refer to it as 'just a discomfort')
- Radiation (ischaemic pain may radiate to the arms, neck, jaw, gums or abdomen and sometimes these may be the only sites)
- Precipitating factors (ischaemic pain is often triggered by exertion, walking uphill, cold air and meals; enquire about rest pain and nocturnal pain)
- Relieving factors (rest, nitrate spray)

Ask about associated symptoms
- Dyspnoea, orthopnoea, paroxysmal nocturnal dyspnoea and ankle swelling
- Syncope or presyncopal symptoms (aortic stenosis)

Ask about risk factors for CHD
These include a family history (especially at an early age), smoking, hypertension, dyslipidaemia and diabetes.

Elicit beliefs, concerns and expectations (page 105)
Elicit a social and occupational history (Box 4.2)
Consider the differential diagnosis of acute chest pain
This includes dissecting aortic aneurysm (classically radiating to the back), pericarditis, pulmonary embolus, pneumonia, dyspepsia, cholecystitis, shingles and musculoskeletal pain (including viral disease and costochondritis).

Assume that investigations do not suggest cardiac pain. How would you manage this patient's cardiac risk factors?

(Secondary prevention of CHD is discussed through pages 146–150)

Lifestyle measures

He should be encouraged not to smoke. Exercise, weight reduction and a low saturated fat/low salt/high fruit and vegetable diet are important. Oily fish and a 'Mediterranean' diet may be beneficial.

Antihypertensive therapy

His hypertension should be managed according to British Hypertension Society Guidelines (Case study 5.17). An angiotensin converting enzyme inhibitor (ACEI) would be a suitable antihypertensive, especially were he to have evidence of diabetic nephropathy. The LIFE study (Case study 5.17) demonstrated the benefits of the angiotensin II receptor blocker losartan in selected high risk individuals.

The Heart Outcomes Prevention Evaluation Study (HOPE, also discussed in Case study 6.13) showed the beneficial effects of the ACEI ramipril on cardiovascular events in patients over 55 years of age with vascular disease (previous coronary artery disease, cerebrovascular disease or peripheral vascular disease) *or* diabetes *plus* an additional cardiovascular risk factor. Ramipril led to a 22% reduction in adverse events (death, myocardial infarction, stroke) with highly significant statistical results (narrow confidence intervals which did not encroach on the line of no significance). The benefits appeared to be *independent* of blood pressure lowering.

Lipid lowering therapy

The WOSCOPS trial confirmed the benefit of primary prevention with statins and this included a subgroup of diabetic patients with hypertriglyceridaemia. Statins may also have endothelial stabilising effects. Meta-analysis of primary prevention trials has shown that statins reduce the risk of CHD by 34%. The Prospective Study of Pravastatin in Elderly at Risk (PROSPER) showed unequivocal benefit of statin therapy in elderly people with CHD or at risk from smoking, hypertension or diabetes.

The Heart Protection Study (HPS) showed that lowering cholesterol reduces cardiac and stroke risk by approximately one-third in patients at high risk of cardiovascular disease (over 20 000 patients aged 40–80 years were randomised and included those with a history of

CHD, non-coronary occlusive vascular disease or cerebrovascular disease) irrespective of their age, sex or even baseline cholesterol level. Benefits were seen in patients with pre-treatment cholesterol levels as low as 3.5 mmol/L. The HPS argues for statin treatment in patients with coronary heart disease, cerebrovascular disease (TIA and stroke), peripheral vascular disease or diabetes.

Glycaemic control

The risk of a cardiovascular event in a diabetic patient without a history of cardiovascular disease is similar to that of a non-diabetic patient with a previous coronary event, arguing for meticulous glycaemic control and cardiovascular prophylaxis in diabetic patients.

Antiplatelet therapy

Numerous trials now support primary prophylaxis with aspirin in *high risk* patients (Case study 5.17), including the Hypertension Optimal Treatment (HOT) trial.

Case Box 4.4   Coronary Risk Prediction Charts for Primary Prevention

1. The Joint British Societies – British Cardiac Society, British Hypertension Society (BHS), British Hyperlipidaemia Association, British Diabetic Association (now Diabetes UK) – Coronary Risk Prediction Charts may be used to estimate 10 year CHD absolute risk (coronary death, non-fatal MI, new angina).
2. Based on the Framingham estimates, the charts aid decisions about intervention with lifestyle measures, antihypertensive therapy or lipid lowering therapy, but should not replace clinical judgement.
3. The charts contain tables for gender, non-diabetes/diabetes status (refers to type 2), smoking status (current or significant lifetime exposure) and age. No estimate is available for people aged over 75 years. 10 year risk estimation is defined according to the point at which the coordinates for systolic blood pressure and total cholesterol : high density lipoprotein (TC : HDL) meet. The initial blood pressure and random (non-fasting) TC : HDL ratio are used to estimate risk. HDL is assumed to be 1 mmol/L if unavailable.
4. If blood pressure is persistently ≥ 160/100 mmHg or there is target organ damage, then antihypertensive therapy is indicated irrespective of CHD risk. The BHS treatment thresholds for intervention are detailed in Case study 5.17.
5. Individuals (up to age 70) with a 10 year risk ≥ 30% (red area) and a serum total cholesterol ≥ 5.0 mmol/L (or LDL ≥ 3 mmol/L) despite at least 3 months of lifestyle measures should be considered for statin therapy. However, treatment thresholds and

target levels are frequently revised, and HOPE and PROSPER support statin therapy regardless of lipid profile or age. Individuals with a 10 year risk ≥ 15% (orange area) should be targeted for treatment when resources allow, according to the National Service Framework, since treatment may be too costly for the health service.

6. The charts are based on groups of people with untreated blood pressures and lipid profiles. In patients already receiving antihypertensive therapy for a whom a decision as to whether to start lipid lowering therapy is to be made (and vice-versa), the charts may be a guide but unless a pre-treatment risk level is available it is generally safer to assume that risk is higher than the predicted value.

7. The charts are not suitable for individuals with pre-existing CHD or other major atherosclerotic disease or existing disease which puts them at high risk, such as familial dyslipidaemias, chronic renal failure or diabetic nephropathy.

8. CHD risk is higher than predicted in the charts for those with a family history of premature CHD (first degree relative: male < 55 years, female < 65 years), those with ECG evidence of LVH, those with raised triglycerides, those not yet diabetic but with impaired fasting glucose, type 1 diabetic patients, those who have recently stopped smoking or started antihypertensive treatment, those approaching the next age category, women with a history of premature menopause and some ethnic minorities.

What do you know about the molecular pathophysiology of coronary artery disease and acute coronary syndromes (ACS)?

Evolution of vulnerable lesions

Chronic minimal injury to the endothelium (endothelial dysfunction) is physiological. It occurs at bends and bifurcations of vessels and is the result of turbulent blood flow. It is enhanced by hypertension. It is also induced by hypercholesterolaemia, tobacco toxins, advanced glycation end products in diabetes and possibly infection.

Endothelial dysfunction encourages low density lipoprotein (LDL), laden with cholesterol, to enter the subendothelial space and bind to subendothelial extracellular matrix. Here, LDL becomes trapped and subsequently oxidised by resident cells including endothelial cells, smooth muscle cells and macrophages.

Oxidised LDL stimulates monocyte chemotaxis by stimulating chemokine monocyte chemotactic protein 1 (MCP-1) synthesis and release from resident cells. MCP-1 attracts circulating monocytes which adhere to the endothelial wall (facilitated by adhesion molecules) and enter the subendothelial space. Oxidised LDL also stimulates resident cells to produce macrophage colony stimulating factors (M-CSFs) which encourage differentiation of monocytes into macrophages. The role of macrophages in endothelial dysfunction may be, in part, to limit excess lipoprotein accumulation.

Increasingly, atherogenesis is viewed as a chronic inflammatory disease in which macrophages and other inflammatory cells of the immune system respond to endothelial injury. T helper lymphocytes almost certainly release interleukin 2 in response to macrophages acting as antigen presenting cells (page 196).

Macrophages internalise oxidised LDL (the apolipoprotein B100 protein on the LDL molecule's surface is recognised by macrophage receptors) to become *foam cells*, so named because they have a foamy appearance when laden with fat. Foam cells eventually undergo necrosis and discharge their fat, together with necrotic debris, into the extracellular space.

Early lesions, containing foam cells rich in lipid droplets, are common in people under the age of 30. They may progress to lesions associated with extracellular lipid. The earliest atherosclerotic lesion, the *fatty streak*, has begun to form an extracellular connective tissue matrix through the extracellular fat, and represents a dynamic balance between entry and exit of lipoprotein, and between development and breakdown of matrix. Essentially, if more lipoprotein exits the fatty streak than enters (by, for example, risk modification), scarring with minimal risk results. If more lipoprotein enters the fatty streak than exits, vulnerable lesions form.

Vulnerable lesions are soft with a high extracellular lipid and macrophage content and a thin fibrous cap. Disruption of these lesions leads to thrombus formation.

Vulnerable plaque disruption

Angiographically small plaques are often the most vulnerable to disruption, provoking thrombus formation with stenosis or total vessel occlusion.

Plaque disruption may be: 1. Passive, in which the thin fibrous cap, infiltrated by foam cells, mechanically erodes, fissures or ruptures. Frequently this is between the plaque and the vessel wall or at the plaque's 'shoulder'. 2. Active, in which macrophages within plaques degrade extracellular matrix and cap by phagocytosis or secretion of proteolytic enzymes such as matrix metalloproteinases.

Acute thrombosis

Tissue factor (TF) is exposed after plaque rupture and initiates the extrinsic coagulation pathway (page 465).

Vasoconstriction

Finally, platelet induced vasoconstriction can exacerbate vessel occlusion.

Clinical correlation

Angina results when myocardial oxygen demand outweighs the supply that stenosed vessels can provide. In ACSs there is invariably some degree of plaque disruption with superimposed thrombosis and vasoconstriction. The type of ACS depends upon the lesion, the degree of natural reversibility from spontaneous thrombolysis and the degree of safety netting from collateral vessels. Myocardial infarction in patients with no antecedent ischaemia is often more catastrophic.

Which mechanisms normally protect against myocardial ischaemia?

● Arteriole dilatation, in response to increased energy consumption, mediated by metabolic signals from the myocardium and amplified by nitric oxide ● Collateral blood vessel formation, stimulated by angiogenic signals from the myocardium. ● Arterial pressure, which increases in diastole when most subendocardial coronary perfusion occurs. ● Preconditioning.

What do you understand by the term preconditioning?

This refers to the protective effect of brief (minutes) periods of ischaemia in limiting the adverse effects of subsequent ischaemia. The mechanism of this postulated concept is uncertain.

What do you understand by the terms stunning and hibernation?

Contractile recovery from brief ischaemia is usually rapid. *Stunning* refers to delayed contractile recovery, and represents the combined insults of ischaemia and reperfusion which itself releases damaging bursts of oxygen free radicals. Patients are at risk of ventricular arrhythmias and heart failure. *Hibernation* refers to a reduction in contractile performance due to postulated downregulation of myocardial metabolism. In contrast to stunning, it may be protective, limiting the heart's metabolic needs in response to ischaemia. Hibernating myocardium is viable and its contractility can improve following coronary revascularisation.

What do you understand by the terms stable and unstable angina?

● *Stable angina* is characterised by a pattern of symptoms occurring predictably on exertion.
● *Unstable angina* refers to symptoms of recent onset, symptoms increasing in frequency, severity or duration, or symptoms occurring at rest. It suggests plaque instability, and is a medical emergency. All patients with newly diagnosed cardiac pain should presumptively be considered to have unstable disease and be referred for objective assessment of myocardial ischaemia.

What are the objective tests for myocardial ischaemia?

1. *Exercise tolerance testing (ETT)* with a standardised treadmill.

2. *Myocardial perfusion imaging* with a radioisotope such as thallium. An area of reduced perfusion at stress that normalises with rest indicates ischaemia, whilst a fixed perfusion effect indicates permanent damage. Perfusion imaging is useful in patients with uninterpretable ECGs (e.g. left bundle branch block (LBBB)), and in patients unable to exercise.
3. *Stress echocardiography* may show wall motion abnormalities under dobutamine stress.
4. *Coronary angiography* is the gold standard investigation for demonstrating coronary anatomy, and is used where diagnostic uncertainty remains and coronary revascularisation would be contemplated.

What are the arguments for medical treatment, coronary artery bypass grafting (CABG) and percutaneous coronary intervention (PCI) in stable angina?

Treatment of stable angina aims to limit chest pain and prevent cardiovascular events. Treatment principles are given in Box 4.5.

Box 4.5	Treatment Principles in Chronic Stable Angina

Medical therapy

Antiplatelet therapy, *beta-blockers* and *statins reduce cardiac events*, but only beta-blockers also have antianginal effects. The HOPE study (page 141) showed the benefit of ACEIs in patients at high cardiovascular risk, but further studies are needed before ACEI can be recommended in patients with angina alone. Nicorandil may also reduce coronary events. *Nicorandil* has nitrate-like properties and activates potassium channels, thereby acting as a balanced coronary and peripheral vasodilator, and reduces both cardiac preload and afterload. *Beta-blockers, calcium channel blockers* (CCBs) and *nitrates* provide *symptomatic benefit*. Verapamil and diltiazem are first choice CCBs in patients in whom beta-blockade is not possible since they are rate limiting, but diltiazem should be used with caution in heart failure, and under cardiologist supervision with beta-blockers (verapamil avoided here) since the combination may impair left ventricular function and cardiac conduction. Amlodipine and nifedipine do not limit heart rate and may precipitate reflex tachycardia and angina (especially during exercise) but may be used safely in combination with a beta-blocker. Tolerance is a major limitation to the use of nitrates.

Coronary artery bypass grafting (CABG)

Trials in the 1970s showed CABG to be more effective in symptom relief than medical therapy. CABG provides a better prognosis in high-risk patients with left main stem or triple vessel disease or two vessel disease involving the proximal left anterior descending artery.

Percutaneous coronary intervention (PCI)

PCI, which includes *percutaneous transluminal coronary angioplasty* (PTCA) and *stenting*, is less invasive than CABG but confers a higher rate of angina recurrence. The re-stenosis rate is lower with stents (10–20%) than with PTCA. Adjunctive glycoprotein IIb/IIIa inhibitors have reduced the risk of acute vessel occlusion and the need for rescue CABG. Clopidogrel has been widely used following PCI, with the combined use of aspirin and clopidogrel (in the short term at least) reducing thrombotic complications after stenting. Patients with chest pain post-stent insertion should be readmitted for ECG and tropinin analysis and possible angiography. PTCA provides better antianginal effects than medical therapy, but neither PTCA nor medical therapy has a clear advantage over the other in terms of outcome. Future meta-analyses will need to take account of more widespread use in recent years of both statins and stents.

What is meant by the term acute coronary syndrome (ACS)?

The term refers to a spectrum of presentations caused by myocardial ischaemia that includes unstable angina, non-Q wave myocardial infarction and ST elevation myocardial infarction. The one umbrella term reflects the common molecular pathophysiology of plaque disruption, platelet activation, intravascular thrombosis and impaired myocardial blood supply.

Non-Q wave myocardial infarction may present similarly to unstable angina but theoretically unstable angina is not accompanied by a rise in cardiac enzyme concentration. Sensitive troponin assays, confirming cell necrosis, have shown that many patients presenting with unstable angina do in fact sustain myocardial necrosis.

How are acute coronary syndromes stratified and managed?

1. Immediate management of ST elevation myocardial infarction is with antiplatelet therapy, thrombolytic therapy (not indicated for LBBB or posterior infarction) or PCI and, where not contraindicated, beta-blockade.
2. Unstable angina and non-Q wave myocardial infarction may be stratified as high, intermediate or low risk based on symptoms, initial ECG and serum markers, and risk stratification has been used to determine optimal therapy (Box 4.6).

What types of myocardial infarction are there and which ECG leads are affected in each?

Anterior, anterolateral, inferior and posterior:

- II, III, aVF are inferior leads—right coronary artery (RCA) territory
- I, aVF, V5, V6 are lateral leads—left circumflex artery (LCA) territory
- V1–V5 are anterior leads—left anterior descending (LAD) territory
- V1 may provide a mirror image of a posterior infarction.

Box 4.6	Treatment Principles in Non-Q Wave Myocardial Infarction/Unstable Angina

High risk

Patients have ST depression (or transient elevation) on ECG and raised troponins (T > 0.1 µg/L or I equivalent). Age, comorbidity, arrhythmias, haemodynamic instability, rest pain or early pain post infarction also indicate high risk. In addition to routine medical managment, including aspirin and beta-blockers, patients benefit from glycoprotein IIb/IIIa inhibitors (pages 464–465, 472), and low molecular weight heparin (but not thrombolysis) and should proceed to coronary angiography with a view to PCI during admission (with adjunctive glycoprotein IIb/IIIa inhibitors, heparin and antiplatelet therapy, including clopidogrel). The ideal duration for continuing clopidogrel after an ACS or PCI is unclear.

Intermediate risk

Patients may have T wave abnormalities or moderately increased troponins (T 0.01–0.1 µg/L) and should undergo exercise or pharmacological stress testing to further stratify risk. Angiography may be considered.

Low risk

Patients are generally younger with no history of rest pain, a normal ECG and no troponin rise (T < 0.01 µg/L). Stress testing is ideally performed during admission and, if measuring, patients are managed out of hospital.

What do you know about right ventricular infarction (RVI)?

The V4R lead placed on the right side of the chest symmetrical to where it is usually placed may help diagnose RVI. V4R should be performed in the setting of an acute inferior territory infarct when it may reveal ST segment elevation absent in its usual V4 placement.

RCA occlusion usually threatens the inferior wall of the heart. Unlike LAD territory, which supplies much of the anterior wall (scarring of which impairs left ventricular function), RCA territory supplies the AV node in 80% of cases (the circumflex artery supplying it in the remaining 20%) and RCA infarcts tend to cause bradyarrhythmias. Temporary pacing is often life saving but because these arrhythmias often represent reversibly ischaemic penumbra, long-term pacing is not inevitable.

ST elevation in V4R implies involvement of the right ventricular branch (RVB) of the RCA. This occurs if the RCA occlusion is proximal to its RVB offshoot. An infarcted right ventricle will impair left heart filling and cause hypotension. Bradyarrhythmias will also cause hypotension, as will a more extensive infarct with left ventricular involvement, as will hypotensive drugs such as beta-blockers. Unlike most causes of hypotension in the setting of acute myocardial infarction, RVI demands high filling pressures. Fluids, rather than diuretics, are needed to maintain right ventricular output and left ventricular filling.

Which complications may follow myocardial infarction?

- Arrhythmias (heart block especially in inferior infarction)
- Heart failure/acute pulmonary oedema (especially in anterior infarction)
- Papillary valve rupture and mitral regurgitation
- Septal rupture
- Thromboembolism (atrial fibrillation or mural thrombus)
- Pericarditis/Dressler's syndrome (pericarditis, pleurisy and pyrexia).

Discuss secondary prevention after myocardial infarction (Box 4.7)

Box 4.7	Secondary Prevention after Myocardial Infarction

1. *Antiplatelet therapy* (aspirin 75–150 mg daily) and *beta-blockers* should be continued indefinitely in all patients unless there are contraindications.
2. *ACEIs* should be started in all patients with anterior infarction or left ventricular dysfunction unless contraindicated. All patients should have an echocardiogram following myocardial infarction to assess left ventricular function and to exclude mural thrombus. The HOPE study (page 141) showed the broader benefits of ACEIs in patients at high cardiovascular risk.
3. There is no conclusive evidence for calcium channel blockers in secondary prevention. Antiarrhythmic drugs other than beta-blockers have exhibited harm or no overall benefit.
4. Mobilisation should start on days 2–3, along with risk factor modification, lifestyle assessment and introduction to *cardiac rehabilitation*.
5. *Blood pressure* targets for secondary prevention have not been established as they have for primary prevention, although the British Hypertension Society targets (Case study 5.17) are widely applied.
6. The evidence for *statin* therapy in the secondary prevention of cardiovascular disease is strong.
7. Meticulous *glycaemic control* is essential in diabetes.
8. *Modifiable lifestyle risk factors* (page 141) should be addressed.
9. 'Uncomplicated' patients may be discharged from hospital at day 5. Patients should mobilise at home for the following week, and gradually increase their exercise thereafter.

10. An outpatient visit at weeks 4–6 should include an assessment of symptoms, clinical examination for signs of heart failure, psychological assessment and an exercise tolerance test (ETT) using the Bruce protocol to identify those patients with reversible ischaemia who might benefit from revascularisation.

11. Implantable cardiac defibrillators are considered for certain patients at risk of sudden cardiac death (page 160) and survivors of ventricular fibrillation or ventricular tachycardia, and should also be considered for high risk patients after myocardial infarction. High risk includes a left ventricular ejection fraction ≤ 35%, non-sustained VT (≥ 3 beats) on 24-hour ambulatory monitoring or inducible VT on electrophysiological testing. Antiarrhythmic drugs paradoxically increase risk.

What is the evidence for statin therapy in the secondary prevention of cardiovascular disease?

Evidence comes from numerous secondary prevention trials, notably 4S, CARE and LIPID (see references). Guidelines formerly recommended statin therapy in patients up to age 75 when serum total cholesterol was > 5 mmol/L. Increasing evidence (page 141), suggests that statin therapy benefits patients with lower cholesterol levels and a broader range of high risk patients.

Is there a role for folic acid in cardiovascular disease prevention? See page 472.

CASE STUDY	**4.9 HEART FAILURE**

Instruction: *Please read the following letter from this patient's general practitioner and then conduct an appropriate consultation. You are not expected to examine her.*

Dear Doctor
This 70-year-old lady has become increasingly dyspnoeic over the last 6 months. She has no cough. She has been sleeping with extra pillows for 2 months and her exertional tolerance has worsened. Her full blood picture, urea and electrolytes, glucose, cholesterol, liver function tests and thyroid function tests are normal. Her open access echocardiogram confirmed moderate left ventricular systolic dysfunction. She is currently on 40 mg of frusemide and an ACEI. I would appreciate your assessment.

What is heart failure?

Heart failure is a complex syndrome resulting from any structural or functional cardiac disorder that impairs the ability of the heart to act as a pump. It affects 1–2% of the population (10–20% of the very elderly) and has a poor prognosis.

Case Box 4.9   **Heart Failure History Taking Points**

Questions in heart failure are similar to those for shortness of breath (Case box 4.1). Try to confirm that symptoms are consistent with heart failure from the range of other diagnoses, common differential diagnoses being chronic obstructive pulmonary disease (COPD), recurrent pulmonary emboli, lower respiratory tract infection and pleural effusion/malignancy.

Try to confirm that the symptoms are consistent with heart failure
- *Left ventricular failure (LVF):* dyspnoea, orthopnoea, paroxysmal nocturnal dyspnoea, nocturnal cough, fatigue (signs include a third heart sound, tachycardia, hypotension, bibasal crackles). Remember that symptoms that are worse when lying flat do not necessarily imply LVF. Symptoms from GORD, postnasal drip and bronchial secretions can also be worse supine.
- *Right venticular failure (RVF):* ankle swelling (signs include raised JVP, pulsatile tender hepatomegaly, sacral and peripheral oedema).
- *Biventricular failure:* both sets of symptoms.

Assess symptom severity
The four classes of heart failure symptoms in the New York Heart Association (NYHA) classification may be summarised as follows: I – no limitations; II – slight limitation of physical activity; III – marked limitation of physical activity; IV – symptoms at rest.

Elicit beliefs, concerns and expectations (page 105)
- What are your patient's thoughts about the cause of symptoms, and expectations of treatment?
- What can your patient no longer do that she would like to do?

Elicit a social and occupational history (Box 4.2)
- Does your patient live alone? What family, friends and other supports are there?

Consider the possible causes of heart failure
1. *Coronary heart disease.* Ask about symptoms of angina and risk factors (Case box 4.8).
2. *Pressure overload*, especially due to *hypertension* or *aortic stenosis*. Ask about high blood pressure and valve disease.
3. *Volume overload*, especially due to *aortic or mitral regurgitation*. Ask about valve disease.
4. *Arrhythmias*, especially *atrial fibrillation*. Ask about palpitations.
5. *Cor pulmonale* (right heart failure secondary to lung disease), often due to COPD but sometimes lung parenchymal diseases or pulmonary emboli. Recurrent multiple pulmonary emboli tend to be underdiagnosd in the elderly and its important to ask about stepwise deterioration/breathlessness.

6. Other causes include *infective endocarditis* (valve dysfunction), *cardiomyopathies* (heart muscle disease not due to ischaemia, hypertension or valvular disease), *myocarditis, pericardial disease* and *high output failure* in thyrotoxicosis, anaemia or Paget's disease.

Ask about investigations so far

1. The blood tests her GP has obtained should be routine. Renal function and albumin should always be part of the assessment of patients with 'heart failure', since fluid overload leading to pulmonary oedema can be due to renal failure or bilateral renal artery stenosis or, less commonly, hypoalbuminaemia.

2. The European Society of Cardiology algorithm for heart failure diagnosis recommends ECG, CXR and natriuretic peptide testing (where available) if heart failure is suspected on the basis of symptoms or signs. If these tests are normal, heart failure is unlikely. If abnormal, transthoracic echocardiography (TTE) should be performed. This is a pivotal test, not just in confirming left ventricular systolic dysfunction (LVSD) and determining the left ventricular ejection fraction (LVEF), but also in detecting/excluding valve disease and assessing cardiac dimensions. The LVEF is determined from the LV end diastolic and LV end systolic dimensions. Normally, it is around 65% or greater. In NYHA class IV disease it is generally < 35%. Frequently, echocardiography excludes heart failure, prompting a search for alternative causes of breathlessness and allowing cardiac drugs to be ceased.

What is the pathophysiology of heart failure?

The shape of the normal left ventricle is designed for maximal efficiency of ejection. Remodelling from scarring, hypertrophy (pressure overload) and dilatation (volume overload) compromises this ideal shape, and ushers in a vicious cycle of decreased cardiac output and compensatory neurohumoral stimulation (sympathetic nervous system and the renin–angiotensin–aldosterone system, RAAS) with positive ionotropy, salt and water retention and vasoconstriction. This leads to increased myocardial work, relative hypoxia, cell death and further left ventricular dysfunction. Arrhythmias are more likely. The role of natriuretic peptides (notably B natriuretic peptide – or N-terminal pro-B type natriuretic peptide) in heart failure and their use as diagnostic markers is of ongoing interest.

What pharmacological treatments improve the prognosis in left ventricular systolic dysfunction (LVSD)?

Optimal treatments (Box 4.8) serve to modulate the RAAS and upregulate or re-sensitise beta-receptors.

Box 4.8	Pharmacological Treatment in LVSD

1. *ACEIs* improve outcome and should be used in all patients unless there are contraindications. Angiotensin II receptor blockers (ARBs), which do not inhibit the breakdown of bradykinin and do not cause cough, may be alternatives for patients intolerant of ACEIs. Although few patients are intolerant of both, the combination of hydralazine and isosorbide dinitrate remains an alternative. ACEIs are relatively contraindicated in patients with obstructive valve disease (these and other agents such as calcium channel blockers which reduce afterload can increase the pressure drop across the valve) and extra vigilance is needed if renal artery stenosis is suspected (renal or epigastric bruit, raised creatinine, peripheral vascular disease).

2. *Beta-blockers* have been shown to improve outcome in selected patients with NYHA classes I–III heart failure, and should be considered in patients already being treated with an ACEI. Negative ionotropism has potential for harm and beta-blockers should only be considered in chronic, stable heart failure where there are no clinical or radiological signs of decompensation. The rule is to start with a low dose and build up slowly – 'low and go slow'. Beta-blockers may not improve symptoms despite improving prognosis, a fact that should be shared with patients before treatment.

3. Everyday experience shows that *loop and thiazide diuretics* improve symptoms but there is no evidence they improve outcome. They are used for patients with signs of sodium and water retention.

4. *Low dose spironolactone* should be considered for patients in NYHA classes III and IV already treated with an ACEI and diuretics. Careful monitoring of blood chemistry is mandatory, since hyperkalaemia is a dangerous complication.

5. *Digoxin* should be considered for all patients with heart failure and atrial fibrillation (AF) who need control of the ventricular rate. Digoxin does not offer survival benefit.

What non-pharmacological interventions might you consider for a patient with LVSD?

- Management of other modifiable risk factors (smoking cessation, hypertension, diabetes)
- Stopping drugs which precipitate fluid retention (e.g. NSAIDs, corticosteroids, calcium channel blockers) or depress myocardial function
- Salt restriction (ready to cook meals and convenience foods contain a high salt content)
- Fluid intake restriction to 1.5–2 L daily in advanced heart failure
- Exercise training programmes (avoiding strenuous exercise) in patients with NYHA class II–III disease

- Weight reduction (unless cardiac cachexia)
- Immunisation (influenza)
- The role of CABG in the setting of angina and heart failure remains uncertain.

What is diastolic dysfunction?

Heart failure usually involves contractile or systolic dysfunction of the ventricle (LVSD). Diastolic dysfunction occurs when the *ventricle resists filling*. A stiff ventricle causes compensatory atrial hypertrophy with a fourth heart sound (S4). Causes of diastolic dysfunction are:
- Severe LV hypertrophy (hypertension in the elderly is the commonest cause; aortic stenosis) ● Hypertrophic cardiomyopathy (HCM) ● Restrictive cardiomyopathy.

Most patients, however, with a clinical diagnosis of heart failure but preserved LVSD will have an alternative explanation for their symptoms such as obesity, lung disease or myocardial ischaemia.

CASE STUDY | **4.10 ATRIAL FIBRILLATION (AF) AND CARDIAC RHYTHM DISORDERS**

Instruction: *This patient presented with palpitations. Please take a history from her/him.*

Patient A

A 40-year-old woman with a 1-month history of irregular palpitations at rest and on exertion. She also describes feeling sweaty.

Patient B

An 82-year-old man with a 2-month history of dizzy spells and intermittent, irregular, fast palpitations. Clinically, he appears to be in sinus rhythm with a rate of 50 beats per minute.

Patient C

A 68-year-old man with known ischaemic heart disease and left ventricular impairment with intermittent episodes of fast, regular palpitations over the last month. Each episode lasts between a few minutes and an hour.

Patient D

A 30-year-old woman with a 1-month history of fast, regular palpitations lasting from several minutes to a few hours.

Patient E

A 25-year-old man with a history of feeling his heart 'missing a beat'. Episodes last a few seconds, and often occur before going off to sleep.

Case Box 4.10   Cardiac Rhythm Disorders History Taking Points

Palpitations are a common complaint. Many patients will not have a proven cardiac arrhythmia. Anxiety is a common cause. In general, older patients are more likely to have underlying structural cardiac disease provoking atrial fibrillation (AF) or less commonly non-sustained ventricular tachycardia (NSVT), and younger patients are more likely to be describing sinus tachycardia (often due to anxiety or exertion but medical causes include thyrotoxicosis and phaeochromcytoma) or supraventicular tachycardia (SVT). Venticular ectopic beats (VEBs) are very common.

Try to establish the following about the palpitations:
1. Are the palpitations *regular or irregular* (AF, VEBs)?
2. Are the palpitations *fast* (tachyarrhythmia—sinus tachycardia, AF, SVT, VT, atrial flutter) *or slow* (bradyarrhythmia—heart block, slow AF) *or normal*? Ask your patient to tap out the beat.
3. Are attacks *intermittent* (AF, VEBs, SVT, NSVT) *or persistent* (persistent AF)?
4. If intermittent, is the *onset abrupt* (paroxysmal AF, SVT, NSVT)?
5. If intermittent, what is the *duration* of attacks?
6. If intermittent, what is the *frequency* of attacks?
7. For *how long* have the attacks been occurring (since childhood in many SVTs)?
8. If intermittent, are there any *triggers* or *relieving factors* (exercise, caffeine, alcohol, drugs)?

Ask about associated symptoms
Chest pain, dyspnoea or syncope

Take a history for the common causes of AF
- Coronary heart disease (risk factors, previous events)
- Hypertension (most recent blood pressure)
- Mitral valve disease (previous rheumatic fever)
- Alcohol intake
- Hyperthyroidism (Case study 11.1).

If you suspect AF, ask about complications
History of heart failure or stroke

Take a full drug history
Elicit beliefs, concerns and expectations (page 105)
Do symptoms limit your patient? If so, how?
Elicit a social and occupational history (Box 4.2)

How would you investigate and manage:

Patient A?

> She most likely has AF due to thyrotoxicosis. An ECG and thyroid function tests will confirm, and should prompt referral to an endocrinologist. A non-selective beta-blocker would be suitable for rate control and may alleviate other thyrotoxic symptoms. Antithrombotic therapy should be started.

Patient B?

> As well as routine biochemistry, he should have a 12-lead ECG and 24-hour Holter monitoring (or a patient activated event recording device if episodes are sufficiently infrequent that a 24–48-hour recording is unlikely to detect one). He likely has sick sinus or brady-tachycardia syndrome. Episodes of dizziness or presyncope are more likely due to bradyarrhythmias than AF, although his palpitations could well be fast, paroxysmal AF or even NSVT, both common in patients with ischaemic/degenerating conducting pathways. Treatment for brady-tachycardia syndrome is commonly with a permanent pacemaker, together with an antiarrhythmic (beta-blocker or amiodarone) and antithrombotic therapy.

Patient C?

> Episodes of fast, regular palpitations may be due to SVT or VT, but in an elderly patient with ischaemic heart disease VT is much more likely. He requires rapid diagnosis and, if VT, treatment with an implantable cardiac defibrillator (ICD). Antiarrhythmic therapy (beta-blocker or amiodarone) would be second choice.

Patient D?

> This woman is more likely to have SVT. The ECG may show evidence of Wolff–Parkinson–White (WPW) syndrome but will likely be normal. Holter monitoring will be necessary unless there is a clear precipitant such as caffeine or alcohol.

Patient E?

> This man describes occasional ventricular or supraventricular ectopics and can probably be reassured if there are no clinical signs of heart disease such as hypertrophic cardiomyopathy.
>
> Note that when palpitations are the primary symptom, the most useful tests are a 12-lead ECG and an ECG monitoring device (and exercise ECG testing if symptoms are produced on exercise). Echocardiography is unlikely to add information if clinical examination and the ECG are normal.

How would you differentiate between VEBs and AF?

> Exercise decreases the frequency of 'benign' VEBs but has no effect on AF. Multiple or frequent VEBs on an ECG which represent an

'irritable myocardium' with underlying ischaemia may worsen with exercise or progress to VT.

What types of AF are there?

- *Paroxysmal* (reverts spontaneously to sinus rhythm)
- *Persistent* (reverts with electrical/pharmacological cardioversion)
- *Permanent*/chronic (does not revert).

Confusingly, some authorities refer to persistent AF as sustained AF, and permanent AF as persistent AF!

What are the main risk factors for AF?

- Coronary heart disease ● Valvular heart disease
- Hypertensive heart disease ● Alcohol ● Thyrotoxicosis
- Infection (e.g. pneumonia) ● Pulmonary embolus ● Many patients have no clear cause (lone AF).

What is the mechanism of AF?

Multiple wavelets of electrical activity arc around the atrium, some circling back on themselves (re-entry) but mostly pursuing altering courses. Atrial enlargement helps to sustain AF by accommodating more wavelets.

What are the complications of AF?

- Heart failure ● Thromboembolism, especially stroke.

How would you control heart rate in AF (and when would you consider cardioversion)?

This depends on the type of AF.

Paroxysmal AF

Infrequent, well tolerated attacks may not require rate control treatment. Beta-blockers or digoxin are first line drug choices.

Persistent AF

Cardioversion is more likely to be successful in:

- Younger patients
- Patients with structurally normal hearts
- AF of short duration (< 3 months).

Any precipitating factors should of course be identified and treated.

Cardioversion is less likely to achieve reversion to or maintenance of sinus rhythm in:

- Older patients
- Patients with a left atrial diameter of > 4.5 cm on echocardiography
- Chronic AF.

Cardioversion may be attempted by direct current under deep sedation/general anaesthetia or pharmacologically. Class 1C antiarrhythmics may be used if there is no ischaemic heart disease or LVSD. Amiodarone may be used if there is ischaemic heart disease or LVSD. Amiodarone, sotalol or other class 1C antiarrhythmics may help maintain sinus rhythm.

If AF is known to have been present for 2 days or less, cardioversion may be attempted immediately, otherwise anticoagulation and deferred cardioversion is needed.

Permanent AF

Haemodynamic compromise in AF results principally from an uncontrolled ventricular rate. A rate of < 90 at rest and < 180 on exercise is desirable. Digoxin is effective in preventing resting tachycardia but unsuccessful during exercise. Alternative choices include a beta-blocker (especially if there is associated hypertension or ischaemic heart disease), a rate limiting calcium channel blocker such as verapamil, or radiofrequency ablation of the AV node and permanent pacing.

What do you know about antithrombotic therapy in AF?

Patients with all types of AF are at risk of thromboembolism and should receive antithrombotic therapy.

The risk of stroke in non-valvular AF is around 5% per year, but varies according to specific risk factors. The risk in patients with rheumatic heart disease is much higher.

Systemic anticoagulation with warfarin has been shown to reduce the risk of stroke by about 60%, compared to only around 20% risk reduction with aspirin. However, these data are based on trials comparing each treatment with placebo. In a systematic review of head to head comparison between aspirin and warfarin for non-rheumatic AF, the benefit of warfarin appeared to be less significant, particularly when weighed against its increased risk of side effects. Further large scale randomised trials are needed to resolve the question of anticoagulation therapy in non-valvular AF, but:

1. Most physicians would *consider warfarin* where *AF is associated with one or more additional risk factors for thromboembolism.* The main risk factors are:

   ● Age > 75 years
   ● Valvular heart disease (especially rheumatic mitral valve disease)
   ● Previous transient ischaemic attack (TIA) or stroke
   ● Heart failure
   ● Large (thrombogenic) left atrium
   ● Ischaemic heart disease
   ● Hypertension
   ● Diabetes mellitus.

An international normalised ratio (INR) of 2–3 should be the target for thromboembolic prophylaxis. Warfarin appears to be especially beneficial in older patients, but some patients may be unsuitable for anticoagulation, such as patients at risk of falls (including patients with severe arthritis who are rendered unsteady), patients with advanced dementia, patients at high risk of gastrointestinal bleeding and patients for whom INR monitoring is impractical.

Echocardiography is not always necessary where there is a clear reason for starting warfarin irrespective of the result, but may be useful to establish other information such as the degree of LVSD or the pressure drop across a diseased valve.

2. Patients under 60 years of age with *lone AF* (no additional risk factor) may not benefit from warfarin but should at the very least receive antiplatelet therapy. Echocardiography is essential to exclude left atrial enlargement and valvular disease.

3. Lone AF in patients over 60 years of age is unusual ('if you look hard enough there is likely to be a risk factor') and many physicians anticoagulate patients with AF in the 60–75 year age group even when no additional risk factor is identifiable.

How may SVT arise in Wolff–Parkinson–White (WPW) syndrome?

WPW syndrome is due to an accessory conducting pathway that bypasses the AV node (AVN).

The accessory pathway may not always conduct and so the ECG may be intermittently normal. When it does conduct, impulses reach the ventricle from both the accessory pathway and the AVN. Impulses via the accessory pathway are faster than those through the AVN, giving rise to the delta wave on the ECG (*pre-excitation*). This does not usually provoke tachycardia.

There may, however, be retrograde conduction through the accessory pathway. This can arise during the transient window of opportunity when the accessory pathway is refractory (having delivered its impulses to the ventricle), and the slower AVN pathway is still conducting. At this time, AVN impulses may loop back up into the accessory pathway, setting up a loop of continuous conduction which results in a *re-entrant* supraventricular tachycardia (SVT). This antegrade conduction through the AV node and retrograde conduction through the accessory pathway is called *orthodromic* and produces a narrow complex tachycardia. More rarely, conduction is down the accessory pathway (*antedromic*) producing a wide complex tachycardia. These types of SVT are referred to as *atrioventricular re-entrant tachycardias (AVRTs)*. A wide complex tachycardia could also represent bundle branch block (BBB) or VT.

SVT often responds to conventional therapy with adenosine, verapamil or beta-blockers.

Why is digoxin contraindicated in WPW syndrome?

AF occurs in up to 15% of patients with WPW. Digoxin must never be used because it decreases the refractory period of the accessory pathway and allows rapid antegrade conduction from atrium to ventricle. The very fast ventricular rate may degenerate to ventricular fibrillation.

What other 'SVTs' are there?

The AVN itself often comprises a slow pathway and a fast pathway. Other SVTs may arise from the ability of the AVN to conduct in an antegrade direction down one of its pathways and in a retrograde direction through the other, giving rise to atrioventricular nodal re-entrant tachycardias (AVNRTs).

SVT is common in patients without structural aberrations in whom there may be numerous triggers such as caffeine or alcohol.

What do you know about broad complex tachycardias?

The difficulty is in distinguishing VT from SVT with aberrant conduction such as left bundle branch block (LBBB). VT is suggested by:

● QRS > 140 milliseconds
● Capture or fusion beats (intermittent sinoatrial beats, or sinoatrial beats fused with ventricular beats)
● Concordance in precordial leads (all of the V lead complexes point in the same direction)
● Absence of BBB on a previous ECG in sinus rhythm
● History of ischaemic heart disease (the strongest predictive factor).

What are the causes of sudden cardiac death in young people?

The majority is attributable to coronary artery disease.

In some cases there is no evidence of a structural cardiac abnormality and the cause of death is unascertainable at autopsy. The term sudden arrhythmic death syndrome (SADS) is sometimes used, and the underlying causes of sudden death in individuals with morphologically normal hearts include the ion channelopathies:

1. *Long QT syndrome* (LQTS), an inherited repolarisation disorder causing QT prolongation and risk of ventricular arrhythmias (torsade de pointes 'twisting of points'). Torsade de pointes may also be caused by metabolic disturbances and drugs.
2. *Brugada syndrome* (BS), a disorder of cardiac activation causing RBBB and ST elevation in V1–3 with a risk of polymorphic VT.
3. *Progressive cardiac conduction disease*, a disorder causing variable degrees of heart block.

4. *Catecholaminergic polymorphic ventricular tachycardia*, a disorder of cellular calcium handling causing exertional ventricular arrhythmias.

These are potentially inherited disorders and relatives of affected family members may be at risk.

Rare genetic conditions causing structural cardiac abnormalities may also be associated with sudden death or be identified in relatives of SADS victims. These include:

● Hypertrophic cardiomyopathy (Case study 5.14) ● Dilated cardiomyopathy (page 247) ● Arrhythmogenic right ventricular cardiomyopathy (ARVC) ● Mitral valve prolapse (Case study 5.7) ● Wolff–Parkinson–White syndrome (WPW, page 158) ● Myotonic dystrophy (Case study 6.32).

How might family members of victims be evaluated?

The history of the affected family member and the family history (especially with respect to unexplained syncope, sudden death, muscle weakness and congenital deafness) should be sought. Ideally, first degree relatives should be evaluated for symptoms and examined, and the following investigations may be undertaken:

● 12-lead ECG ● Echocardiogram ● Holter monitoring ● Exercise ECG testing.

Further testing relating to Brugada syndrome, ARVC and WPW include cardiac magnetic resonance imaging, ajmaline provocation testing and adenosine provocation testing.

Genotyping of families with LQTS, BS and HOCM may allow confirmation of diagnosis and clarification of carrier status, and may sometimes guide therapy—for example beta-blockers and/or implantable cardiac defibrillators in LQTS. Limited knowledge of the full genetics of these disorders, however, renders negative results unhelpful.

What kinds of pacing do you know about?

There is a code to pacing with three letters:

● 1st letter = paced chamber (atrium A, ventricle V or dual D)
● 2nd letter = sensed chamber (A, V or D)
● 3rd letter = mode of pacing (inhibited I, triggered T or dual D).

VVI pacing via a temporary pacing wire placed into the right ventricle after inferior myocardial infarction is often needed. A single electrode senses QRS, a single electrode paces QRS and pacing is inhibited if QRS is sensed, i.e. on demand pacing only. The operator may adjust the rate at which pacing is triggered. If the heart rate falls from 60 to

59 and the pacer is set to trigger at < 60, V will take over. In other words, a small change in intrinsic heart rate can result in a large change physiologically. If the patient's intrinsic heart rate happens to be around 60, continual switching in and out of pacing can be very uncomfortable. VVI pacing can cause cannon waves (page 222).

AAI pacing is similar but paces the right atrium and is inhibited if P waves are sensed. It is used in sick sinus node syndrome and requires normal conducting pathways from the AVN onwards. The advantage is that it provides the physiological atrial 'kick' or systole.

DDD is also encountered frequently. Dual chamber pacing is more physiological and in patients with heart block and P wave activity has largely superseded single chamber pacing.

All modes may include R. R implies rate responsive—movement is sensed and the pacing rate increases if the pacer 'thinks' the patient is exercising.

What do you understand by the term pacemaker syndrome?

This may arise when retrograde conduction produces atrial contraction against a closed AV valve. This leads to decreased ventricular filling and decreased cardiac output with presyncopal symptoms.

| CASE STUDY | 4.11 DIZZY SPELLS AND ATTACKS OF ALTERED CONSCIOUSNESS |

| Box 4.9 | Initial Questions |

1. Ask exactly what your patient means by 'dizziness', 'giddiness', 'lightheadedness', 'faintness', or 'blackouts'. Patients often use these terms interchangeably. It is very important to *exclude* any *sensation of movement* (*vertigo*, discussed on pages 273–275).
2. Try to differentiate between the two main causes of collapse: a *syncopal episode* (Case box 4.11A) or a *seizure* (Case box 4.11B).
3. Consider various other medical disorders such as transient ischaemic attacks (Case study 4.12) or hypoglycaemia. Instability, not due to presyncope or vertigo, is common in elderly people, multifactorial (page 275) and may lead to falls.

Despite a comprehensive history of events, the diagnosis in patients with discrete episodes of loss of consciousness can remain a challenge because of the periodic and unpredictable nature of symptoms. The diagnostic work up of such patients can include erect and standing blood pressures, ECG recording, ambulatory ECG/blood pressure monitoring, echocardiography, tilt table testing, carotid ultrasound scanning, neuroimaging and electroencephalography (EEG) (including sleep deprived or prolonged EEG monitoring).

Instruction: *This 38 year old woman has been complaining of recurrent dizzy spells. Please take a history from her. You are not expectd to examine her.*

Case Box 4.11(A) Syncope History Taking Points

Presyncope refers to symptoms without progression to collapse. *Syncope* refers to transient loss of consciousness associated with loss of muscle tone, and is due to inadequate blood flow to the brain. If a fall in blood pressure is prolonged, seizure-like activity may occur. The following are causes of syncope:

Neurocardiogenic (vasovagal) syncope

This is the most common cause in young people. It usually occurs in the *upright* position, when patients typically describe a feeling of *warmth* or *sweating* and a sense of 'greying out'. There may also be *brief visual blurring* and *hearing loss* before the *collapse*. These symptoms reflect falling blood pressure and overactivity of compensating nerves and muscles. There is usually sufficient warning to *avert injury*. Patients are usually unresponsive for less than one minute, although they may feel fatigue for some hours afterwards. Naive bystanders may try to 'help' by sitting a patient up, thus delaying otherwise *rapid recovery* or precipitating a further attack. Whilst on the ground a patient may appear *pale, clammy and sweaty*, and sometimes the limbs may jerk ('syncopal seizure'). The heart rate may slow markedly, but more commonly increases. Vasovagal syncope may be situational, triggered by coughing, micturition or defaecation. It may also occur more commonly if sleep deprived, fasting, anaemic (heavy menstruation), anxious (impending injections, dental work) or in a hot atmosphere. It may occur 'out of the blue'. There is often a long history of a *tendency* to 'faints'. The mechanism may involve excessive pooling of blood in the lower limbs because of venous abnormalities or centrally mediated abnormal regulation of venous tone.

Irregularities of heart rate or rhythm

Ask particularly about *coronary heart disease symptoms* and *risk factors* (Case box 4.8) and *palpitations* prior to the blackout (Case box 4.10).

Cardiac lesions which obstruct blood flow

Ask about a history of valvular heart disease.

Orthostatic (postural) hypotension
This refers to a reduced ability to maintain blood pressure whilst standing, and tends to occur with *advancing age*. It may be triggered or compounded by *drugs*. Always ask about *diabetes* (autonomic neuropathy).

Postural tachycardia syndrome
This is due to an excessive increase in heart rate whilst standing but with little reduction in blood pressure. Patients experience *dizziness*, '*near faints*', *fatigue* and *exercise intolerance*.

Other than vasovagal episodes, what causes of syncope are there?

Irregularities in heart rate or rhythm

- Bradyarrhythmias, including Stokes–Adams attacks (syncope due to transient heart block with very little warning, sudden collapse and post-collapse flushing) and carotid sinus hypersensitivity
- Tachyarrhythmias, including paroxysmal atrial fibrillation, supraventricular tachycardias (SVTs) and non-sustained ventricular tachycardias (NSVTs)
- Sick sinus syndrome.

Cardiac lesions which obstruct blood flow

- Decreased left ventricular outflow (aortic stenosis, hypertrophic obstructive cardiomyopathy, large myocardial infarct)
- Decreased left ventricular inflow (mitral stenosis, atrial myxoma or valve thrombus)
- Decreased pulmonary inflow into the left heart (massive pulmonary embolus)
- Decreased right ventricular outflow (pulmonary stenosis)
- Decreased venous return (cough, micturition, Valsalva manoeuvre)
- Pericardial disease.

Postural hypotension (failure of vascoconstriction)

- Drugs (e.g. antihypertensives, levodopa) ● Hypovolaemia
- Autonomic neuropathy (e.g. diabetes mellitus, amyloidosis).

Instruction Patient B: *This 40-year old man describes episodes of loss of consciousness. Please take a history from him. You are not expected to examine him.*

Case Box 4.11(B) **Seizure History Taking Points**

A description of episodes is essential (information from a witness usually integral):

1. Ask about the *frequency of episodes* (a seizure diary is useful) and *duration of epidodes*
2. Take a detailed *description of symptoms* before and after attacks from the patient

3. Request a detailed description of what was *observed* before, during and after attacks from a witness
4. Ask about the duration of individual symptoms
5. Find out whether or not any injury was sustained
6. Ask about tongue biting or loss of sphincter control.

Ask about the following *predisposing* factors:
- Birth injury ● Stroke ● Head injury ● Space occupying lesion
- Meningitis/encephalitis.

Ask about the following *precipitating or trigger* factors:
- Sleep deprivation ● Drugs/alcohol ● Flashing lights ● Stress
- Menstruation.

How would you define a seizure?

A seizure is a clinically apparent episode of aberrant, paroxysmal neuronal discharge. The term epilepsy refers to recurrent seizures.

How do you classify seizures?

Seizures may be:

1. Partial, arising from a focal cortical lesion, frequently the temporal lobe. Partial seizures may be:
   (i) Simple (no loss of consciousness)
   (ii) Complex (loss of consciousness)
   (iii) Partial evolving to secondary generalised.
2. Generalised, with bilateral cortical discharges. These may be convulsive or non-convulsive. Generalised seizures may be:
   (i) Absence (previously called 'petit mal')
   (ii) Myoclonic, with single or multiple jerks in the limbs
   (iii) Tonic, tonic-clonic or clonic (previously called 'grand mal')
   (iv) Atonic, a type of drop attack with sudden loss of posture.

What do you know about the different stages of a seizure?

Broadly, there are three phases to a seizure:

1. An initial phase, sometimes called an aura, taking almost any form

There may, for example, be a strange *epigastric sensation*. In *complex partial seizures*, which can have a protracted aura, patients often describe a feeling of familiarity with the situation (*déjà vu*) or failure to recognise their surrounding (*jamais vu*), or *strange smells or tastes* (olfactory or gustatory aura).

In *primary generalised seizures* the aura may be very short or there may be no warning at all.

In absence seizures and atonic drop attacks there is no warning and in the latter the sudden fall to the ground can cause serious injury.

2. A phase of loss of awareness (not necessarily collapse!) or consciousness

Patients are inaccessible, failing to respond to other people. Patients are usually amnestic for events in this phase. Witnesses, in addition to being unable 'to access' the patient, may observe:

- *Abnormal behaviour* in complex partial seizures. Lip smacking or chewing movements or other 'automatisms' (repetitive stereotyped semipurposeful movements) are frequently seen in partial complex seizures. Complex partial seizures may last for seconds, minutes, hours or rarely days ('epilepsy partialis continuum').
- *Abnormal movements.* A jerk of one arm, for example, may be the result of abnormal discharge in the contralateral motor gyrus.
- *A brief (5–10 seconds) absence*, in which the patient appears to be daydreaming. The eyelids may flutter. There is rapid recovery.
- A full blown *convulsion*, usually lasting minutes, in which the eyes roll up and there is a period of rigidity ± cyanosis (tonic phase) followed by a generalised jerking (clonic) phase, during which there may be tongue biting, vomiting and incontinence.

3. A postictal phase

Patients may be aware that *something* has happened, but remain confused for a few hours afterwards, and amnestic for seizure events.

Following partial complex seizures, patients sometimes recall bizarre experiences of alterations in perception. These include visuospatial abnormalities such as macropsia or micropsia (a sense of the world around them enlarging or shrinking), altered time perception and 'magical thinking'.

The variety of experiences is almost endless, and may culminate in referral to a psychiatrist.

Three further noteworthy points about complex partial seizures

1. Symptoms depend on the lobe/s affected (pages 287–289).
2. Complex partial seizures are considerably less common than psychiatric conditions with psychotic features.
3. Violent behaviour is sometimes attributed to complex partial seizures. This is in fact rare, and when patients do exhibit aggressive behaviour, it is invariably non-directional.

How are seizures diagnosed?

Central to diagnosing a seizure is an accurate history of the episode. All patients merit neuroimaging and an EEG (a normal EEG does not exclude epilepsy!). Magnetic resonance imaging is increasingly the preferred modality. It will detect most lesions, including mesial temporal sclerosis which can underlie complex partial seizures of the temporal lobe.

EEG waveforms include:

- Alpha: normal, 8–12 Hz ● Beta: fast normal or abnormal, > 12 Hz
- Theta: slow, usually abnormal, 5–7 Hz ● Delta: very slow, abnormal, < 4 Hz.

Common EEG abnormalities include:

- Focal abnormalities, usually implying a structural lesion
- Sharp/spiked complexes, which may indicate epilepsy
- Diffuse slow wave activity, often seen in encephalitis.

What do you know about the use of antiepileptic drugs (AEDs)?

1. Most neurologists would not institute an AED after a single episode unless an underlying lesion is identified.
2. Most AEDs aim to inhibit excitatory neurotransmitters such as gamma-aminobutyric acid (GABA). Older AEDs include phenytoin, carbamazepine and sodium valproate and remain first line drugs for generalised seizures.
3. Vigabatrin was one of the first new generation AEDs but is limited by visual field defect side effects, which may be irreversible. It may also cause psychosis or depression.
4. Lamotrigine may be used as monotherapy in partial seizures, and may act synergistically with valproate when either drug alone is ineffective. Rash is a major side effect of lamotrigine which can be limited by slow initiation of the drug.
5. Gabapentin may be used to treat partial seizures, and is also used in neuropathic pain.
6. Topiramate is an effective AED in many seizures but can cause reversible cognitive slowing.
7. Levetiracetam is a novel, effective AED with a unique mode of action, mimimal side effects or drug interactions, and used as add-on therapy by many neurologists.

What other treatment considerations are important?

1. Risk advice is essential, particularly with respect to driving, occupation (such as operating machinery or working at heights), sport (such as never swimming alone) and hot water. Patients should learn to switch on cold taps first when showering. Burns units frequently admit patients with epilepsy!
2. Special considerations include preconception advice, pregnancy (the slightly higher risk of teratogenicity from drugs must be weighed against the risk of seizures to mother and fetus), lactation and drug interactions.

| CASE STUDY | 4.12 TRANSIENT ISCHAEMIC ATTACKS (TIAs) |

Instruction Patient A: *This 72-year-old gentleman was recently unable to speak. The attack lasted around 2 minutes, during which he could hear what others were saying* *and knew how he wished to reply, but could not speak words which expressed his thoughts, or, if he began to, could not complete his sentences and found himself substituting incorrect words. His vision, hearing and limb movements were unaffected. Please take a history from him.*

Instruction Patient B: *This 58-year-old man with a history of angina has had four episodes where his right hand becomes 'clumsy', during which he is unable to do up his shoelaces or grip objects properly. Please take a history from him.*

Case Box 4.12   **Transient Ischaemic Attacks History Taking Points**

Symptoms

Symptoms attributable to a TIA relate to a *specific area of brain.* Commonly encountered symptoms such as light-headedness, altered consciousness and confusion do not have a focal origin and are *not* suggestive of a TIA. Diagnosis of a TIA remains essentially clinical and the following features are characteristic:

- Symptoms are almost invariably of *sudden onset.*
- The deficit tends to be *maximal at the onset* with progressive resolution over minutes or hours.
- Attacks are *self-limiting.*
- Symptoms are characteristically *'negative'* — e.g. loss of movement rather than unwanted movement.
- Symptoms are *attributable to focal areas of brain* such as motor cortex or language areas. *Carotid artery territory (anterior circulation) TIAs* may produce weakness or sensory symptoms in the contralateral upper limb, lower limb or face, dysphasia or amaurosis fugax. *Vertebrobasilar territory (posterior circulation) TIAs* may produce diplopia, ataxia, dysphagia, unilateral or bilateral weakness or sensory symptoms.
- Most patients do not experience significant headache but mild headache is not unusual. Severe headache during the attack should prompt an alternative diagnosis.
- Loss of consciousness is highly unusual, except in a small number of cases of vertebrobasilar TIA. A history of sudden, transient loss of consciousness suggests a global problem such as a seizure, which can occasionally herald the onset of a stroke but seldom a TIA.

Important history taking points

1. Single or recurrent event/s?
2. Mode of onset — sudden or insidious?
3. Progression of symptoms — maximal at onset, progressive or fluctuating?
4. Resolution and time it took. Did the patient seek medical attention and what was done?

5. Nature of deficit—focal (motor, sensory, language or visual) or global?
6. Absence or presence of headache?
7. Absence or presence of loss of consciousness?
8. Past medical history (TIAs are usually a manifestation of generalised vascular disease)—stroke or other cardiovascular disease, hypertension, diabetes, dyslipidaemia, smoking?
9. Drug history—oral contraceptive pill in young females?
10. Family history of cerebrovascular or cardiovascular disease?

What other conditions can produce focal neurological symptoms and resemble a TIA or stroke?

- Migraine with aura (particularly if no headache)
- Focal seizure or focal weakness (Todd's paresis) following a seizure
- Intracranial space occupying lesion (haemorrhage, tumour)
- Disorders causing vertigo
- Metabolic disturbances (usually global disturbance)
- Demyelination
- Meningitis or encephalitis.

What are the important aspects of examination for a patient with a suspected TIA?

Most patients will have no neurological findings between attacks. Examination is directed towards eliciting clinical evidence of a predisposing cause:

- Blood pressure
- Vascular bruits (carotid or vertebrobasilar, but also renal or femoral for evidence of diffuse vascular disease)
- Cardiac examination for atrial fibrillation or murmurs.

What investigations would you recommend for a patient with a suspected TIA?

Investigations are directed at establishing a predisposing cause:

1. Blood tests—full blood picture, urea and electrolytes, coagulation profile. In young patients or if clinically suspected, thrombophilia and vasculitis screening may be warranted.
2. ECG.
3. Chest X-ray.
4. Carotid duplex scanning is required in all patients with symptoms referable to a cerebral hemisphere or in patients with amaurosis fugax.
5. Echocardiography is indicated in patients with atrial fibrillation or ECG disturbances or if examination findings detect a murmur, signs of heart failure or signs of infective endocarditis. It is also mandatory in patients with multiterritory symptoms or peripheral embolism. Transoesophageal echocardiography (TOE) is indicated

if a cardiac origin is strongly suspected but not confirmed by transthoracic echocardiography (TTE).

6. Neuroimaging is not necessarily undertaken in patients with a history of brief (< 1 hour) symptoms, and the decision may be determined by resource implications. The advent of magnetic resonance imaging (MRI) has demonstrated the high prevalence of 'silent strokes'.

Investigations are increasingly undertaken in rapid access outpatient cerebrovascular clinics but high-risk patients who may warrant immediate admission to hospital include those with recurrent TIAs and those on anticoagulant therapy.

What secondary prevention measures would you recommend for a patient after a suspected TIA?

The risk of stroke after a TIA is highest in the first year and patients remain at increased risk without secondary prevention.

1. All patients not anticoagulated should take an *antiplatelet agent*, e.g. aspirin 75–325 mg daily. If symptoms resolve within one hour it may be assumed that they were of ischaemic rather than haemorrhagic origin and antiplatelet therapy may be commenced before brain imaging. The role of alternative antiplatelet agents is inconclusive. Clopidogrel, which has proven efficacy in preventing cardiac events (CURE study, see references) may be considered as monotherapy in patients intolerant of aspirin or as adjunctive therapy in patients with recurrent TIAs already taking aspirin. Many physicians treating patients without an embolic source would increase the dose of aspirin from 75 mg to 150 mg daily and introduce clopidogrel at 75 mg daily. The role of dual antiplatelet therapy after a first event is not established.

2. *Anticoagulation* in cerebrovascular disease (CVD) is discussed in Case study 6.13.

3. *Antihypertensive therapy* should be considered for all patients with CVD (Case study 6.13).

4. *Statins* should be considered for all patients with CVD (Heart Protection Study, pages 141–142).

5. All patients should be assessed for other cardiovascular risk factors and advised/treated appropriately – *smoking cessation, meticulous glycaemic control, low cholesterol/salt diet, exercise.*

6. *Carotid endarterectomy* should be considered for symptomatic carotid stenosis > 70%.

7. Folate supplementation may be protective (page 472).

Refer also to Case study 6.13.

| CASE STUDY | **4.13 HEADACHE** |

Instruction: *This 26-year-old man has developed right sided headaches over the last 3 months. Please take a history from him.*

| Case Box 4.13 | **Headache History Taking Points** |

Simplified International Headache Society Classification of Headache
Primary headaches
1. Migraine, without or with aura
2. Tension type headache (TTH), episodic or chronic
3. Cluster headache and chronic paroxysmal hemicrania
4. Miscellaneous headaches unassociated with a structural lesion

Secondary headaches
5. Headache associated with head trauma including acute and chronic post-traumatic headache
6. Headache associated with vascular disorders including subarachnoid haemorrhage
7. Headache associated with non-vascular intracranial disorders including idiopathic ('benign') intracranial hypertension, intracranial infection and intracranial neoplasm
8. Headache associated with substances or their withdrawal including acute alcohol induced headache, alcohol withdrawal headache and medication overuse headache
9. Headache associated with non-cephalic infection
10. Headache associated with a metabolic disorder
11. Headache or facial pain associated with disorders of the cranium, neck, eyes, nose, sinuses, teeth, mouth or other facial or cranial structures, including headache of cervical spine origin, acute glaucoma and acute sinus headache
12. Cranial neuralgias including postherpetic and trigeminal neuralgia
13. Headache not classifiable.

Important headache history taking points
1. How *recently* did attacks begin (days, weeks, months or years ago) and have they *changed* over time
2. *Frequency* of attacks: episodic (e.g. daily, weekly, monthly, cyclical) or unremitting. A headache diary is useful
3. Details about the *onset* of attacks—presence or absence of aura, time of day, associated sleep disturbance, after intercourse or exertion, etc.
4. *Duration* of each headache, with and without treatment

5. *Character* (*quality and intensity*) of the headache (dull ache, lancing pain, etc.) and associated symptoms such as nausea, vomiting or photophobia. Note that more than one type of headache may occur.
6. *Site and spread* of headache and whether unilateral or bilateral
7. *Predisposing* or *trigger* or aggravating factors such as foods, work, sneezing, coughing or bending
8. *Relieving* factors such as a dark room
9. *Family history* of headache
10. *What does the patient do* during the headache and what activities are limited by it?
11. *Investigations* and *treatments* in the past.
12. *State of health between attacks*

How do you distinguish between migraine with and without aura?

1. Patients with migraine without aura (common migraine) report recurrent headaches, often unilateral or throbbing, often with marked restriction of usual activities during attacks, with preference for a quiet, dark room. There may be nausea, vomiting and sometimes visual symptoms. Attacks typically last from 4 to 72 hours. Patients are symptom free between attacks.
2. Patients with migraine with aura (classic migraine) report, in addition, reversible focal neurological disturbances such as hemianopia or unilateral paraesthesia of their face, arm or hand. A spreading scotoma may occur but 'spots in front of the eyes' or visual blurring are not diagnostic. An aura only occurs in some attacks in this subgroup of migraine sufferers. Some patients develop an aura without headaches, but the differential diagnosis must include transient ischaemic attacks.

List some predisposing factors for migraine

● Stress, anxiety, depression ● Menstruation ● Oral contraceptive pill (contraindicated in migraine with aura) ● Trauma ● Inactivity.

List some common migraine triggers

● Relaxation after stress (Friday night/weekend migraine)
● Missing meals or mild dehydration
● Missing sleep and excess sleep
● Long distance travel
● Alcohol, caffeine, cheese, chocolate, citrus fruit
● Sudden unaccustomed exercise.

What first line treatments may be used in the primary prophylaxis of migraine?

● Beta-blockers ● Amitriptyline ● Pizotifen.

What is tension type headache (TTH)?

This is a band-like headache or a feeling of pressure, and rarely significantly disabling. It may spread to or from the neck, and may be associated with stress or cervical or cranial musculoskeletal abnormalities. It seldom lasts more than a few hours and may be episodic or chronic, the latter occurring on most days.

The differential diagnosis often includes pain from other cranial or facial structures, and medication overuse headache (MOH). MOH is caused by a wide range of analgesics which paradoxically exacerbate symptoms when used regularly.

What is a cluster headache?

This is more common in males and smokers, and may occur at the same time each day for a few weeks. It may recur annually. It typically lasts less than an hour but is intense and disabling, often associated with unilateral lacrimation, rhinorrhoea and conjunctival injection.

List some serious causes of headache

- Intracranial tumours (symptoms of raised intracranial pressure, e.g. morning headaches exacerbated by coughing, personality change, seizures, etc.)
- Meningitis (fever, neck stiffness, altered consciousness)
- Subarachnoid haemorrhage (explosive headache)
- Temporal artertis (> 50 years, scalp tenderness, jaw claudication, mild systemic symptoms)
- Primary open angle (acute) glaucoma
- Idiopathic ('benign') intracranial hypertension (page 525)
- Subacute carbon monoxide poisoning.

CASE STUDY | **4.14 JOINT SYMPTOMS**

Instruction: *Please read the letter from this patient's general practitioner and then conduct an appropriate consultation. You are not expected to examine her.*

Dear Doctor
This 46-year-old lady has been complaining of worsening polyarthralgia in her hands and wrists for 6 months. Her rheumatoid factor is positive. Her blood results are appended. I would be grateful for your further assessment. [FBC, U&E, LFTs and rheumatoid factor are appended. The abnormalities are a borderline normochromic normocytic anaemia, an elevated creatinine of 135 mmol/L and a weakly positive rheumatoid factor.]

This is a difficult question because there are potentially a large number of diseases to explore. It highlights the importance of a structured approach to joint symptoms.

Case Box 4.14 **Joint Symptoms History Taking Points**

Determine any past medical history.

Symptoms
1. Check that the *pain* is *localised to joints*, and not diffuse. The latter could imply a chronic pain syndrome such as fibromylagia. Myalgic symptoms can occur in rheumatoid arthritis (RA).
2. Determine as precisely as you can *which joints* are affected.
3. Is there *joint stiffness* as well as pain? *Morning stiffness*, improving with exercise, characterises an inflammatory arthropathy. Mechanical pain is usually relieved by rest.
4. It is essential to know early on if there is *joint swelling* (polyarthritis) as well as pain (polyarthralgia) and stiffness. Any soft tissue swelling is highly suggestive of inflammatory joint disease.
5. The next step is to test each differential diagnosis in turn by asking about symptoms from the diagnostic criteria given in Chapter 9. In this middle-aged female you should consider rheumatoid arthritis (her RF is positive) and SLE (given the raised creatinine) first. The normochromic normocytic anaemia supports an inflammatory condition but does not help diagnostically.

For rheumatoid arthritis, ask about:
● Morning stiffness > 1 hour ● At least three types of joint being affected (although monoarticular RA can occur) ● Hand joint involvement ● Symmetrical involvement ● Nodules.

For SLE, ask about:
● Rashes ● Sunlight sensitivity ● Mouth ulcers ● Symptoms of Raynaud's phenomena ● Chest pains (pleuritic) ● Seizures or changes in behaviour, including symptoms of depression.

Elicit beliefs, concerns and expectations (page 105)

Elicit a social and occupational history (Box 4.2)

How would you assess functional status in rheumatoid arthritis?
Refer to pages 489–490.

How would you manage joint symptoms in rheumatoid arthritis/SLE?
Refer to Case studies 9.1 and 9.3.

CASE STUDY	4.15 BACK PAIN

Instruction: *This 68-year-old gentleman was referred to the haematology clinic with back pain. Please take a history from him.*

Case Box 4.15	Back Pain History Taking Points

- Back pain can be due to a problem in the back or referred from elsewhere such as the genitourinary system.
- Whereas simple mechanical back pain is very common in young to middle-aged patients with lumbosacral, buttock or thigh symptoms, 'red flags' to back pain should be explored.

Red flags to back pain
1. Age > 55
2. 'Non-mechanical' back pain with no clear aggravation by movement or change with posture
3. Thoracic pain
4. Systemic symptoms such as weight loss or loss of appetite
5. Past history of carcinoma (especially colorectal, breast, renal, thyroid)
6. Patient with HIV infection
7. Drug history, especially repeat prescriptions for corticosteroids
8. Neurological symptoms and signs. Any history of bladder or bowel symptoms should also be elicited in determining whether or not back pain is a neurosurgical emergency.

Always ask how your patient is coping at home and whether or not it is affecting work. Be alert to depression.

What is myeloma?

Myeloma refers to a malignant clone of plasma cells producing high concentrations of a single specific (monoclonal) immunoglobulin— IgG, IgA or pure light chain. Myeloma tends to occur in the 50–70 year age group.

What are the clinical consequences of myeloma?

- Back pain/bone pain due to lytic lesions, seen best on a skeletal survey
- Hypercalcaemia
- Anaemia (normochromic normocytic due to chronic disease and bone marrow infiltration)
- Renal failure (due to any combination of hypercalcaemia, light chain proteinuria, urate nephropathy, sepsis, amyloid deposition)

- Infection, often a consequence of hypogammaglobulinaemia of non-clonal immunoglobulins
- Bone marrow failure.

Which markers may be used to assess disease load?

- Lactate dehydrogenase ● Uric acid ● β_2 microglobulin.

How is myeloma diagnosed?

Diagnosis is suggested by serum protein electrophoresis and immunoglobulin levels. These may not detect light chain disease and urine should always be examined for Bence Jones proteinuria. Diagnosis is confirmed by bone marrow examination, plasma cells comprising > 10–15% of all cells.

What other paraprotein diseases are there?

- Waldenström's macroglobulinaemia (IgM)
- Monoclonal gammopathy of uncertain significance (MGUS)

CASE STUDY	4.16 OSTEOPOROSIS

Instruction: *Please read the letter from this patient's general practitioner and then conduct an appropriate consultation. You are not expected to examine her.*

Case Box 4.16	Osteoporosis History Taking Points

Your assessment in this case should aim to elicit:

1. Details about the fall. You need to determine what sort of force was involved and why she fell. A history suggesting, for example, a seizure, would redirect your consultation.
2. What she was told by the A&E staff. Did they comment on her X-ray?
3. What she understands about why she has been referred.
4. Her past medical history. Ask specifically about thyrotoxicosis.
5. Any drug treatments, in particular repeated courses of corticosteroids for conditions like asthma, chronic obstructive pulmonary disease or inflammatory bowel disease.
6. Any history of smoking or heavy alcohol ingestion.
7. Any family history of osteoporosis.
8. Any symptoms consistent with osteoporosis—menopausal symptoms at an early age (or hysterectomy), back pain, kyphosis or loss of height.
9. Ask how these, and the recent fracture, may have impacted on her personal/social circumstances.
10. Her risk factors for osteoporosis. These are described below.

Dear Doctor
Thank you for seeing this 62-year-old lady who was recently
discharged from A&E with a left Colles' fracture following a fall
at home. I wonder if she should have a DEXA scan.

The optimal management of and screening approach to osteoporosis
is not yet clear.

How would you define osteoporosis?

The definition is based on the standard deviation (SD) of bone mineral
density (BMD), called a T score, in relation to the young normal mean
BMD:

- Osteoporosis is defined as < 2.5 SD below the mean.
- Osteopenia is defined as between 1 and 2.5 SD below the mean.

The definition is arbitrary. The natural history of BMD is that it
increases in early life, peaking in the third decade or so before a steady
lifetime decline. The young normal mean has been derived from BMD
measurements on large representative population samples.

An adequate diet and weight bearing exercise are essential for
achieving optimal peak BMD.

How would you measure BMD?

A dual energy X-ray absorption (DEXA) scan is the current gold
standard. Heel ultrasound has also been used.

A DEXA scan is expensive with a long waiting time. If this lady's wrist radiograph had shown osteopenia, wouldn't you treat her anyway?

Radiographs are unreliable. It is likely from the history that she would
benefit from treatment but optimal management would include a
baseline BMD measurement both to confirm osteoporosis and serve
as a baseline for assessing response to treatment.

That sounds sensible in theory, but DEXA scans have enormous resource implications. Who should get one?

This is a two pronged question. We have to consider what is
happening now and what may happen in the future.

1. Currently, those deemed at risk of osteoporosis are targeted for
   bone densitometry (Box 4.10), and, if osteoporosis is confirmed,
   proceed to treatment. Some physicians start treatment prior to
   confirmation, especially for vertebral fractures since these are
   strongly attributable to osteoporosis.
2. In the next few years, we may see population screening, especially
   for the older female population.

Who are those at risk?

1. For hip fractures, hip BMD may be helpful and clinical factors are
   good indicators of risk:

Box 4.10	**Clinical Indications for Bone Densitometry (adapted from guidelines produced by the Royal College of Physicians)**

1. Personal history of low trauma fracture such as distal forearm, spine or hip
2. X-ray evidence of osteopenia or vertebral collapse detected incidentally or in the investigation of loss of height or thoracic kyphosis
3. Maternal history of hip fracture
4. Low body mass index ($< 19 \ kg/m^2$)
5. Corticosteroid treatment (7.5 mg prednisolone for a cumulative period of > 3 months)
6. Oestrogen deficiency (premature menopause < 45 years, primary hypogonadism, secondary amenorrhoea lasting > 6 months)
7. Conditions predisposing to secondary osteoporosis, including malabsorption syndromes, organ transplantation, eating disorders, chronic renal failure, primary hyperparathyroidism, hyperthyroidism, Cushing's syndrome, prolonged immobilisation, male hypogonadism

---

● Low body weight   ● Previous fracture > 40 years of age
● Maternal hip fracture   ● Current smoking   ● Tendency to fall.
Approximately 70% of patients who sustain a hip fracture have osteoporosis.

2. For vertebral and wrist fractures, which affect a generally younger age group, clinical factors are not so important but include a previous fracture and early menopause. Site-specific BMD is the best predictor (osteophytes and aortic calcification may affect reliability), but peripheral BMD by forearm and heel ultrasound has also been used.

Are there any other investigations you might consider?

Over 90% of women will have no secondary cause. Investigations in selected patients in whom a secondary cause is suspected include:

● Follicle stimulating hormone (FSH) levels (to detect menopause in hysterectomised women with conserved ovaries—osteoporosis risk higher despite ovarian presence)
● ESR and immunoglobulin electrophoresis (myeloma)
● U&Es/LFTs (chronic renal failure/liver disease)
● Thyroid function tests (hyperthyroidism)
● Testosterone levels (male hypogonadism)
● Full blood picture (malabsorption).

Why are postmenopausal women at particular risk of osteoporosis?

Loss of inhibition from endogenous oestrogens leads to increased osteoclastic bone resorption. Overall bone turnover is increased, but the rate of resorption exceeds that of formation for some 5–10 years. Following this, the rate of bone loss reverts to that normally associated with ageing.

What treatment options are available for osteoporosis?

Hormone replacement therapy (HRT)

Oestrogen, in the form HRT, is especially beneficial in the perimenopausal/early postmenopausal years. It prevents bone loss in the immediate postmenopausal period and can also increase BMD in older females. Preventing an annual rate of bone loss of 0.5% over a number of years has been shown to reduce all fractures by 50%. The benefits of HRT are lost soon after stopping treatment.

Selective oestrogen receptor modulators (SERMs)

SERMs are still in their infancy. They are tissue specific, having both oestrogenic and antioestrogenic effects. They may confer BMD and cardiovascular benefit without breast and uterine risk. Raloxifene has been shown to increase BMD at the spine and hip in postmenopausal women and reduce the risk of vertebral fractures. Raloxifene is licensed in the UK for the prevention and treatment of osteoporosis in postmenopausal women.

Bisphosphonates

Bisphosphonates are widely used for prevention and treatment of osteoporosis in postmenopausal females, corticosteroid induced osteoporosis (CIO) in males and females and osteoporosis in males. Numerous bisphosphonates are available, but indications for which they are licensed vary slightly. Bisphosphonates unequivocally reduce overall fractures rates but randomised controlled trials of different bisphosphonates have shown different benefits and optimal results at differing sites. This may reflect the different population samples between trials.

Disodium etidronate is taken on a cyclical basis for 2 weeks in every 13, so that bone resorption rather than formation is preferentially reduced. Calcium supplementation is taken daily for the 11 intervening weeks. Alendronate and risedronate have more potent antiresorptive effects and are taken daily at lower doses, although alendronate may be taken weekly. They can attenuate postmenopausal bone loss, especially in the early postmenopausal period, and reduce fracture rates at vertebral and non-vertebral sites in established osteoporosis.

Bisphosphonates are generally poorly absorbed and need to be taken on an empty stomach, the patient abstaining from food for 30 minutes. Alendronate and risedronate may both cause erosive oesophagitis and patients are advised to take these drugs with water and not to lie down afterwards. Benefits can be demonstrated within 1 year of treatment.

Calcium and vitamin D₃ supplementation

Calcium and vitamin D_3 supplementation have been examined in several randomised controlled trials. Again, conflicting results may merely represent wide differences in population samples studied. Most current guidelines suggest that treatment with both (at doses of around 1200 mg calcium and 800 IU vitamin D3/calitriol daily, e.g. calcichew D3 forte, one tablet twice daily) is good practice for those at risk such as elderly patients.

Other

Current drug treatments generally inhibit osteoclasts, but drugs promoting osteoblast activity may appear in the future.

General lifestyle advice is appropriate for all patients at risk. Smoking and excessive alcohol intake should be discouraged. Weight bearing exercise such as walking is beneficial and non-weight bearing exercise may also reduce fracture risk by improving strength and coordination and reducing the risk of falls. Physiotherapy can help at-risk patients in reducing falls and help with pain management.

Patients with osteopenia and a previous fracture may also be considered for these treatment options.

What other potential benefits and risks of HRT are there?

1. As well as reducing bone loss, HRT is an effective means of controlling the vasomotor and genital symptoms associated with the menopause.
2. There is a higher relative risk of breast cancer but the absolute increased risk appears to be small. Current recommendations are to stop HRT after 5–10 years of treatment, although the increased risk of breast cancer attributable to HRT is thought not to begin until around 50 years of age.
3. Oestrogen only HRT tablets or patches may be used in hysterectomised patients, but preparations opposed with progesterone should otherwise be used to limit endometrial hyperplasia and the risk of endometrial malignancy. Amenorrhoea need not be awaited before starting HRT. Cyclical (sequential) hormone regimens are generally used in perimenopausal women and continuous combined regimens in postmenopausal women. Continuous combined treatment is associated with a high risk of irregular bleeding in perimenopausal women but should not cause induced bleeding in postmenopausal women. Postmenopausal bleeding generally necessitates investigation to exclude endometrial malignancy.
4. HRT increases the relative risk of venous thromboembolism, but again the absolute risk is low, and possibly offset by the

favourable effects of HRT on lipid profiles and potential cardiovascular benefit.

5. Studies are inconclusive as to whether HRT reduces (or even increases) cardiovascular risk. There is no current evidence to support the use of HRT in either the primary or secondary prevention of coronary heart disease, and no evidence that HRT reduces stroke risk. A systematic review and meta-analysis has suggested that HRT may have a role in lowering the risk of dementia and cognitive decline but further evidence is needed to establish this.

6. HRT does not cause weight gain.

Note: Some of the questions and answers herein are adapted from lectures given by Professor David Reid, University of Aberdeen, who has made significant national and international contributions to osteoporosis research and understanding.

CASE STUDY | **4.17 VISUAL LOSS AND OTHER VISUAL SYMPTOMS**

Instruction: *This 70-year-old man has complained of deteriorating vision over the last few months. Please ask him some questions.*

What are the causes of a cataract?

Cataracts are the commonest cause of remediable visual disability in the UK.

1. They are usually age related (the lens also becomes less pliable with age and less able to accommodate).
2. Diabetes is the next commonest cause, most commonly producing early onset age related types but occasionally 'snowflake' dots of cortical opacification.
3. All other causes are much rarer and include Wilson's disease (stellate cataracts), hypoparathyroidism, congenital causes (familial, myotonic dystrophy, infection), drugs (steroids) and trauma (including radiation damage).

Where do cataracts arise?

One of two lens changes may occur:

1. Opacification of the posterior cortical zone (posterior subcapsular cataract). A clinical analogy is that of whitewash behind a window. There is a 'dirty window' sensation, which can create 'glare' on a sunny day or from car headlights at night.
2. Yellowing of the nucleus (nuclear sclerosis). The clinical analogy is more that of a rippled window.

| Case Box 4.17 | **Visual Loss History Taking Points** |

Visual loss may be acute or gradual, and affect one or both eyes. It may be due to any of the following:

Disorders of the neuro-ophthalmological pathways
These are discussed in Chapter 6, section 1

Gradual loss of central vision in one or both eyes
- Cataract (page 181)
- Age related macular degeneration (Case study 10.10)

Gradual loss of peripheral vision in one or both eyes
- Primary open angle glaucoma (see below)
- Retinal detachment (Case study 10.9)
- Retinitis pigmentosa (Case study 10.6)

Acute loss of central vision in one eye
- Optic neuritis (Case study 10.4)

Acute loss of vision in variable distribution in one eye
- Central/branch retinal vein occlusion (Case study 10.7)
- Central retinal artery occlusion (Case study 10.8)
- Retinal detachment
- Retinal haemorrhage

Patients frequently complain of *spots* in their vision. It is important to differentiate between:
1. Flashing lights (a sign of incipient retinal detachment, page 533)
2. Floaters (opacities in the vitreous, page 533)
3. Haloes (a waterlogged cornea breaks up white light as does the sky after a rainstorm, and because of the shape of the cornea the 'rainbow' is round. It may be a sign of incipient acute glaucoma)

How may a cataract be treated?

Routinely, phacoemulsification with a lens implant can be performed as day surgery and is increasing 'sutureless'. YAG laser capsulotomy is also used to eradicate a posterior capsule opacity. In many cases, patients want more than anything to be able to read and the risks of surgery must be taken into account. A bright light close to a book should improve the vision of an eye with a cataract, but will not improve vision in retinal disease such as age related macular degeneration (ARMD). This is often a useful test for dual pathology, because fundoscopy may be precluded by the presence of a cataract.

How does primary open angle glaucoma (POAG) present?

This disease presents insidiously, often without symptoms until considerable ocular damage has been sustained. Haloes are a feature of acute closed angle glaucoma. Patients may present because of visual field loss but are frequently referred from optometrists following the detection of raised intraocular pressure (IOP).

There are three cardinal features of POAG:

1. Raised IOP > 21–22 mmHg (> 30 mmHg warrants urgent referral to an ophthalmologist)
2. A cupped optic disc with an increased cup : disc (C : D) ratio
3. Visual field loss.

Raised IOP with normal visual fields and discs is called ocular hypertension.

How does POAG arise?

The mechanisms behind this triad of features can be explained as follows:

1. The pathophysiological changes in POAG have traditionally been attributed to raised IOP causing damage to the optic nerve head (optic disc). Increasingly, however, vascular and toxic damage to the optic nerve fibres are thought to contribute, and 'POAG' with normal IOP is recognised. Doubtless ageing has a role, and the optic nerve, which at birth contains approximately 10^6 neurons, loses about 10^4 of these per year.
2. A normal optic disc contains a central cup, an indentation or cavity from which the blood vessels emanate. It is normally shallow and the ratio of the cup diameter to the disc diameter is normally around 1 : 3. But optic discs are like shoe sizes, varying between individuals and, when examining C : D ratios, asymmetry between the eyes and progression over time is more important than a 'snap shot' appearance. As POAG progresses, neurons are lost and the cup becomes a deepening cave into which the blood vessels appear to dive.
3. The classical field defect in POAG is an arcuate scotoma of peripheral visual loss, with relative preservation of macula or central vision (visual acuity may be 6/6) (Fig. 4.5). There are two considerations when explaining this. The first is that the ratio of visual receptors (R) to their attached neurons (N) running to the optic disc is much greater at the periphery (R : N approximately 8 : 1) than at the macula (R : N 1 : 1). For every neuron lost from peripheral vision, multiple receptors are lost. Secondly, the organisation of nerve fibres is such that those from the macula run directly to the optic disc whilst those from the periphery must 'arc' around the macula, tending to reach the disc at its vertical north and south poles. These poles tend to be damaged first in POAG, resulting in arcuate scotomas. Patients may start bumping into things.

Fig. 4.5 *Cupping of the optic disc and arcuate scotoma in primary open angle glaucoma*

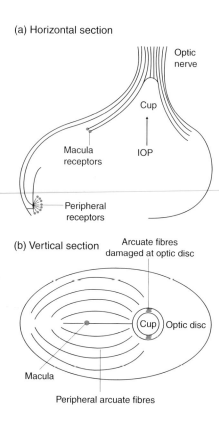

(a) Horizontal section

(b) Vertical section

What are the visual requirements for driving?

Visual acuity driving requirements for driving a private car are based on the number plate test. A 79.4 mm number plate should be read (binocular vision with correction for any refractive errors) at 20.5 m.

What are the causes of a painful, red eye?

A distinguishing feature between most of the serious, sight-threatening causes of red eye from non-threatening conjunctivitis is that in the former the redness dominates at the corneoscleral limbus (where blood vessels emerge from the depths of the eye). This is sometimes called ciliary injection. Further, serious causes are usually painful.

The uveal tract comprises the anterior uvea (iris and ciliary body) and the posterior uveal tract (choroid — the vascular layer which supplies the outer pigment retina).

Uveitis/iritis

Uveitis may affect the anterior or posterior uvea or both (panuveitis). Uveitis typically produces a *painful, watery, photophobic red eye with blurred vision* due to the presence of inflammatory cells.

The *pupil is small and in spasm in iritis* and adhesions between the iris and anterior lens capsule (posterior synechiae) may render it *irregularly shaped*. There may be *keratitic precipitates* (clumps of white cells on the inner lining of the cornea and floating in the anterior chamber appear like dust in a beam of light) and precipitation of neutrophils in the anterior chamber may result in a hypopyon.

Anterior uveitis is classically associated with HLA B27 conditions like ankylosing spondylitis (up to 20% of patients), Reiter's syndrome and psoriatic disease. It occurs in most patients with Behçet's disease (a multisystem vasculitis also causing oral and genital ulceration). Inflammatory bowel disease, sarcoidosis and TB can cause anterior or posterior uveitis (chorioretinitis), as can a wide range of other infections including toxoplasmosis, toxocariasis, HIV and the herpes simplex and zoster viruses.

Acute (closed angle) glaucoma

This is caused by sudden closure of the drainage angle and is more common in long sighted people with short eyeballs and may be precipitated by dilating drops and mydriatics such as tricyclics. The cornea is steamy/cloudy/stormy with a mid-dilated unreactive pupil, and the anterior chamber is narrow. It is an emergency.

Keratitis

The cornea may be damaged by trauma (corneal abrasions or penetrating eye injury), foreign bodies and infection.

Keratitis and ulceration due to herpes simplex or zoster may assume a punctate or dendritic pattern. Keratitis usually presents with pain, redness and lacrimation. Bacterial ulceration may result in a hypopyon. Keratitis may also arise as a sterile immunological response to antigens. An example is marginal keratitis where staphyloccal exotoxin triggers marginal inflammation of the cornea with ciliary injection. It is often due to staphylococcal overgrowth in patients with blepharitis. When assessing a corneal problem, the eye should be examined completely with appropriate stains, and a safe rule is that topical steroids should never be commenced without ophthalmological recommendation.

Scleritis

Scleritis may be a feature of vasculitis, sarcoid, rheumatoid disease, SLE, inflammatory bowel disease and ankylosing spondylitis.

Patients with rheumatoid disease may also develop *scleromalacia perforans*, a necrotising scleritis, which gives the eye a grey-blue tinge. The grey-blue tinge results from thinning of the sclera, faintly exposing the choroid pigment beneath. Osteogenesis imperfecta, Ehlers–Danlos syndrome and Marfan's syndrome may also cause blue sclera.

Episcleritis produces superficial redness, usually without significant pain. It may be associated with rheumatoid disease but is usually an idiopathic self-limiting condition.

| CASE STUDY | 4.18 DIABETES MELLITUS |

Instruction: *This 62-year-old gentleman with diabetes is very knowledgeable about his disease. Please take a history from him to determine more about his condition.*

This is a very open question. There is potentially a lot to discuss, and what the examiners would look for is your awareness of the protean manifestations of diabetes.

Case Box 4.18   Diabetes History Taking Points

Your history should aim to both elicit clinical details about his diabetes and place these details in the context of any other medical conditions and his day to day life. Clinical areas to cover include:

- The mode of presentation of diabetes
- The duration of diabetes
- The type of diabetes and its mode of treatment (now and previously)
- Symptoms of hyperglycaemia or hypoglycaemia
- Frequency of admission to hospital
- His knowledge of his level of control
- His knowledge of and symptoms of complications — cardiovascular, renal, eye, foot, autonomic, sexual
- His motivation and education with respect to treatment, diet, lifestyle, foot care, self-monitoring, hypoglycaemic awareness and intercurrent illness
- Attendance at annual screening.

How is diabetes defined?

The World Health Organization 2000 diagnostic criteria are as follows:

1. For asymptomatic patients, two diagnostic blood glucose measurements (Box 4.11) on separate days.
2. For symptomatic patients, one diagnostic blood glucose measurement.
3. Impaired fasting glucose (IFG) is defined as a fasting venous plasma glucose within the range ≥ 6.1 to < 7.0 mmol/L. Such patients should have an OGTT.

Box 4.11   Diagnostic Blood Glucose Measurements

- Fasting venous plasma glucose ≥ 7 mmol/L
- Random venous plasma glucose ≥ 11.1 mmol/L
- 2 hour venous plasma glucose ≥ 11.1 mmol/L in 75 g oral glucose tolerance test (OGTT).

4. Impaired glucose tolerance (IGT) is defined by a 75 g OGTT as a fasting venous plasma glucose < 7.0 mmol/L and a 2 hour value ≥ 7.8 mmol/L and < 11.1 mmol/L.

How is diabetes classified?
- Type 1 diabetes usually (but not always) presents in children or young adults and is due to autoimmune pancreatic beta cell (insulin secreting) destruction. Patients require insulin.
- Type 2 diabetes (majority of patients) is due to peripheral insulin resistance and relative insulin deficiency. Patients are generally middle aged/elderly and many are obese.
- Diabetes may be secondary to diseases such as haemochromatosis and Cushing's syndrome, or part of a genetic syndrome such as maturity onset diabetes of youth.

What are the symptoms of newly diagnosed diabetes?
- Thirst, polyuria, dehydration, weight loss and vomiting, associated with glycosuria ± ketonuria are classic symptoms in Type 1 diabetes. Dehydration, weight loss and ketonuria are indications for immediate insulin therapy.
- People with Type 2 diabetes are frequently asymptomatic.

What are your initial priorities in assessing a newly diagnosed patient with diabetes?
1. The first and most important decision is whether or not immediate rehydration and/or insulin are needed, as determined by the presence of vomiting, dehydration and/or ketonuria. Thirst, polyuria and the initial blood glucose level do not correlate well with the need for immediate hypoglycaemic treatments.
2. A patient who is dehydrated or vomiting should be admitted to hospital as an emergency for rehydration and initial intravenous insulin treatment.
3. Patients with marked weight loss and persistent ketonuria are likely to have Type 1 diabetes, and should be commenced on insulin urgently in an outpatient setting if this is practicable.
4. People with Type 1 diabetes will invariably proceed to insulin.
5. People with Type 2 diabetes may be managed initially by dietary modification followed by oral agents if blood glucose levels remain elevated. Many eventually require insulin to obtain glycaemic control.

What baseline work-up would you consider for your patient with diabetes?
Baseline work-up for all diabetic patients includes measurement of weight, height, body mass index (BMI—kg/m^2) and urinalysis, and:

Assessment of level of control
- HbA1c.

Assessment for complications

- Blood pressure
- Cardiovascular risk (past history of macrovascular disease, family history, smoking, blood pressure, lipid profile, proteinuria
- Renal failure (serum creatinine and urinary albumin : creatinine ratio)
- Retinopathy
- Foot disease (signs of neuropathy, peripheral vascular disease or ulceration).

Diabetes education

- Education about diabetes, its complications, type of treatment and treatment goals.
- Dietary advice, with referral to a dietician. Generally, over 50% of intake should comprise carbohydrate, especially from complex carbohydrate foods rich in natural fibre such as fruit and vegetables. The fat intake should comprise unsaturated fats. All people with diabetes should be encouraged to eat regular meals.
- Lifestyle advice including exercise and attenuating modifiable cardiovascular risk factors.
- Foot care information/involvement of chiropodist if needed.
- Self-monitoring with urine or blood glucose testing—where appropriate.
- Recognition and management of hypoglycaemia.
- Intercurrent illness managment.
- Support groups including 'Diabetes UK'.
- Driving. Patients on hypoglycaemic treatment (oral or insulin) have a responsibility to inform the DVLA.

The above may be coordinated by a specialist diabetic service with whom patients are registered on a regional diabetic register. Annual reviews should assess the overall level of control (HbA1c), assess for the presence of symptoms or complications as outlined above and reinforce diabetic education. The level of integration of care between primary and secondary care varies from region to region.

How would you screen for and manage diabetic complications?

Cardiovascular risk

- The British Hypertension Society Guidelines (Case study 5.17) suggest an optimal blood pressure target of < 140/80 mmHg (measured in clinic) for diabetic patients. The UK Prospective Diabetes Study (UKPDS) highlighted the importance of tight blood pressure control in Type 2 diabetes. The choice of antihypertensive agent should be individually determined, but many physicians favour angiotensin-converting enzyme (ACE) inhibitors as first line therapy (page 141).

● Diabetic dyslipidaemia tends to produce hypertriglyceridaemia, hypercholesterolaemia and low levels of high density lipoprotein (HDL). Covert hypothyroidism may coexist with diabetes and produce dyslipidaemia. Statin therapy is discussed on page 141.

Renal disease

Nephropathy is suggested by isolated proteinuria. There is usually concurrent retinopathy. Microalbuminuria (30–300 mg/24 hours or 20–200 mg/min, the best screening test being measurement of a spot albumin : creatinine ratio) is a marker of nephropathy and predicts macroalbuminuria and progression of nephropathy in both Type 1 and Type 2 diabetic patients (Case study 3.17).

Meticulous glycaemic and blood pressure control is pivotal in slowing progression of renal disease. ACEIs slow progression of albuminuria in both Type 1 and Type 2 diabetes and angiotensin II receptor blockers are renoprotective in early and late nephropathy due to Type 2 diabetes. The mechanism of renoprotection may be independent of blood pressure lowering (Case study 3.17).

Eyes

Diabetic retinopathy is discussed in Case study 10.1.

Feet

Annual screening should assess fine touch sensation using 10 g monofilaments, vibration sensation and pulses (manual or Doppler) and look for evidence of ulceration, callus formation, deformity or Charcot's joints.

Autonomic neuropathy

Clinical manifestations include postural hypotension, gastroparesis and vomiting, diarrhoea, bladder dysfunction and erectile dysfunction.

What do you know about current drug treatments for glycaemic control?

The *current treatments* for glycaemic control are described below and in Box 4.12; *management steps in Type 2 diabetes* are outlined below.

● In Type 2 diabetes, hypoglycaemic agents may be used as monotherapy, in combination or with insulin.
● Traditionally, metformin has been first line therapy in overweight patients and sulphonylureas have been used in normal or underweight patients. However, metformin is increasingly used as first line therapy in all patients with Type 2 diabetes in whom it is not contraindicated—on the pathophysiological basis that Type 2 diabetes involves insulin resistance as well as beta cell failure, and because of the benefits of metformin monotherapy in the UK Prospective Diabetes Study (UKPDS).
● Most patients eventually require combination therapy, which can be as metformin and a sulphonylurea, but modern regimens now

Box 4.12	Drug Treatments for Glycaemic Control

1. *Insulin* is now largely biosynthetic and of human sequence or modified human sequence (insulin analogues) and is available in ultra short acting (analogues), short acting, intermediate acting, long acting and mixed preparations. Twice daily injection of a mixed short and intermediate acting preparation is a common regimen, as are 'basal-bolus' regimens combining newer long-acting insulins (with more predictable and sustained absorption from subcutaneous tissue) with short-acting boluses at mealtimes.

2. *Sulphonylureas* potentiate insulin release and are generally used for Type 2 patients who are not overweight (they may cause weight gain). Hypoglycaemia is an important side effect.

3. *Metformin*, which increases peripheral sensitivity to insulin, is the drug of first choice for Type 2 overweight (BMI > 25) patients. Hypoglycaemia is not a side effect. Lactic acidosis is a rare but serious side effect, seen principally in patients with renal failure, alcoholism or with cardiovascular shock, in whom the drug is contraindicated. Creatinine should remain < 150 µmol/L.

4. *Thiazolidinediones* do not stimulate insulin secretion but mimic its action on carbohydrate and lipid metabolism through increasing insulin sensitivity. They activate peroxisome proliferator activated receptor gamma (PPARγ), which controls the expression of genes regulating metabolism. They are currently used in the UK only in combination with a sulphonylurea or metformin. They are contraindicated in cardiac failure and liver disease.

5. *Prandial glucose regulators* (short acting secretagogues) induce rapid postprandial insulin secretion and need to be taken with meals, i.e. thrice daily.

6. *Alpha glucosidase inhibitors*, which attenuate carbohydrate absorption by reducing conversion of complex sugars to simple sugars, may be used in patients intolerant of metformin, but can cause gastrointestinal side effects with excessive flatulence.

include the addition of a thiazolidinedione to monotherapy or the addition of a prandial glucose regulator. Of the prandial glucose regulators, nateglinide is licensed for use in combination with metformin, whereas repaglinide is licensed as monotherapy or in combination with metformin.

● Acarbose, an alpha glucosidase inhibitor, is often used with two other drugs as triple therapy. In practice, patients requiring this level of oral hypoglycaemic treatment probably require insulin.

New techniques have been developed which may allow patients to assess their glycaemic control without the need for fingertip blood sampling. These include devices for sampling from less densely innervated sites and which can operate with smaller volumes of blood, and non-invasive sensing by a process of 'reverse ionophoresis'.

What do you know about the pathogenesis of diabetic complications?

Advanced glycation end products (AGEPs) are of pathogenic importance. Glucose binds with protein to produce glycated proteins such as glycosylated haemoglobin HbA1c. The property of these proteins is altered by, for example, crosslinks, and this is very important for molecules which are not readily renewed such as collagen, which become advanced glycation end products.

What do you know about diabetic control and treatment targets?

Overall glycaemic control is best measured by HbA1c measurement. The HbA1c level achieved in the intensive treatment arm of the two major randomised control trials that showed the benefit of good blood glucose control was 7%. However, these studies suggested a continuous benefit at lower levels. The extent to which rigorous control is pursued in the individual should depend upon many patient factors such as motivation, practicality and overall life expectancy. HBA1c should not be measured at intervals of less than 3 months.

1. The Diabetes Control and Complications Trial (DCCT) demonstrated unequivocal benefit of tight glucose control on complications in Type 1 diabetes but at the cost of a higher risk of hypoglycaemia.
2. The UK Prospective Diabetes Study (UKPDS) was a 20-year study of over 5000 patients with Type 2 diabetes. The endpoint data showed important relative risk reductions in microvascular complications (mainly retinopathy), myocardial infarction, stroke and diabetes related death in patients randomised to tight glycaemic or tight blood pressure control, with blood pressure control having the greatest effect on macrovascular outcomes. The UKPDS also noted that in Type 2 diabetics, the HbA1c concentration tended to rise by 1% every 5 years even in tightly controlled patients, perhaps reducing our temptation to 'blame' patients or doctors for disease progression.

CASE STUDY | **4.19 OBESITY**

Instruction: *This young woman is overweight. Please take a history from her.*

What causes obesity?

Most cases of obesity are in part because energy intake exceeds expenditure. Despite a drive to reduce calorie intake, physical

| Case Box 4.19 | Obesity History Taking Points |

- Family history
- Dietary history including 'junk' foods
- Physical exercise undertaken
- Attempts at weight loss
- Menstrual history
- Symptoms of hypothyroidism (Case study 11.2)
- History of cardiovascular disease (hypertension, dyslipidaemia)
- History of snoring (obstructive sleep apnoea)
- History of DVT
- History of diabetes
- History of gallstones
- History of back pain
- Previous pregnancy complications
- Previous anaeasthetic complications
- Drug history
- Effects on self-esteem
- Expectations of patient.

exercise undertaken by many people in the Western world has diminished. This is the double-edged sword of safer, easier lives. There is also a strong genetic basis in many cases, and many candidate genes are being studied.

Secondary causes of obesity include:

● Hypothyroidism ● Cushing's syndrome ● Polycystic ovarian syndrome ● Insulinomas ● Hypothalamic and pituitary disease ● Drugs (e.g. corticosteroids, antithyroid drugs, sulphonylureas, antipsychotics) ● Genetic syndromes (e.g. Laurence–Moon–Biedl syndrome) ● Leptin deficiency or leptin receptor defects.

What are the risks of obesity?

- Low self esteem and depression ● Discrimination
- Cardiovascular disease (hypertension, dyslipidaemia)
- Worsening of COPD and asthma ● Obstructive sleep apnoea
- Venous thromboembolism ● Type 2 diabetes ● Biliary disease
- Intertrigo ● Soft tissue infection ● Varicose veins ● Back pain
- Osteoarthritis ● Hepatic steatosis ● Increased risk of falls
- Stress incontinence ● Oligomenorrheoa and infertility ● Risks from the contraceptive pill ● Pregnancy complications
- Anaesthetic risks.

There may also be an increased risk of many types of cancer.

What investigations would you consider?

● Weight and height (Box 4.13) ● Waist circumference ● Blood pressure ● Urinalysis for glycosuria ● Thyroid function tests

Box 4.13	Body Mass Index (BMI)

$BMI = kg/m^2$

- < 18.5 = underweight
- $18.5-24.9$ = normal range
- $25-29.9$ = overweigt/pre-obese
- ≥ 30 = obese

- Lipid profile ● Fasting plasma glucose ● Other hormonal tests as directed by the history.

What do you know about abdominal obesity and the hypertriglyceridaemic phentoype?

Abdominal obesity, which is closely associated with intra-abdominal or visceral fat (which can be distinguished from subcutaneous fat by imaging) and measured by waist circumference (male > 102 cm, female > 88 cm) or waist : hip ratio, predicts coronary artery disease better than the BMI.

Furthermore, abdominal obesity is associated with insulin resistance and predicts the development of Type 2 diabetes. High waist and fasting triglyceride measurements—the hypertriglyceridaemic waist—is a marker for the metabolic syndrome associated with hypertension, hyperglycaemia, insulin resistance, hyperinsulinaemia and atherogenic dyslipidaemia (including low HDL cholesterol, raised apolipoprotein B and small, dense low and high lipoprotein particles).

What management options are there?

- Weight loss of 0.5–1 kg/week is an ideal, but frequently not attainable, goal.
- Patients should be advised to avoid food with more than 2–3 g fat/100 g.
- Exercise such as brisk walking, swimming or cycling for 30–40 minutes a day on at least 5 days of the week.
- Drug therapy is considered only as an adjunct for patients with a BMI over 30 when other measures have failed.
- Surgery, for example gastric stapling, may be considered for patients with very high BMIs.
- Pancreatic lipase inhibitors reduce fat absorption but cause fatty stools and may reduce absorption of fat soluble vitamins.
- Research has centred on inhibiting appetite pathways. Leptin (a satiety hormone) has been studied but other hormones such as ghrelin (page 551) may be therapeutic targets.

CASE STUDY | **4.20 PYREXIA OF UNKNOWN ORIGIN (PUO)**

Instruction: *This patient has had night sweats with spikes of fever for the last 3 weeks. Please ask her some questions.*

Case Box 4.20   **Pyrexia of Unknown Origin History Taking Points**

- Nature of symptoms and chronology
- Pattern of fever (sustained, intermittent, remittent, relapsing)
- History of invasive (including dental) procedures
- Drug history
- Occupational history
- History of exposure to animals including household pets and farm animals
- History of insect bites
- Food history (poorly cooked meat, etc.)
- History of unwell contacts
- Travel history
- Sexual history
- Intravenous drug history
- Family history.

What are the causes of PUO?

The differential diagnosis is very wide. A mental checklist of important causes (not exhaustive!) may aid history taking.

Localised pyogenic infection

- Intra-abdominal (subphrenic, paracolic/diverticular, hepatic) abscess
- Cholecystitis (right upper quadrant discomfort)
- Osteomyelitis (prostheses; haematogenous spread)
- Septic arthritis (classically exquisitely tender joint)
- Soft tissue infection (especially patients with oedematous legs or peripheral vascular disease, and patients with infected dermatitis)
- Dental abscess (facial pain)
- Sinusitis (facial pain, worse with coughing, bending and lying down)
- Chronic otitis media (otalgia, conductive hearing loss)
- Unresolving pneumonia (especially if underlying obstruction)
- Unresolving urinary tract infection (frequency, dysuria, loin pain)
- Genitourinary infection (vaginal or urethral discharge, dysuria, dyspareunia, pelvic pain, sexual history).

Systemic bacterial infection

- Infective endocarditis (Case study 5.9) ● Salmonellosis (page 134)
- Atypical pneumonia (page 19) ● Brucellosis (unpasteurised milk)

- Leptospirosis (occupational history) ● Listeriosis (dairy products)
- Lyme disease (tick bites).

Mycobacterial infection (Case study 2.5)

Viral infection

- HIV (Case study 4.21) ● Hepatitis B and C viruses (Case study 3.5)
- Epstein–Barr virus.

Systemic fungal infection

- Systemic candidiasis (usually immunocompromised).

Protozoal infection

- Malaria (travel history) ● Giardiasis (common, often asymptomatic or watery diarrhoea/malabsorption) ● Amoebiasis (page 63) ● Toxoplasmosis (cats).

Worms

Toxocariasis (dogs).

Neoplasm

- Lymphoma (night sweats, lymphadenopathy) ● Renal cell carcinoma (haematuria, loin pain or fever) ● Hepatocellular carcinoma (complication of cirrhosis) ● Metastatic disease ● Atrial myxoma.

Autoimmune/connective tissue disorders

- Systemic vasculitides (page 86) ● SLE (Case study 9.3)
- Polymyositis (Case study 9.6) ● Adult Still's disease.

Infections in immunocompromised patients (transplant recipients, HIV infected patients, neutropenic patients) can present in an atypical fashion, as can infections in patients taking antipyretics, corticosteroids or antibiotics.

What causes pyrexia?

The release of certain cytokines and acute phase reactants involved in the immune response.

The following brief revision of immunology in question and answer format helps to explain not just the body's response mechanisms to infection, but also the immune mechanisms which underlie many of the chronic disorders described elsewhere in this book and emerging therapeutic strategies:

How does the immune system first respond to antigens?

The immune system responds to antigens it deems harmful. Antigens may be exogenous such as micro-organisms or endogenous such as tumour proteins, transplant grafts or autoantigens. When an antigen invades a host cell it is processed by that cell such that some antigen

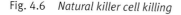

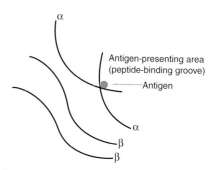

Fig. 4.6   *Natural killer cell killing*   Fig. 4.7   *HLA presentation of an antigen*

molecules are expressed on the host cell's surface. Natural killer cells (NKCs), at a simple level in the immune response, may kill such a cell (Fig. 4.6). NKCs, otherwise known as large granular lymphocytes, are fast, 'tough' and leave a lot of damage in their wake. The NKC response is neither *antigen specific* nor *MHC restricted*.

What is the major histocompatibility complex (MHC)?

Also termed the human leucocyte antigen (HLA) complex, this is a segment of genes on the short arm of chromosome 6 that encode MHC (HLA) proteins. HLA proteins *present* antigens to lymphocytes (Fig. 4.7). Each HLA protein presents a specific antigen and an immune response is only triggered in the presence of the HLA protein. Immune responses involving HLA molecules are therefore said to be *antigen specific* and *MHC restricted*.

Some diseases are associated with certain HLA variants. Examples include the B27 seronegative arthropathies, DR2 with narcolepsy, DR3 with coeliac disease, DR4 with rheumatoid arthritis and B8, DR3 with many organ specific autoimmune diseases.

What is the relationship between: (1) antigen presenting cells (APCs) and cytotoxic T lymphocytes?; (2) APCs and T helper lymphocytes (TH lymphocytes)?

The HLA complex is highly *polymorphic* between individuals, resulting in a unique HLA or tissue type.

1. HLA A, B and C genes encode *HLA class 1 proteins* (containing beta-2 microglobulin), which are present on virtually all cells. Class 1 proteins presenting an antigen send a signal to cytotoxic T lymphocytes (also known as CD8 cells) instructing the cytotoxic T lymphocytes — 'kill me' (Fig. 4.8). Class 1 proteins generally present 'internal' antigens.
2. HLA DP, DR and DQ genes encode *HLA class 2 proteins* which are present only on APCs (mostly macrophages). Class 2 proteins are inducible, their genes upregulated in response to an antigen. Class 2 proteins presenting an antigen send a signal to TH lymphocytes

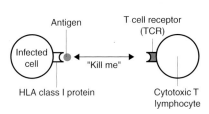

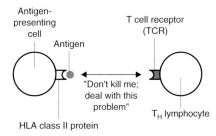

Fig. 4.8　*Cytotoxic T lymphocyte response*　　　Fig. 4.9　*TH lymphocyte response*

(also known as CD4 cells) instructing the TH lymphocytes—'don't kill me but deal with this problem' (Fig. 4.9). Class 2 proteins present processed, 'external' antigens.

Terminology in immunology is often confusing. Cell surface molecules or markers are frequently termed antigens because they are routinely identified by diagnostic antibodies or are involved in self-recognition. Thus, HLA proteins are sometimes referred to as antigens, even though they are not foreign molecules. Further, many important cell surface molecules are described as CD antigens, based on the cluster of differentiation (CD) nomenclature, and are identified by specific monoclonal antibodies.

How do immune signals between APCs and TH lymphocytes induce TH lymphocyte activation?

A specific immune response requires, at its core, activation of TH lymphocytes. Activation signals arise when an APC and a TH lymphocyte join in a cohesive relationship (Fig. 4.10). Two signals are needed for activation:

1. **Signal 1**. The APC ingests a protein antigen, cleaves it into peptides and transports some of those peptides to the cell membrane where they are presented, cradled within the HLA molecule as an HLA–peptide complex, to the T cell receptor (TCR).
2. **Signal 2**. The intimate ligation of signal 1 is not enough to effect an immune response. The TH lymphocyte remains inactive or *naïve*, a state known as *anergy*. Activation of the TH lymphocyte also requires a second, or *costimulatory*, signal. There are many

Fig. 4.10　*TH lymphocyte activation*

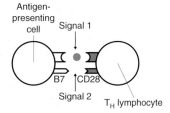

costimulatory molecule interactions, including one called the B7–CD28 interaction.

There must also be immunological 'brakes' to APC–TH lymphocyte activation, otherwise lymphoproliferation would continue unchecked. One such brake is the CTLA4 molecule, induced simultaneously on the surface of activated TH lymphocytes with CD28. CTLA4's action is inhibitory, rather than costimulatory, and it may be aberrant in some lymphoproliferative disorders.

Whilst the HLA system confers interindividual variability, the almost infinite variability of T cell receptors and immunoglobulins within an individual confers the ability to respond to an almost infinite variety of antigens.

What happens to activated TH lymphocytes?

Activated TH lymphocytes are prolific secretors of cytokines including interleukin 2 (IL-2). Cytokines produced during the initial APC–TH lymphocyte interaction provoke proliferation of further TH lymphocytes, which may differentiate into predominantly one of two subsets—TH1 lymphocytes or TH2 lymphocytes. TH1 lymphocytes and TH2 lymphocytes in turn secrete characteristic groups of cytokines.

What are cytokines?

Cytokines are molecules secreted by cells which tell other cells what to do. Molecular biology, and immunology especially, has been revolutionised by the concept of intercellular signals or 'cell talk'. There are a huge array of cytokines, and groups include:

- Interleukins (ILs; 'secreted by leucocytes and acting on leucocytes')
- Interferons (IFNs) ● Tumour necrosis factors (TNFs)
- Chemokines (chemotactic) ● Colony stimulating factors, promoting haematopoiesis ● Growth factors.

Most cytokines have multiple roles or effects. If one cytokine is absent, another may take its place.

Cytokines are only produced by activated cells and are secreted locally. They bind with *cytokine receptors* on cells nearby. Every cell is covered with receptors. The cell membrane can no longer be considered a quiet rural surface. It is a world buzzing with activity, an urban sprawl of business where information technology is at its most advanced!

Which cytokines do TH1 lymphocytes tend to secrete?

IL2, IFNγ. The role of TH1 lymphocytes and these cytokines is proinflammatory (see below).

Which cytokines do TH2 lymphocytes tend to secrete?

ILs 4, 5, 6, 10, 13. The role of TH2 lymphocytes and these cytokines is described below.

What do you know about the TH1 and TH2 responses (Fig. 4.11)?

TH1 response

The TH1 response is also called the *cell mediated immune* response. It tends to be *proinflammatory*. TH1 lymphocytes secrete cytokines which stimulate macrophages, which in turn synthesise and secrete inflammatory cytokines (IL1, IL6 and notably TNF-α), mediating the *acute phase response*. Ultimately, this response can lead to chronic inflammation and, if unchecked, healing with fibrosis mediated by fibroblast stimulating cytokines such as transforming growth factor beta (TGF-β).

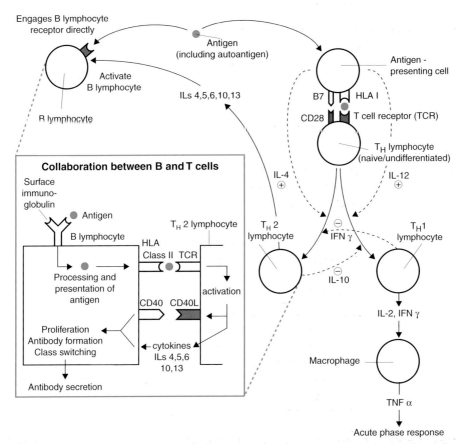

Fig. 4.11   *TH1 lymphocyte and TH2 lymphocyte pathways. IL12, produced by APCs, encourages TH1 lymphocyte production. IL4, produced by both APCs and TH2 lymphocytes, encourages TH2 lymphocyte production. IFNγ, produced by TH1 lymphocytes, tends to inhibit TH2 lymphocyte production, promoting the established TH1 response. IL10, produced by TH2 lymphocytes, tends to inhibit TH1 lymphocyte production, promoting the established TH2 response*

This immune response typifies many bacterial and other infections and antitumour activity and can perpetuate autoimmune disease.

Inflammation is the body's response to many insults. Many systemic changes associated with proinflammatory cytokines are recognised. These changes, collectively termed the *acute phase response*, include the hepatic synthesis and release of acute phase proteins — complement proteins, coagulation proteins (including activated protein C), transport proteins and C reactive protein (CRP). Some acute phase proteins such as albumin decrease in concentration. Other acute phase phenomena include fever, tachycardia, anorexia, rising concentrations of 'stress' hormones such as cortisol and catecholamines, decreased insulin-like growth factor 1 (IGF-1), anaemia of chronic disease, leucocytosis, thrombocytosis, catabolism and cachexia.

Monoclonal antibodies against TNF-α have been used to modify the proinflammatory response in chronic inflammatory diseases such as Crohn's disease and rheumatoid arthritis.

TH2 response

The TH2 response normally serves to regulate the intensity of the TH1 response, dampening down the tendency to inflammation by the negative stimulus of IL-10.

Furthermore, TH2 lymphocytes collaborate with B lymphocytes in the production of specific antibodies.

For this collaboration to occur, two signals are again required. Signal 1 is between the B lymphocyte expressed antigen and the T cell receptor. Signal 2 is a costimulatory signal, in this case between the CD40 surface molecule and its ligand CD40L on the TH2 lymphocyte.

B lymphocytes may be stimulated directly by antigens to produce antibodies, but more commonly antibody production results from collaboration between TH2 lymphocytes and B lymphocytes.

TH2 lymphocyte cytokines also induce class switching, enabling recombination of immunoglobulin (Ig) genes and production of different Ig classes. There is TH2 lymphocyte collaboration for each class of and specific antibody produced, but TH2 cytokines are notoriously important in parasitic infections when high levels of IgE are required to eliminate antigen. Asthma and atopic diseases are characterised by an excessive TH2 response.

What is meant by cell mediated immunity (CMI) and humoral immunity (HI)?

CMI refers to immunity dependant on specifically primed cells, and includes T lymphocyte toxicity, the TH1 proinflammatory cascade and TH2–B lymphocyte collaboration. HI involves antibody production.

What do you know about cytokine receptors?

Cytokine receptors comprise a number of polypeptide subunits with intra- and extracellular domains. One subunit, the common gamma chain (γc), is common to receptors to several IL cytokines. Whilst cytokines will stand in for absent colleagues, cytokine receptors have no backup. Mutations of γc occur in *X-linked severe combined immunodeficiency* (SCID), with loss of function of several cytokine receptors. In SCID the signals of ILs 'fall on deaf ears' and severe immunodeficiency results. 'Combined' implies that both T and B cell receptors are affected.

A stimulated receptor is the starting point on a relay to the inner world of an effector cell. Just as there are a huge array of cytokines and cytokine receptors, there are a huge array of *intracellular pathways*. One such pathway is the Jak (**Ja**nus **k**inase) and STAT (**s**ignal **t**ransducers and **a**ctivators of **t**ranscription) pathway. Jaks are tyrosine kinases associated with the intracellular domains of cytokine receptors. After cytokine binding, a phosphorylation cascade of Jaks and STATs occurs enabling STATs to translocate to the nucleus, bind to DNA and act as transcription factors. As expected, mutations of Jak are another cause of SCID.

What are chemokines?

Attracting leucocytes to tissues is essential for an effective inflammatory response. Attraction is the role of *chemokines*, chemoattractant cytokines. There are many chemokines, belonging to different families. Generally, alpha chemokines attract neutophils and macrophages and beta chemokines attract eosinophils, basophils, monocytes and many lymphocytes. *Chemokine receptors* are present on all leucocytes.

Chemokines are allies with *adhesion molecules* called *selectins* and *integrins* in seducing leucocytes down extravasation pathways from blood into tissues. Chemokine imbalance probably has a role in inflammatory disease. Chemokine receptor variants have a role in some infectious diseases. CXCR4 and CCR5 are coreceptors that are needed for entry of the human immunodeficiency virus into TH lymphocytes and macrophages respectively. Homozygous mutations of these receptors confer some immunity to acquisition of HIV and heterozygous mutations confer a likelihood of slower progression to acquired immunodeficiency syndrome (AIDS).

What do immunoglobulins do?

During development in the bone marrow, virginal B cells contain 'unmutated' immunoglobulin V region genes. These genes undergo appropriate somatic mutation in response to antigen encounters in peripheral lymphoid sites, and B cells subsequently survive as memory cells in the lymph nodes or circulation, or undergo isotype class switching to become antibody producing plasma cells. Immunoglobulins (or antibodies) *precipitate antigens* and *activate complement proteins*, the role of complement being to eliminate precipitated antigens and immune complexes.

What are cryoglobulins?

A cryoglobulin is simply any antibody which precipitates in the cold (at < 4°C). It dissolves when warmed to 37°C. Cryoglobulins may be immunoglobulin (Ig)G, M or A, and may be *monoclonal* IgM or G, tending to form precipitates (cryo-precipitation), *mixed* (usually monoclonal IgM directed against polyclonal IgG) or *polyclonal* (mixtures of polyclonal IgM and G). Mixed and polyclonal cryoglobulins tend to form immune complexes with antigens.

Cryoglobulins, especially monoclonal, are often associated with lymphoproliferative disease and polyclonal with autoimmune disease such as SLE and infections such as hepatitis C. Cryoglobulinaemia may result in vasculitis, occlusive vascular disease and Raynaud's phenomenon.

What are cold agglutinins?

These are IgM antibodies which cause red blood cells to aggregate at < 37°C. They may be found in *Mycoplasma, Coxsackie* and malarial infections and in lymphoproliferative disease, especially lymphoma. It is not surprising (given that both cryoglobulins and cold agglutinins are merely Igs secreted from plasma cells) that cryoglobulinaemia and cold agglutination are much more common in diseases of plasma cell proliferation. They merely represent a proportion of the Ig production in these diseases. They may also be found in otherwise healthy people, especially elderly people.

What are complement proteins?

The complement system is a cascade of plasma proteins, synthesised in the liver, whose role is to *remove antigen precipitates and immune complexes* (antigen–immunoglobulin complexes). The complement system may be activated by one of two routes, the *classical pathway* or the *alternative pathway*. The common result of both pathways is cleavage of the complement protein C3.

C1 (esterase) inhibitor deficiency causes hereditary angioedema, in which attacks of non-inflammatory oedema are triggered by an excess of the complement protein C2.

What are hypersensitivity (HS) reactions?

These are excessive immune responses.

Type I HS: anaphylaxis

Antigens react with IgE on mast cells leading to release of vasoactive substances including histamine and leukotrienes. Reactions usually begin within minutes of exposure in previously sensitised individuals.

Type II HS: antibody dependent cytotoxicity

Cell surface antigens react with circulating antibody triggering complement activation, e.g. transfusion reactions, hyperacute transplant rejection.

Type III HS: immune complex mediated

Circulating antigens react with circulating antibodies, e.g. extrinsic allergic alveolitis, deposition of complexes in blood vessels of kidneys, joints and skin as in serum sickness, postinfectious glomerulonephritis.

Type IV HS: Cell-mediated immunity (CMI): delayed hypersensitivity

Antigens, in association with HLA class 2 molecules on APCs, are presented to already sensitised (memory) TH lymphocytes, e.g. the tuberculin reaction, contact dermatitis, graft versus host disease (GVHD) and graft rejection.

How does allergy arise?

Allergic diseases are increasing in prevalence in the Western world. Atopy refers to the predisposition to generate allergic antibodies (IgE) in response to environmental triggers.

Understanding how the immune system responds to foreign antigens—by presentation to naïve TH lymphocytes and differentiation either to a TH1 response driving cell mediated inflammation or to a TH2 response driving B lymphocytes to switch to IgE production—is central to understanding the allergic process.

The optimal scenario is a well balanced ability to produce TH1 and TH2 responses. Allergy is increasingly regarded as a TH2 weighted imbalance. Atopic predisposition seems to start in early life, with impaired IFN-γ production. Exposure to bacteria in early life may increase IFN-γ levels and lends weight to the 'hygiene' hypothesis, in which reduced exposure to bacteria, antibiotics and certain infant diets result in persistence of a dominant TH2 pathway. Mycobacterial species are known to stimulate powerful IFN-γ production and research has focused on bacterial vaccines to promote switching from TH2 to TH1 pathways.

What do you understand by the terms tolerance and autoimmunity?

Immune responses to antigens and autoimmune responses to auto (self) antigens involve the same mechanisms. What is remarkable is how the immune system determines what is foreign and what is self. It does not normally respond to self-antigens, and this state of affairs is called *tolerance*.

Tolerance is not fully understood. It begins in embryonic life, when lymphocytes 'learn' to react to antigens during their production in the thymus, bone marrow and lymphoid organs. Their developing cell receptors undergo random gene rearrangement in preparation for the diverse array of exogenous antigens in postembryonic life, and every T lymphocyte has a specific T cell receptor (TCR) encoded by a specific T cell gene rearrangement. Understandably, during development, TCRs will encounter self-antigens. At this stage, any strong interactions between TCR and self-antigen will lead to de-selection—lymphocytes with a tendency to 'friendly fire' are destroyed by apoptosis, or programmed cell death.

However efficient this process, it is never enough to prevent some self-reacting lymphocytes from 'qualifying'. These dangerous cells, and their clonal offspring, must be kept in check by the immune system for the rest of an individual's life. One safeguard is called *anergy*. Anergy ensures the lack of response to a self-antigen by an autoimmune T cell unless a second, costimulatory signal is present. Most cells in the body are not competent to deliver such a signal. Another protective mechanism is *ignorance*. Frequently, autoimmune lymphocytes never encounter their respective self-antigens because the latter are 'hidden' behind cellular or vascular barriers. Equally, apoptosis ensures that, unlike necrotic cell death, antigenic intracellular contents do not spill out into the face of danger. Even these stealthy safeguards may fail. The result is autoimmune disease.

How does transplant rejection occur?

Transplant immunology is discussed on page 98.

How might immunodeficiency arise?

- *Primary non-specific immunodeficiency*, e.g. complement deficiency, neutrophil disorders.
- *Primary specific immunodeficiency*, e.g. severe combined immune deficiency (SCID), MHC class 1 or 2 deficiencies ('bald' lymphocyte syndrome), X-linked agammaglobulinaemia (B cells unable to produce immunoglobulin), hyper-IgM syndrome (failure of class switching from IgM producing B cells), common variable immune deficiency (IgA deficiency the commonest).
- *Secondary immunodeficiency*, e.g. secondary complement deficiency (SLE, postinfectious GN, bacterial endocarditis), secondary immunoglobulin deficiency (B lymphocyte lymphoproliferative diseases, splenectomy, nephrotic syndrome), hypergammaglobulinaemia (monoclonal lymphoproliferative diseases in which a single B lymphocyte clone 'crowds out' normal B lymphocytes or polyclonal hypergammaglobulinaemia as in chronic infection/inflammation/autoimmune disease), T lymphocyte deficiency due to T lymphocyte lymphoproliferative diseases, immunosuppressant drugs, human immunodeficiency virus (HIV) infection.

| CASE STUDY | 4.21 HUMAN IMMUNODEFICIENCY VIRUS (HIV) INFECTION |

Instruction: *This young man has been diagnosed with HIV. Please ask him some questions.*

| Case Box 4.21 | Human Immunodeficiency Virus Infection History Taking Points |

- Duration of diagnosis and how it came to be diagnosed
- Likely mode of transmission (vaginal or anal sexual intercourse, contaminated needles from intravenous drug misuse, vertical transmission). Less common causes include needlestick injuries, acquisition from infected breast milk and previous blood transfusions, particularly in haemophiliac patients
- Modification of risk transmission behaviour
- Ethnic background (HIV-2 is common in parts of Africa)
- List of symptoms and opportunistic diseases treated to date
- Combination therapy regimen
- Side effects of treatments
- A thorough social history.

Describe the structure of the HIV virion?

HIV is a retrovirus comprising two RNA copies of the genes env, gag and pol: env encodes glycoprotein gp160 which includes the gp120 surface molecule and gp41, a transmembrane molecule; gag encodes the capsid molecules p17, p24 and p9; pol encodes the enzymes reverse transcriptase, protease and integrase. There are also regulatory genes.

How does the virus replicate?

Gp 120 binds to CD4 surface antigens on T cells and macrophages. Binding and entry of the HIV virion is further facilitated by chemokine coreceptors. Binding leads to a conformational change in the envelope molecules, exposing gp41 which has a hydrophilic sharp tip which can penetrate the host cell. Once the viral capsid enters the host cell, reverse transcriptase converts the RNA genome into double stranded DNA. DNA is then integrated into the host genome under the control of viral integrase. The integrated gene is treated by the host as a normal gene, transcribed and translated into a new virion which subsequently buds out of the cell.

Replication is rapid, with perhaps 10^9 host cells being infected daily, especially at lymph node sites.

What is the serological response to HIV infection?

A T cell mediated cytotoxic response and a humoral response with antibody production against envelope and core genes.

Why are the clinical features of opportunistic disease in HIV often atypical?

The eloquent workings of the immune system are illustrated best when at fault. HIV, which parasitises the cell mediated immune (CMI) system, affirms that it is ravished defence rather than microbiological attack which causes the clinical manifestations of HIV disease and acquired immunodeficiency syndrome (AIDS). Just as an extravagant CMI enhances the inflammatory cascade (the acute phase response and inflammed pharynx cause fever and pain in a common cold, not the furtive adenovirus), so impoverished CMI attenuates it. Whilst meningococcal meningitis in immunocompetent individuals rapidly results in severe headache with a life threatening acute phase response, cryptococcal meningitis in HIV infected individuals may be insidious with minimal signs despite a cerebrospinal fluid overrun with organisms.

Broadly, the CMI system evolved to fight viruses and fungi, and humoral immunity to fight bacteria.

What is the natural history of HIV infection?

The Centers for Disease Control (CDC) in the USA divides HIV infection into four stages:

1. Primary HIV infection

This is the stage of seroconversion, usually occurring in the first 3 months of infection. It may be symptomless, but non-specific constitutional symptoms or a glandular fever like illness may occur. Neurological autoimmune diseases may occur such as Guillain–Barré syndrome, chronic inflammatory demyelinating polyneuropathy, myopathies, transverse myelitis or aseptic meningitis.

2. Asymptomatic phase

Patients may remain asymptomatic for over 10 years. Viral load falls and CD4 counts are generally $> 350 \times 10^6$ cells/μL.

3. Persistent generalised lymphadenopathy (PGL)

This may be the presenting feature of HIV infection. It persists for > 3 months and in at least two extra-inguinal sites.

4. Symptomatic infection

This comprises:

- 4A: HIV wasting syndrome (AIDS defining) and constitutional disease
- 4B: HIV encephalopathy (AIDS defining) and neurological disease
- 4C: Minor opportunistic infections and major AIDS defining opportunistic infections
- 4D: AIDS defining cancers.

Stage 4 results from increased viral replication at previously latent sites, and the exact triggers for this are unknown. As the CD4 count declines, characteristic diseases emerge. For example, *Pneumocystis carinii* pneumonia (PCP) may occur with CD4 counts above 200×10^6 cells/μL whilst mycobacterial TB (MTB), Kaposi's sarcoma and non-Hodgkin's lymphoma tend to occur with counts below 200×10^6 cells/μL. Cerebral toxoplasmosis, cytomegalovirus (CMV) infections, *Mycobacterium avium* complex (MAC) and cryptococcal meningitis tend to occur with very low CD4 counts.

Most neurological HIV disease occurs in advanced infection and includes encephalopathy, subcortical dementia and progressive multifocal leucoencephalopathy (PML). Cerebral toxoplasmosis is usually the result of reactivation of latent infection. Ring enhancing lesions are seen on the CT brain scan, although the differential diagnosis of this should include cerebral lymphoma. CMV may cause retinitis, encephalitis, ventriculitis and polyradiculopathy.

What conditions define AIDS?

AIDS defining conditions without laboratory evidence of HIV include:

● Progressive multifocal leucoencephalopathy (PML)
● *Pneumocystis carinii* pneumonia (PCP)
● Oesophageal, tracheal, bronchial or lung candidiasis
● Extrapulmonary cryptococcosis
● Cytomegalovirus (CMV) infection outwith the lymphoreticular system
● Mucocutaneous herpes simplex virus (HSV) infections > 1 month
● Oesphageal or pulmonary HSV
● Cerebral toxoplasmosis
● Disseminated *Mycobacterium avium/kansaii*
● Cryptosporidiosis with diarrhoea > 1 month
● Lymphoid intestinal pneumonia in a child < 13 years
● Kaposi's sarcoma in a patient < 60 years
● Primary cerebral lymphoma in a patient < 60 years.

AIDS defining conditions with laboratory evidence of HIV include:

● HIV wasting syndrome
● HIV encephalopathy
● *Pneumocystis carinii* pneumonia (PCP)
● Oesophageal candidiasis
● Cytomegalovirus (CMV) infection
● Cerebral toxoplasmosis
● Mycobacterial tuberculosis (MTB)
● Disseminated mycobacterial disease other than MTB
● Isosporiasis with diarrhoea > 1 month
● Recurrent *Salmonella* septicaemia
● Disseminated histoplasmosis or coccidioidomycosis
● Recurrent pneumonia within 1 year
● Recurrent/multiple infections in child < 13 years
● Kaposi's sarcoma

- Primary cerebral lymphoma
- Non-Hodgkins lymphoma—diffuse, undifferentiated B cell, or unknown phenotype
- Invasive cervical cancer.

These AIDS defining clinical lists are used by the World Health Organisation. The CDC defines AIDS as a CD4 count $< 200 \times 10^6$ cells/μL.

What do you know about PCP?

Most patients develop PCP without prophylaxis. PCP causes a dry cough and severe hypoxia for the degree of symptoms. Chest X-ray appearances range from mild interstitial pneumonitis to severe alveolar opacification.

Whilst the differential diagnosis includes atypical pneumonia, a careful history usually reveals other signs of immune compromise such as oral candidiasis. Lymphopenia is common.

PCP may be confirmed by Giemsa staining or PCR analysis of induced sputum or bronchoalveolar lavage fluid.

Co-trimoxazole is the treatment of choice. Secondary prophylaxis is essential and primary prophylaxis is recommended when the CD4 count falls below 200×10^6 cells/μL.

What do you know about mycobacterial disease in HIV?

MTB (Case study 2.5) is a potent stimulator of cell mediated immunity and thus may accelerate HIV replication in infected cells. This is also true of some other HIV opportunistic infections such as syphilis.

TB may be reactivated in HIV or may occur as a primary infection. It behaves like TB in immune competent hosts in early HIV infection and the Mantoux test (page 27) becomes positive. A wide variety of pulmonary or extrapulmonary presentations occur in advanced HIV infection when the Mantoux test is often negative. Multi-drug resistant TB is common and has a high mortality.

MAC (page 207) and other mycobacteria present in a wide variety of ways, often with symptoms of dissemination.

What do you know about antiretroviral treatment?

This is specialised treatment. The two broad categories of drug are:

1. *Reverse transcriptase inhibitors (RTIs)*, which prevent conversion of viral RNA to DNA. Only DNA can be incorporated into the host genome. Nucleoside RTIs inhibit reverse transcriptase (RT) and act as DNA chain terminators. Non-nucleoside RTIs bind to RT at a site distant to the active site but lead to conformational changes in RT which render it inactive.
2. *Protease inhibitors*, which bind competitively to the substrate site of viral protease.

Combination therapy has significantly reduced HIV resistance, maintaining viral RNA load at undetectable levels and dramatically reducing rates of progression to AIDS. The optimum time to start antiretroviral therapy is still not known.

| CASE STUDY | 4.22 TIREDNESS |

Instruction: *This nurse has been referred to your medical outpatient clinic because she feels tired all the time, worse after physical activity. Her routine bloods are normal. Please take a history from her.*

Case Box 4.22   Tiredness History Taking Points

Tiredness or lethargy is a common complaint, often without an identifiable physical cause. Excluding common medical causes is the first priority, but the history taking skills on pages 103–110 are paramount in identifying possible non-medical reasons, including 'stress'. *Three key areas* to explore are:

1. What exactly the patient means by tiredness
Patients may complain of feeling 'tired all the time', having 'no energy' or feeling 'exhausted'. It is important to try to establish:
(i) *What is meant* by tiredness (e.g. a general feeling of fatigue after minimal activity, or weakness in specific muscle groups)
(ii) Whether symptoms are present *all the time* or are episodic. If episodic, do they occur at *specific times* of the day (e.g. rheumatoid arthritis causes morning stiffness which improves with activity whilst mechanical back pain may be worse towards the end of a working day) or after *specific activities* (e.g. myasthenia gravis causes fatiguable weakness in specific muscle groups)?
(iii) The *duration* of symptoms
(iv) The mode of *onset* of symptoms (insidious or sudden, following a specific illness?).

2. How it affects the patient
(i) Activities they cannot do now which they could do before
(ii) How it affects work
(iii) How it affects home life
(iv) Whether or not there are any factors the patient can identify which contribute to the way they feel.

3. Symptoms which might suggest important causes
(i) *Anaemia* (Case study 8.14): pallor, per rectal or vaginal bleeding, menstrual blood loss, diet
(ii) *Hypothyroidism* (Case study 11.2): preference for warmth, weight gain, dry skin, hair thinning

(iii) *Obstructive sleep apnoea* (Case study 2.9): history of snoring, overweight/obese

(iv) *Heart failure* (Case study 4.9): dyspnoea, orthopnoea, paroxysmal nocturnal dyspnoea, ankle swelling

(v) *Chronic lung disease*, e.g. COPD (Case study 2.1), asthma (Case study 4.2), pulmonary fibrosis (Case study 2.6): cough, wheeze, dyspnoea

(vi) *Inflammatory bowel disease* (Case study 4.6): altered bowel habit with presence of blood, mucus or pus

(vii) *Diabetes mellitus* (Case study 4.18): family history, polyuria, polydipsia, recurrent fungal infections

(viii) *Addison's disease* (Case study 11.7): postural dizziness, nausea, pigmented skin creases, vitiligo

(ix) *Chronic renal failure* (Case study 3.17): nocturia, oliguria, fluid retention

(x) *Colorectal cancer* (Case study 4.7): altered bowel habit, per rectal bleeding, weight loss

(xi) *Lung cancer* (Case study 2.2): cough, haemoptysis, weight loss, smoking history

(xii) *Myopathy/polymyalgia rheumatica* (Case study 6.31): persistent proximal muscle weakness

(xiii) *Myasthenia gravis* (Case study 6.30): fatiguable weakness in certain muscle groups

(xiv) *Periodic paralysis* (very rare): episodic marked generalised weakness

(xv) *Depression*: sleep disturbance, change in appetite or weight, loss of libido

(xvi) *Chronic fatigue syndrome*: fatigue after minimal activity, prodromal viral illness

(xvii) *Iatrogenic*: e.g. beta-blockers.

List some features of depression

- Depressed mood
- Loss of enjoyment, interest or pleasure in activities
- Diminished ability to concentrate (subjective or observation by others)
- Feelings of worthlessness or excessive and inappropriate feelings of guilt
- Change in weight or appetite
- Sleep disturbance (difficulty getting off to sleep and/or wakening through the night and/or early morning wakening)
- Thoughts of death, suicidal ideation/attempts/specific plans
- Fatigue or loss of energy
- Agitated behaviour or reduced activity
- Feelings of hopelessness (despondence) and a bleak, pessimistic outlook.

What is chronic fatigue syndrome (CFS)?

CFS typically follows an upper respiratory tract infection with incomplete recovery. Many viruses have been implicated as possible causes. There are many possible symptoms, but profound fatigue, worsened by minimal physical or mental exertion, is central. CFS is more common in females but there is no clear link with occupation or social class. Investigations are usually non-specific, although altered lymphocyte function, hypocortisolism and other altered blood parameters have been described in some patients. There may be full recovery, but symptoms may relapse and remit or persist as a chronic illness.

REFERENCES AND FURTHER READING

HISTORY TAKING SKILLS

Neighbour R. The inner consultation. Lancaster: MTP Press; 1987.

Tate P. The doctor's communication handbook. Oxford: Radcliffe Press; 1984.

COPD

COPD Guidelines Group of the Standards of Care Committee of the BTS. BTS Guidelines for the management of chronic obstructive pulmonary disease. Thorax 1997; 52 (suppl 5): S1–S28.

ASTHMA

British Thoracic Society. Guidelines on asthma management. Online. Available: www.brit-thoracic.org.uk.

DYSPEPSIA

British Society of Gastroenterology (includes guidelines on dyspepsia management). Online. Available: www.bsg.org.uk.

Dent J, Brun J, Fendrick AM et al. An evidenced based appraisal of reflux disease management – the Genval workshop report. Gut 1999; 44 (suppl 2): S1–16.

ABDOMINAL PAIN

Lafferty K. Understanding abdominal pain. Practitioner 2001; 245: 156–161.

COELIAC DISEASE

Primary Care Society for Gastroenterology. Follow up care of adult celiac disease. 2001. Online. Available: www.pcsg.org.uk

Van de Wal Y, Kooy Y, van Veelen P et al. Selective deamidation by tissue transglutaminase strongly enhances gliaden-specific T cell reactivity. J Immunol 1998; 161: 1585.

INFLAMMATORY BOWEL DISEASE

Rampton D. Management of Crohn's disease. Br Med J 1999; 319: 1480.

Rampton D. A GP guide to inflammatory bowel disease. Practitioner 2001; 245: 224–229.

COLORECTAL CANCER

Schofield JH. Screening. ABC of colorectal cancer. Br Med J 2000; 321: 1004–1006.

PRIMARY PREVENTION OF CHD

General

Department of Health. National service framework for coronary heart disease. London: Department of Health; 2000.

Wood D, Durrington P, Poulter N et al, on behalf of the British Cardiac Society, British Hyperlipidaemia Association, British Hypertension Society and British Diabetic Association. Joint British recommendations on prevention of coronary heart disease in clinical practice. Heart 1998; 80 (suppl 2): S1–29.

Antithrombotic therapy

Antithrombotic Trialists Collaboration. Collaborative meta-analysis of randomised trials of antiplatelet therapy for prevention of death, myocardial infarction, and stroke in high risk patients. Br Med J 2002; 324: 71–86.

A randomised, blinded, trial of clopidogrel versus aspirin in patients at risk of ischaemic events (CAPRIE). Lancet 1996; 348:1329–1339.

Hypertension

Hansson L, Zanchetti A, Carruthers SG et al. Effects of intensive blood pressure lowering and low dose aspirin in patients with hypertension: principal results of the Hypertension Optimal Treatment (HOT) randomised trial. HOT Study Group. Lancet 1998; 351: 1755–1762.

Ramsay LE, Williams B, Johnston GD et al. British Hypertension Society guidelines for hypertension management 1999: summary. Br Med J 1999; 319: 630–635.

ACEI (high cardiovascular risk)

Mindlen F, Nordaby R, Ruiz M et al. The HOPE (Heart Outcomes Prevention Evaluation) Study Investigators. Effects of an angiotensin converting enzyme inhibitor, ramipril, on cardiovascular events in high risk patients. N Engl J Med 2000; 342: 145–153.

Lipid lowering therapy (primary prevention)

Heart Protection Study Collaborative Group. MRC/BHF Heart Protection Study of cholesterol lowering with simvastatin in 20536 high risk individuals: a randomised placebo controlled trial. Lancet 2002; 360: 7–22.

La Roas JC, He J, Vapputuri S et al. Effect of statins on risk of coronary heart disease. A meta-analysis of controlled trials. JAMA 1999; 82: 2340–2346.

Shepherd J, Blauw GJ, Murphy M et al. Pravastatin in elderly individuals at risk of vascular disease (Prospective Study of Pravastatin in Elderly at Risk PROSPER): a randomised controlled trial. Lancet 2002; 360: 1623–1630.

Shepherd J, Cobbe SM, Ford I et al. Prevention of coronary heart disease with pravastatin in men with hypercholesterolaemia. West of Scotland Coronary Prevention Study group (WOSCOPS). N Engl J Med 1995; 333: 1301–1307.

PATHOPHYSIOLOGY OF CHD

Fuster V, Fayad ZA, Juan J. Acute coronary syndromes: biology. Lancet 1999; 353 (suppl II): 5–9.

Haffner SM, Lehto S, Ronnema T et al. Mortality from coronary heart disease in subjects with type 2 diabetes and in non-diabetic subjects with and without prior myocardial infarction. N Engl J Med 1998; 339: 229–234.

STABLE ANGINA

Bucher HC, Hengstler P, Schindler C et al. Percutaneous transluminal coronary angioplasty versus medical treatment for non-acute coronary heart disease: meta-analysis of randomised controlled trials. Br Med J 2000; 321: 73–77 (Editorial 62–63).

Maliq I, Berger A. Science commentary: Coronary angioplasty and stenting. Br Med J 2002; 325: 519–520.

The IONA Study Group. Effect of nicorandil on coronary events in patients with stable angina: The Impact Of Nicorandil in Angina randomised trial. Lancet 2002; 359: 1269–1275.

Scottish Intercollegiate Guidelines Network (SIGN). Coronary revascularisation in the management of stable angina pectoris. Edinburgh. SIGN. 1998. Online. Available: www.sign.ac.uk

ACUTE CORONARY SYNDROMES/MYOCARDIAL INFARCTION

British Cardiac Society Guidelines and Medical Practice Committee and Royal College of Physicians Clinical Effectiveness and Evaluation Unit. Guideline for the management of patients with acute coronary syndromes without persistent ECG ST segment elevation. Heart 2001; 85: 133–142.

Connolly DL, Lip GYH, Chin SP. Antithrombotic strategies in acute coronary syndromes and percutaneous coronary interventions. (ABC of antithrombotic therapy). Br Med J 2002; 325: 1404–1407.

The Clopidogrel in Unstable Angina to Prevent Recurrent Events (CURE) Trial Investigators. Effects of clopidogrel in addition to aspirin in patients with acute coronary syndromes without ST-segment elevation. N Engl J Med 2001; 345: 494–502.

ISIS-2 (Second International Study of Infarct Survival) Collaborative Group. Randomised trial of intravenous streptokinase, oral aspirin, both, or neither among 17 187 cases of suspected acute myocardial infarction: Lancet 1988; 2: 349–360. [There were many thrombolysis trials (e.g. GUSTO, GREAT), references to which may be found in guidelines. The Task Force on the management of acute coronary syndromes of the European Society of Cardiology. Management of acute coronary syndromes in patients presenting without persistent ST elevation. Eur Heart J 2002; 23: 1809–1840.

Watson DS, Chin BSP, Lip GYH. Antithrombotic therapy in acute coronary syndromes (ABC of antithrombotic therapy). Br Med J 2002; 325: 1348–1351. This article embraces guidance on the use of glycoprotein IIb/IIa inhibitors issued by the National Institute of Clinical Excellence. These are beneficial as adjuncts to high and low risk PCI (e.g. EPIC, CAPTURE) and as primary treatment in acute coronary syndromes (e.g. PRISM-PLUS, PURSUIT).

WHO Consultation on Obesity. Preventing and managing the global epidemic. Geneva: World Health Organization; 1997.

HIV

Adler MW. ABC of AIDS. Development of the epidemic. Br Med J 2001; 322: 1226–1229 (includes Centers for Disease Control and Prevention's outline of HIV staging).

Mindel A, Tenant-Flowers M. ABC of AIDS. Natural history and management of early HIV infection. Br Med J 2001; 322: 1290–1293 (contains World Health Organization's list of AIDS defining conditions).

CARDIOVASCULAR SYSTEM AND NERVOUS SYSTEM

5. CARDIOVASCULAR SYSTEM

EXAMINATION: CARDIOVASCULAR SYSTEM

Inspection

Hands

Look for:

1. *Finger clubbing*, characterised by fluctuant nail beds (page 9), increased angle between the nail plate and posterior nail fold, and increased nail curvature (page 443). Cardiac causes include cyanotic heart disease and infective endocarditis.
2. *Cyanosis* due to right to left cardiac shunts.
3. *Peripheral stigmata of infective endocarditis* (Case study 5.9) — Osler's nodes, Janeway lesions, splinter haemorrhages, digital infarcts.

Face and neck

1. Examine the tongue for *central cyanosis*.
2. Note any *pallor* or abnormal skin markings, specifically a *malar flush*. A malar flush may be a sign of pulmonary hypertension and you should especially consider mitral stenosis as a cause.

Jugular venous pulse (JVP)

Usually a glance is enough, but occasionally you will be asked to examine the JVP specifically. You should be able to differentiate arterial from jugular venous pulsation, recognise normal waveforms (Fig. 5.1, Box 5.1) and recognise and interpret certain abnormal waveforms (Box 5.2).

The right internal jugular vein should be used in preference to the left. This runs a relatively straight course medial and deep to the sternomastoid, from behind the

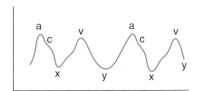

Fig. 5.1   *Normal waveforms of the JVP*

'**a**': represents atrial contraction; it is presystolic

'**c**': is a flicker in the x descent and represents closure of the tricuspid valve whose leaflets bulge back towards the right atrium during ventricular systole

'**x**': represents the tricuspid valve drawing away from the right atrium, as the right ventricle empties in systole; it is synchronous with the carotid pulse

'**v**': represents venous return to the right atrium whilst the tricuspid valve is still closed; it is *not* synchronous with ventricular systole

'**y**': represents opening of the tricuspid valve and blood rushing from the right atrium into the right ventricle just prior to the 'kick' of atrial contraction

Box 5.2 Abnormal Waveforms of the JVP (Fig. 5.2)

Loss of 'a' wave

In *atrial fibrillation* the 'a' wave is lost because effective atrial contraction is lost.

Systolic 'V' wave

In *tricuspid regurgitation* the *'x' descent is lost* and replaced by very prominent upright systolic waves—representing blood shooting back up into the neck as the right ventricle contracts. These systolic waves are synchronous with the carotid pulse and are called *systolic 'V' waves (terminology not to be confused with 'v' waves)*. They are sometimes called *'cV' waves*. Frequently 'V' waves may be seen rising up to the earlobes.

Prominent 'a' wave

In *tricuspid stenosis* there is a prominent 'a' wave because the atrium is contracting against resistance. Prominent 'a' waves may also occur when there is pulmonary stenosis or pulmonary hypertension of any cause resulting in right ventricular overload.

'Giant a' or 'cannon' wave

'Giant a' or 'cannon' waves occur when the atrium contracts against a closed ventricle. This situation arises notably in *complete heart block*.

Kussmaul's sign

Kussmaul's sign is a paradoxical rise in the JVP on inspiration and is seen in *constrictive pericarditis*. It is due to the inability of the right heart to accommodate the blood volume of venous return without a marked rise in filling pressure. Kussmaul's sign may also be seen in restrictive cardiomyopathy and severe heart failure of any cause.

Raised venous pressure

Raised venous pressure (> 4 cm) may occur in *congestive biventricular cardiac failure, pericardial effusion* and *tamponade*. In all of these the arterial blood pressure may be low and in large effusions and tamponade the apex beat absent. A raised JVP, hypotension and an absent apex beat is known as Beck's triad.

Non-pulsatile raised neck veins

Non-pulsatile raised neck veins are a sign of *superior vena cava obstruction*. In addition to facial congestion, veins of the hands and arms and under the tongue may be distended.

---

sternoclavicular joint to the angle of the jaw. The JVP reflects right atrial pressure. Unlike the arterial pulse it has two main waves, the *'a' wave* and the *'v' wave*, and has a definite upper level, which falls during inspiration as venous return is increased by a suction effect of the lungs. The venous pulse is better seen than felt, whereas the arterial pulse may be readily felt with light palpation. You should be able to comment on the height of the JVP in centimetres above the manubriosternal angle with the patient reclined at 45 degrees. Normal is up to 3–4 cm.

Chest wall

Look for evidence of previous surgery:

1. A *median sternotomy scar* consistent with coronary artery bypass grafting, open mitral valvotomy or valve replacement, aortic valve surgery or mediastinal surgery.
2. A *left lateral/inframammary thoracotomy scar* consistent with closed mitral valvotomy.
3. Scar of (and palpable) permanent pacemaker or implantable cardiac defibrillator.

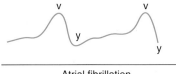

Atrial fibrillation

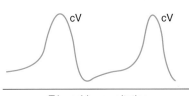

Tricuspid regurgitation

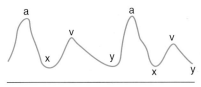

Tricuspid stenosis or
pulmonary hypertension

Fig. 5.2   *Some abnormal waveforms of
the JVP*

Palpation

Arterial pulse

1. Note the heart rate and rhythm (abnormalities are discussed in Case study 4.10).
2. Palpate the carotid pulse as part of your routine assessment. The percussion wave is the dominant wave transmitted along elastic arterial walls. The dicrotic notch (difficult to detect) is a normal blip on the downstroke of the percussion wave representing aortic valve closure. Abnormalities in arterial pulse character are shown in Box 5.3.

Apex

Aim to locate the *apex beat*, normally palpable in the *fifth intercostal space* at the *midclavicular line*, and determine if it is displaced. An absent apex beat may be a sign of obesity, emphysema, pericardial effusion or dextrocardia. Many terms have been used to describe abnormalities in apex beat character (Box 5.4).

Right ventricular parasternal lift

Also known as a *right ventricular heave* or a *left parasternal heave*, this is detected by placing your palm over the left lower parasternal edge. It will palpably (and visibly) lift if there is right ventricular hypertrophy, which itself is usually a consequence of pulmonary hypertension (page 229) of any cause.

Palpable heart sounds and murmurs ('thrills')

Thrills are palpable murmurs caused usually by blood being squeezed through a narrow aperture. They are the tactile manifestation of murmur energy.

1. If you feel a systolic thrill at the apex think of mitral regurgitation.
2. If you feel an upper parasternal thrill think of aortic stenosis (right parasternal edge) or pulmonary hypertension (left parasternal edge).

Blood pressure

Take (or ask for) the blood pressure at this point. *This is essential.* You must be able to use a conventional sphygmomanometer with standard or large cuffs.

1. Check that the sphygmomanometer is set to zero.
2. Ensure you have the correct cuff size. Obese patients need a large cuff. A standard cuff will exert greater pressure to compress the artery and give falsely elevated readings.
3. Inflate whilst palpating the brachial artery to obtain the systolic pressure by palpation. Inflate 20–30 mmHg above where you no longer feel pulsation, then

Box 5.3   Abnormalities in Arterial Pulse Character

Slow rising, plateau pulse

A slow rising, 'plateau' or 'anacrotic' pulse is characteristic of *aortic stenosis*. The pulse is slow rising with a delayed percussion wave and sometimes a palpable judder on the upstroke. Characteristically there is a narrow pulse pressure.

Collapsing pulse

A collapsing pulse has a very brisk upstroke followed by its 'collapse'. It occurs when there is 'run off' from the aorta as in *aortic regurgitation*, an *arteriovenous fistula* or a *patent ductus arteriosus*. Characteristically there is a wide pulse pressure (the difference between systolic and diastolic pressure). A collapsing pulse may be visible at the brachials or the carotids and is best felt by raising the patient's arm, your left hand feeling their brachial artery and your right hand feeling their radial pulse 'slap' against your fingertips or palm.

A *large volume, hyperkinetic pulse* may occur in any cause of high cardiac output such as thyrotoxicosis, Paget's disease or severe anaemia. A *small volume collapsing pulse* is associated with ventricular run off states such as mitral regurgitation or a ventricular septal defect. There is a quickly rising percussion wave but it is small.

Pulsus alternans

Pulsus alternans refers to alternating large and small beats and is a sign of poor left ventricular function. It is common in *aortic stenosis* and *left ventricular failure*.

Pulsus paradoxus

Pulsus paradoxus refers to an excessive fall in pulse pressure (> 10 mmHg) during inspiration. It is not, in fact, paradoxical, but an exaggeration of normal physiology. It is difficult to detect, but may occur in *cardiac tamponade, pericardial constriction* or *acute severe asthma* compromising venous return.

Jerky pulse

A *jerky pulse* may be a sign of *hypertrophic cardiomyopathy*. Ventricular ejection is in 'stops and starts'.

Box 5.4   Apex Beat Abnormalities

- **Double impulse**, which may be a sign of *hypertrophic cardiomyopathy*
- **Tapping apex**, which is the palpable equivalent of a loud first heart sound and should alert you to *mitral stenosis*
- **Hyperdynamic/thrusting apex**, which should alert you to *aortic regurgitation*
- **Sustained apex beat**, which should alert you to *aortic stenosis*
- **Heaving apex**, which is a sign of left ventricular hypertrophy.

Apex beat abnormalities can be difficult. As a rule of thumb, try to determine if the apex beat is displaced or undisplaced and whether or not it is forceful:

Undisplaced apex

This is normal or implies *pressure overload*, as in *aortic stenosis* (the apex is also undisplaced in *mitral stenosis*).

Displaced apex

This implies *volume overload*, as in *aortic regurgitation* and *mitral regurgitation*.

slowly deflate the cuff until you feel the pulse return.

4. Use the bell or diaphragm, re-inflating the cuff back to 20–30 mmHg above the estimate of systolic pressure by palpation. Deflate slowly, 2 mmHg/sec.

5. The point at which you hear the first Korotkoff sound is the systolic pressure and the point at which sound disappears (fifth Korotkoff sound) is the diastolic pressure. The fourth Korotkoff sound (muffling) is acceptable in patients in whom sound does not disappear.

6. Record measurements to the nearest 2 mmHg.

7. Tell the examiners that you would also check for a postural fall in blood pressure.

Be alert to a *wide pulse pressure* (aortic regurgitation) and a *narrow pulse pressure* (aortic stenosis).

Be aware of the significance of differences greater than 15–20 mmHg in blood pressure between upper and lower limbs and always palpate pulses for *radiofemoral delay*, otherwise silent but significant aortic coarctation is missed.

*One of your aims in cardiovascular examination to this point should be to try to diagnose any valve abnormality **before** you auscultate. Ideally, auscultation should confirm already aroused suspicions. Common examples are given in Box 5.5.*

Percussion

Percussion of the cardiac border or cardiac dullness adds little to clinical assessment. Omit unless other signs suggest the presence of a pericardial effusion.

Auscultation

1. Start at the *apex* with the diaphragm followed by the bell (applied very softly) of your stethoscope, then *move through the areas shown* in Figure 5.3.

2. Next listen at the *apex* with your patient in the *left lateral position* and at the *aortic and pulmonary areas* with your patient *sitting forward*. Which you do first depends upon where you think the pathology lies, but be seen to do both. *In both positions listen in expiration 'breathe in, and out, and hold your breath...and breathe again' and in inspiration if you suspect a right sided (pulmonary or tricuspid) murmur.* Inspiration increases the loudness of right sided murmurs and expiration the loudness of left sided murmurs (see page 226–227).

First heart sound (S1)

This represents mitral valve closure. The intensity may be altered in certain situations (Table 5.1).

Second heart sound (S2)

S2 comprises aortic valve closure (A2) followed by pulmonary valve closure (P2). Normally A2–P2 is slightly split (< 0.05 seconds apart) and A2 comes first—think of the efficient left ventricle contracting swiftly, offloading its stroke volume. Variations are described below:

Box 5.5 Diagnosing Valve Abnormalities before Auscultation	
Sinus rhythm/AF + normal BP + undisplaced apex = mitral stenosis (or normal!)	Small volume pulse + narrow pulse pressure + undisplaced apex = aortic stenosis
Large volume pulse + wide pulse pressure + displaced apex = aortic regurgitation	Displaced apex without signs of aortic regurgitation = mitral regurgitation

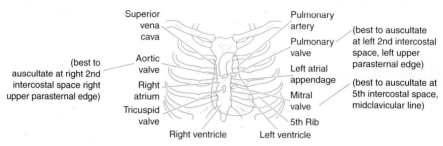

Fig. 5.3   *Surface markings of the heart valves*

TABLE 5.1   **Loud, soft and variable S1**

Loud S1	Soft S1	Variable S1
Tachycardia/hyperdynamic state	Bradycardia	Atrial fibrillation
Short PR interval	Long PR interval, heart block	Complete heart block
Mitral stenosis (mobile valve)	Mitral stenosis (immobile valve)	

1. Wide inspiratory splitting

Inspiration widens the split. The explanation is shown in Box 5.6.

2. Wide expiratory splitting

This occurs when *right ventricular emptying is further delayed*, as in right bundle branch block or pulmonary stenosis *or* when *left ventricular emptying is fast*, as in mitral regurgitition, because some blood is ejected back into the left atrium.

3. Wide and fixed splitting

This occurs in atrial septal defects.

Physiological splitting (Box 5.6) occurs because right ventricular systole is delayed due to increased right sided flow caused by inspiration. In the presence of a shunt the right side of the heart is already maximally overloaded so that systole cannot be delayed further and the second heart sound is 'fixed'.

4. Reversed splitting

Reversed splitting occurs when *left ventricular emptying is delayed*, as in left bundle branch block, aortic stenosis or hypertrophic

---

Box 5.6   Wide Inspiratory Splitting

Reduced intrathoracic pressure on inspiration 'sucks' blood into the pulmonary vessels of the lungs. There is increased venous return and increased blood flow through the right side of the heart as this blood is sucked through, which delays right ventricular emptying and so delays P2. Decreased blood flowing out of the lungs into the left side of the heart gives rise to earlier left ventricular emptying and an earlier A2. The diminished cardiac output during inspiration also explains why during inspiration blood pressure falls (and heart rate rises to compensate). The converse of these rules applies in expiration.

TABLE 5.2   Loud and soft S2

Loud S2	Soft S2
Tachycardia	Aortic stenosis
Systemic hypertension (loud A2)	
Pulmonary hypertension (loud P2)	

obstructive cardiomyopathy, *or* when *right ventricular emptying is fast*, as in right ventricular pacing.

Causes of a loud and soft S2 are given in Table 5.2.

Extra heart sounds
● *Ejection clicks* may occur in aortic stenosis or pulmonary stenosis.
● An *opening snap* may occur in mitral stenosis (Case study 5.1).
● A *third heart sound (S3)* is due to rapid left ventricular filling in early diastole. It occurs in healthy children/young adults, hyperdynamic states, heart failure and mitral regurgitation.
● A *fourth heart sound (S4)* is due to vigorous atrial contraction filling a stiff ventricle. It may occur in systemic hypertension, aortic stenosis, left ventricular hypertrophy or amyloid heart disease, and is always pathological.
● A *pericardial knock* (page 248) is a third heart sound equivalent, present in constrictive pericarditis.
● A *midsystolic click* may occur in mitral valve prolapse (Case study 5.7)
● Metallic *prosthetic sounds* are discussed in Case study 5.8.

Pericardial friction rub
This is a scratching sound heard best with the diaphragm. It is a sign of pericarditis.

Murmurs
Specific murmurs are described in individual case studies. Be seen to time any murmur with the carotid pulse.

1. Murmurs and respiration
(i)   Right sided heart murmurs are louder in inspiration because in inspiration blood flow increases through the right side of the heart (Box 5.6).
(ii) Left sided heart murmurs are louder in expiration because in expiration blood flow increases through the left side of the heart (Box 5.6).

2. Murmurs and radiation
As a general rule, aortic murmurs tend to radiate more than mitral murmurs. This said, the quality of a murmur is invariably more helpful than its location. You are the same person wherever you go—murmurs are no different!

3. Murmurs and dynamic auscultation
Subtle murmurs may be enhanced by certain manoeuvres. Tell your examiner that you would consider them but *never ask a patient to perform these unless directed to do so by examiners*:

(i)   **Valsalva manoeuvre**. During the *strain phase* there is raised intrathoracic pressure which reduces venous return, cardiac filling and hence output. Blood pressure falls and heart rate rises to compensate. Most murmurs are quieter because there is less blood flowing within the heart. The murmur of hypertrophic obstructive cardiomyopathy is louder because reduced cardiac filling in diastole worsens the subsequent dynamic obstruction. A mitral valve prolapse murmur is also louder because prolapse is enhanced when the heart is underfilled. During the *release phase* there is overshoot correction of blood pressure, which falls, and heart rate rises.

(ii) **Position**. Standing reduces cardiac filling (same rules as Valsalva). Squatting/passive leg raising increases cardiac filling (opposite rules to Valsalva).

(iii) **Exercise**. Isotonic (e.g. jogging) or isometric (e.g. hand grip) exercise may be used. Generally exercise increases blood flow through the heart.

Additional points

Complete cardiovascular system examination includes assessment of lower limb pulses and examining for pulmonary, sacral and lower limb oedema.

CASE STUDY | **5.1 MITRAL STENOSIS**

Instruction: *This 65-year-old lady is thought to have a heart murmur. She is short of breath on exercise. Please palpate and auscultate her heart, tell the examiners what signs you find, and discuss your proposed management.*

RECOGNITION

There may be a *malar flush* (a sign of pulmonary hypertension). A *prominent 'a' wave* in the JVP is present if there is pulmonary hypertension, but only in sinus rhythm (see explanation on page 222) and even then can be difficult to detect. A *left thoracotomy scar* suggests a previous mitral valvotomy.

The patient may be in sinus rhythm or in *atrial fibrillation*.

The *apex is tapping, and undisplaced* in pure mitral stenosis (in mixed mitral valve disease mitral regurgitation may dominate, giving rise to a thrusting, displaced apex). You may feel a *left parasternal heave* and a *palpable P2* if there is pulmonary hypertension.

Auscultation usually reveals a *loud S1* (mobile valve only) because the mitral valve leaflets close against high left atrial pressure generated by the stenotic valve. It is this which gives rise to the tapping apex. There may be a *loud S2 (P2 component)* if there is pulmonary hypertension. Often there is an *opening snap*. This is a high pitched sound caused by high left atrial pressure snapping open the valve (a bit like the wind suddenly catching sails), and therefore only heard when the valve is mobile and pliable—not if it is calcified. It is difficult to hear!

There is a *low pitched, rumbling, mid-diastolic murmur loudest at the apex in the left lateral position in held expiration*. In sinus rhythm, there may be presystolic accentuation of the murmur resulting from the forceful contraction of a pressure-overloaded left atrium.

INTERPRETATION

Confirm the diagnosis

Encountering the 'full-house' of signs is improbable, and even when present they are difficult to elicit. Many physicians say they have never heard an opening snap; a very loud murmur may obscure other auscultatory findings; atrial fibrillation renders heart sounds and murmurs difficult to time. Interpretation can be especially difficult if there is mixed mitral valve disease. At this point, many candidates fail themselves, believing the signs too confusing and their diagnosis to be wrong. Try to keep a sense of logic:

● *Remember to try to diagnose valve lesions before you apply your stethoscope — paying particular regard to pulse character, blood pressure and whether or not the apex is displaced.*
● *Remember that the character of a murmur is often more helpful than its location.* The murmur of mitral stenosis is almost unmistakable once engrained in your mind. You may think it like heavy rain on a tin roof, the rumble of a tube train or a buffalo stampede!
● Simply 'blurting out' a diagnosis about which you are unsure is hazardous. Describing your findings, even if your diagnosis is incorrect, will allow the award of some points.

Assess severity

Signs of severity include:
● Signs of pulmonary hypertension. Interpreting them requires knowledge of the pathophysiological sequence of backward pressure events (Box 5.7). See also page 12.
● The shorter the interval between S2 and the opening snap, the higher the left atrial pressure.
● The longer the diastolic murmur, the greater the severity.

Box 5.7	Sequence of Signs in Pulmonary Hypertension

1. Raised left atrial pressure generates raised pressure in the pulmonary vessels and a *loud (and later palpable) P2* is often the earliest sign.
2. *Pulmonary regurgitation (early diastolic murmur louder in inspiration, sometimes called a 'Graham Steel' murmur)* may follow.
3. This in turn generates right ventricular overload and a *right ventricular heave.*
4. *Tricuspid regurgitation (pansystolic murmur louder in inspiration)* may follow. When tricuspid regurgitation is severe it causes *'V' waves in the JVP* and leads to pulsatile hepatomegaly and peripheral oedema.

Evidence of decompensation

- Pulmonary hypertension may be irreversible, especially where there are signs of right heart overload (Box 5.7).
- Thromboembolic disease, especially stroke.
- Signs of infective endocarditis (Case study 9.1).
- Ortner's phenomenon—hoarseness resulting from an enlarged left atrium exerting pressure on the left recurrent laryngeal nerve supplying the vocal cord.

DISCUSSION

What are the causes of mitral stenosis?

1. Rheumatic heart disease is the commonest cause worldwide. In Australia, for example, where streptococcal infection is highly prevalent within the Aboriginal population, rheumatic heart disease is a major health burden.
2. Congenital.
3. Rarely—left atrial myxomas, SLE, rheumatoid disease, carcinoid.

Two-thirds of patients are female. Stenosis may involve the cusps, commissures or chords.

What are the diagnostic criteria for rheumatic fever?

Rheumatic fever (Table 5.3) and rheumatic heart disease remains common in the underdeveloped world, the latter a common usher for infective endocarditis. In the developed world the legacy of rheumatic fever remains, most commonly as mitral stenosis.

What is your differential diagnosis of a mid-diastolic murmur?

- Left atrial myxoma (fever, constitutional symptoms, raised ESR).
- Austin Flint murmur—the regurgitant jet in aortic regurgitation hits the opening mitral valve (page 234). Usually there are other signs of aortic regurgitation.
- Carey Coombs murmur of rheumatic fever.

What is the commonest presenting symptom of mitral stenosis?

Exertional dyspnoea.

TABLE 5.3   Diagnostic criteria (Jones) for rheumatic fever

Major criteria	Minor criteria
Carditis	Fever
Migratory polyarthritis	Arthralgia
Erythema marginatum	Raised acute phase reactants
Chorea	Prolonged PR interval
Subcutaneous nodules	

Two major *or* one major and two minor criteria *plus* evidence of antecedent group A streptococcal infection are required.

Which investigations might help to assess severity?

- Chest X-ray (enlarged left atrium, carinal angle > 90°, alveolar oedema ± haemosiderosis)
- Echocardiography (valve aperture < 1 cm^2)
- Cardiac catheterisation.

Left ventricular end diastolic pressure (LVEDP) is usually normal in pure mitral stenosis, but left atrial pressure is raised (> 25 mmHg), as are right ventricular and pulmonary artery pressures. The end diastolic gradient (theoretically a gradient is a rate of change and pressure drop is a more accurate phrase) between the left atrial pressure and the LVEDP is a guide to severity and surgery. Surgery would not normally be performed for a drop of < 5 mmHg.

Mitral valve prostheses are slightly obstructive by their nature.

Which treatments should be considered?

1. Percutaneous or open surgical valvotomy.
2. Valvuloplasty, rather than mitral valve replacement, may be possible if the valve is mobile and relatively undistorted, provided there is no/minimal mitral regurgitation and no left atrial thrombus. Otherwise a prosthetic mitral valve is needed.
3. All patients should be considered for anticoagulation if there are no contraindications and receive antibiotic prophylaxis during procedures.

CASE STUDY | **5.2 MITRAL REGURGITATION**

Instruction: *This 66-year-old man is thought to have a heart murmur. Please palpate and auscultate his praecordium and discuss your findings.*

RECOGNITION

There is a *displaced apex beat*, which may be forceful. There may be an *apical thrill*. *S1 is soft*. S3 may be present, due to rapid ventricular filling. There is a *pansystolic murmur at the apex*, often *radiating to the axilla*. Signs of *cardiac failure* may be present. Sometimes the pulse is jerky if a large volume of blood regurgitates into the left ventricle with reduced systolic ejection time.

INTERPRETATION

Confirm the diagnosis

Listen in the *left lateral position* and in *expiration* which accentuates the murmur. The *differential diagnosis* includes:

1. The *pansystolic murmur* of *tricuspid regurgitation*, which is *louder in inspiration*. Look for *'V' waves* in the JVP and a pulsatile liver.

2. The *pansystolic murmur* of a *ventricular septal defect*.
3. The murmur of *aortic stenosis*, which is a harsh, *ejection systolic murmur* which *may radiate to the carotids* and cause a parasternal thrill.

Look for/consider causes

1. Left ventricular dilatation of any cause. Mitral regurgitation is most commonly a consequence of ischaemic heart disease with a dysfunctional left ventricle. Tell the examiners you would ask about coronary heart disease risk factors.
2. Rheumatic heart disease.
3. Connective tissue disease.
4. Mitral valve prolapse *(midsytolic click)*.
5. Complication of mitral valvotomy *(scar)*.
6. Acute mitral regurgitation may be due to papillary muscle rupture (infarction) and infective endocarditis *(Janeway lesions, Osler's nodes, splinter haemorrhages, digital infarcts, fever, splenomegaly)*.

DISCUSSION

What are the treatments for mitral regurgitation?

1. Asymptomatic patients should receive antibiotic prophylaxis during procedures and be followed up with serial echocardiography.
2. Patients with enlarging left ventricular dimensions or a left ventricular ejection fraction (LVEF) < 55% should be considered for surgery.
3. Patients with left ventricular systolic dysfunction (LVSD) should be treated for heart failure but may be considered for surgery depending upon the underlying cause and if left ventricular function will tolerate surgery. Severely symptomatic patients with adequate left ventricular function may be considered for surgery.

CASE STUDY   5.3 AORTIC STENOSIS

Instruction: *Please examine this 72-year-old man's cardiovascular system and discuss your findings.*

RECOGNITION

There is a *low volume, slow rising pulse* with a *narrow pulse pressure*. The *apex is not displaced but heaving* (pressure overload). There is a *harsh ejection systolic murmur (ESM)* — which sounds like sawing wood — with a discernible up-stroke and down-stroke (crescendo-decrescendo). The ESM often *radiates to neck*.

INTERPRETATION

Confirm the diagnosis

The *differential diagnosis of the murmur* includes:

1. *Pulmonary stenosis* (murmur *louder on inspiration, radiates to left clavicle*)
2. *Mitral regurgitation (pansystolic murmur, loudest at apex)*
3. *Hypertrophic (obstructive) cardiomyopathy* (Table 5.4).

Look for/consider causes

- Degenerative aortic valve (elderly)
- Rheumatic heart disease, usually with associated mitral valve disease
- Congenital bicuspid valve (commonly presents in fifth and sixth decades).

Assess severity

The following are signs of severe aortic stenosis:

- Narrow pulse pressure/slow rising pulse ● Soft S2 ● Reversed S2 (page 226) ● Thrill/heave ● Left ventricular failure ● S4.

DISCUSSION

Do you know of any unusual associations with aortic stenosis?

- Angiodysplasia ● Microangiopathic haemolytic anaemia.

How would you differentiate aortic sclerosis from aortic stenosis?

Aortic sclerosis is common in the elderly. The pulse volume tends to be normal, the apex undisplaced and the murmur does not radiate to the carotids.

What are the indications for surgery in aortic stenosis?

- Symptoms (syncope, chest pain or dyspnoea)
- Asymptomatic with mean gradient > 100 mmHg (controversial).

Antihypertensives reducing afterload exacerbate the gradient (pressure drop across the valve) and should be avoided.

TABLE 5.4   **Aortic stenosis and hypertrophic (obstructive) cardiomyopathy (HCM)**

	Aortic stenosis	HCM
Carotid character	Slow rising	Bifid, jerky
Thrill	Upper right parasternal area	Lower left parasternal area
Ejection sound	May be present	Usually absent
Aortic early diastolic murmur	Often present	Rare
Effect of manoeuvres	Fixed murmur	Variable murmur

CASE STUDY	5.4 AORTIC REGURGITATION

Instruction: *Please examine this 64-year-old lady's cardiovascular system and discuss your findings.*

RECOGNITION

There is a *large volume collapsing pulse* (feel for a sharp upstroke at the brachial/carotid arteries) with a *wide pulse pressure*. There is a *displaced apex beat* (volume overload), *thrusting* in character. There is an *early (blowing) diastolic murmur (EDM)* representing the regurgitant jet of blood which may be heard across a 'sash' area extending from the aortic area to the lower left sternal edge. The EDM is *louder in expiration with the patient sitting forward*. There may be an *Austin Flint murmur*, a mid-diastolic murmur which represents the regurgitant jet hitting the opening anterior mitral valve leaflet.

Some eponymous signs of the hyperdynamic circulation heard in aortic regurgitation include:

- *Corrigan's sign*: visible vigorous carotid pulsation
- *De Musset's sign*: head nodding with each pulsation (Abraham Lincoln is said to have had)
- *Quincke's sign*: nail bed capillary pulsation
- *Traube's sign*: pistol shot sounds at the femoral arteries
- *Duroziez's sign*: flow is heard on compressing the femoral artery then auscultating proximally
- *Müller's sign*: uvula pulsation.

INTERPRETATION

Look for/consider causes

- Infective endocarditis (*Janeway lesions, Osler's nodes, splinter haemorrhages, digital infarcts, fever, splenomegaly*)
- Prosthetic valve paravalvular leak—acute or chronic
- Rheumatic heart disease
- Ankylosing spondylitis (*kyphosis, question mark posture*)
- Marfan's syndrome (*tall, long extremities with arm span > height, arachnodactyly, high arched palate*)
- Rheumatoid arthritis (*rheumatoid hands*)
- Syphilitic aortitis (rare).

Assess severity

The following are signs of severe aortic regurgitation:
- Wide pulse pressure ● Soft S2 ● Short EDM (earlier equalisation of aortic and ventricular pressures) ● S3/left ventricular failure
- Austin Flint murmur ● Hill's sign (systolic BP in legs > arms).

DISCUSSION

What are the indications for surgery in aortic regurgitation?

Symptoms. Surgery is the definitive treatment to halt volume overload. The aim is to replace the valve before significant left ventricular dysfunction occurs or before the left ventricular end systolic dimension (LVESD) is > 55 mm. Nifedipine may delay the need for surgery in asymptomatic patients with severe aortic regurgitation but long-term vasodilator treatment is not recommended for patients with significant LV systolic dysfunction. Patients with reduced LV ejection dysfunction should be considered for surgery.

CASE STUDY   5.5   TRICUSPID REGURGITATION AND EBSTEIN'S ANOMALY

Instruction: *Please examine this 48-year-old lady's cardiovascular system and discuss your findings.*

RECOGNITION

There are *'V' waves* in the JVP (pathognomonic of tricuspid regurgitation). There is a *right ventricular/left parasternal heave* and a *pansystolic murmur at the lower left sternal edge* which is *louder on inspiration*. A right ventricular S3 may be heard. Hepatic systolic pulsation and peripheral oedema may be present.

INTERPRETATION

Look for/consider causes

Secondary causes (dilatation of the right ventricle and tricuspid valve) include:

- Secondary pulmonary hypertension due to chronic lung disease (cor pulmonale) or mitral stenosis or in biventricular failure
- Right ventricular infarction
- Eisenmenger's syndrome.

Primary causes include:

- Rheumatic heart disease
- Right sided endocarditis
- Carcinoid syndrome.

DISCUSSION

What do you know about Ebstein's anomaly?

This is congenital, isolated tricuspid regurgitation (without signs of pulmonary hypertension) which leads to cardiomegaly and right sided heart failure. Ebstein's anomaly is characterised by downward displacement of the tricuspid valve into the right ventricle, due to anomalous attachment of the tricuspid leaflets. The abnormally situated tricuspid orifice produces an 'atrialised' portion of right ventricle, which lies between the atrioventricular ring and origin of the valve. The right ventricle is often hypoplastic.

Cyanosis results because of right to left shunting at the atrial level (through a patent foramen ovale or an atrial septal defect).

CASE STUDY 5.6 MIXED VALVE DISEASE

Instruction: *This patient has a mixture of heart valve abnormalities. Please decide which valve abnormality is predominant.*

RECOGNITION

Mixed mitral valve disease

Pulse character, apex, and S1 examination may be used to help determine which is predominant (Table 5.5).

Further, the presence of a S3 would imply the absence of significant stenosis.

Mixed aortic valve disease

Pulse, blood pressure, apex examination and the character of the murmur may be used to determine which of stenosis or regurgitation predominates (Table 5.6).

Consider also the possibility of a prosthetic aortic valve with an ejection systolic flow murmur and an early diastolic murmur suggesting a paravalvular leak.

TABLE 5.5 Determination of predominant mitral valve abnormality

	Mitral stenosis	Mitral regurgitation
Pulse	Small volume	Sharp and rapid
Apex	Not displaced, tapping	Displaced, thrusting
S1	Loud	Soft (± S3)

TABLE 5.6 Determination of predominant aortic valve abnormality

	Aortic stenosis	Aortic regurgitation
Pulse	Slow rising	Collapsing
Blood pressure	Narrow pulse pressure with low systolic pressure	Wide pulse pressure with high systolic pressure
Apex	Not displaced, heaving	Displaced, thrusting
Murmur	Loud and harsh ± thrill	Soft usually

INTERPRETATION

Refer to individual valve lesions.

DISCUSSION

Refer to individual valve lesions.

CASE STUDY   5.7 MITRAL VALVE PROLAPSE (MVP)

Instruction: *This 30-year-old lady is thought to have a heart murmur. Please examine her cardiovascular system and report your findings.*

RECOGNITION

There is a *midsystolic click* followed by a late or midsystolic murmur.

INTERPRETATION

Confirm the diagnosis

Tell the examiners that you would like to perform dynamic auscultation. Squatting brings the click closer to S2 and decreases the duration of the murmur (pages 227–228). The Valsalva manoeuvre and standing have the opposite effect.

Look for/consider causes

MVP is common, affecting between 2 and 10% of the population. Occasionally, it may be associated with Marfan's syndrome (*tall, long extremities with arm span > height, arachnodactyly, high arched palate*), rheumatic heart disease, an ostium secundum atrial septal defect, Ehlers–Danlos syndrome, Ebstein's anomaly or SLE.

DISCUSSION

What complications of mitral valve prolapse may occur?

● Severe mitral regurgitation ● Arrhythmias ● Atypical chest pain ● Transient ischaemic attacks/strokes ● Infective endocarditis (usually only if associated mitral regurgitation) ● Sudden cardiac death.

CASE STUDY   5.8 METALLIC VALVE REPLACEMENT AND PROSTHETIC VALVE DYSFUNCTION

Instruction: *Examine this man's praecordium and auscultate his heart before discussing your findings.*

Mitral valve prosthesis

There is a *midline sternotomy scar*. There is a *metallic S1 click* representing closure of the prosthesis, a *metallic opening snap in* diastole and a *normal S2*. Systolic murmurs are common and do not necessarily indicate valve dysfunction.

Aortic valve prosthesis

There is a *midline sternotomy scar*. *S1 is normal* and is followed by an *ejection click* (often synchronous with S1) representing opening of the prosthesis, an *ejection systolic murmur* and an *S2 click* representing closure of the prosthesis.

An early diastolic murmur and collapsing pulse imply a leaking prosthetic aortic valve.

Both mitral and aortic valves may be prosthetic.

Evidence of decompensation

- Thromboembolic sequelae
- Infective endocarditis (*Janeway lesions, Osler's nodes, splinter haemorrhages, digital infarcts, fever, splenomegaly*)
- Evidence of leakage (may be due to wear and tear or endocarditis)
- Ball embolus
- Valve obstruction
- Haemolysis (aortic valve) with anaemia.

What types of metallic valve do you know of?

- Caged ball devices, e.g. Starr–Edwards. Blood flows around the ball and hence there is a high incidence of haemolysis.
- Pivoted single tilting discs, e.g. Björk–Shiley. Flow is laminar with a lower incidence of haemolysis.
- Double tilting discs, e.g. St Jude.

Mechanical valves are increasingly preferred to bioprosthetic (porcine xenograft/cadaveric homograft) valves because of lower re-operative rates. The endocarditis risk is higher. Bioprosthetic valves may be more suitable for patients in whom anticoagulation would present a risk or where a patient's life expectancy is perceived to be less than that of the expected life of a bioprosthetic valve.

CASE STUDY   **5.9 INFECTIVE ENDOCARDITIS**

Instruction: *Please examine this patient's hands and then auscultate the heart. Discuss your proposed further assessment and management.*

RECOGNITION

Peripheral signs include *anaemia, clubbing, Janeway lesions* (non-tender red palmar macules), *Osler's nodes* (tender nodules of the finger and toe pulps), *splinter haemorrhages* and areas of *digital infarction. A murmur* is present (state location and describe).

Janeway lesions and Osler's nodes are thought to be due to vasculitis or septic embolisation. Splinter haemorrhages are more common. Digital infarction is due to embolisation of end arteries.

INTERPRETATION

Assess other systems

- Roth's spots (retinal vasculitis).
- Fever.
- Splenomegaly, which indicates generalised activation of the reticuloendothelial system and occurs in subacute bacterial endocarditis (SBE).
- Tell the examiners that you would check for haematuria and ask about a history of valvular or congenital heart disease, recent surgery or dental procedures, and recent fevers and rigors.

DISCUSSION

How does endocarditis arise?

Endocarditis probably arises when trauma to a valve leaflet disrupts the endothelium, promoting a microthrombus which acts as a potential culture medium should bacteraemia concurrently occur.

Valve trauma is more likely in the presence of a structurally abnormal valve or where there is turbulent blood flow. High shear stress is more likely in the region of the mitral and aortic valves, the tricuspid and pulmonary valves being colonised with decreased frequency respectively. Once seeded with infection, 'vegetations' tend to appear downstream of the jet of blood flow on the low pressure side of the valve, for example the ventricular side of the aortic valve, normally close to the closure line of the leaflet.

Rheumatic valves are particularly susceptible but any valve disease predisposes to endocarditis. Prosthetic valves are notoriously susceptible to endocarditis. Mitral valve prolapse usually requires concomitant mitral regurgitation for the valve to be susceptible and ostium secundum atrial septal defects almost most never develop endocarditis.

Bacteraemia can occur with very mild trauma, dental interventions being a common source, and can even occur brushing teeth. Areas more heavily colonised with bacteria (oral, gastrointestinal) are more likely to predispose to bacteraemia.

What organisms are responsible?

The profile of organisms varies geographically and changes over time.

Native valve endocarditis tends to be due to viridans streptococci which colonise the oral cavity, lower gastrointestinal tract and genitourinary tract, but may also be due to staphylococci, gram negative bacilli or organisms which are notoriously culture negative such as the HACEK group of organisms (*Haemophilus* species, *Actinobacillus actinomycetemcomitans, Cadiobacterium hominis, Eikenella corrodens, Kingella* species), *Coxiella burnetti, Brucella, Bartonella, Chlamydia*, and fungi and yeasts (*Candida, Aspergillus, Cryptococcus*). One antibiotic dose is sufficient to induce culture negativity and contribute to diagnostic uncertainty.

Prosthetic valve endocarditis may occur *early*, mostly due to staphylococci (*S. aureus, S. epidermidis*) or *late*, with a similar organism profile to native valve disease.

How may endocarditis present?

Viridans streptococci grow slowly and tend to be associated with subacute bacterial endocarditis (SBE), presenting with fevers and weight loss. *S. aureus* tends to cause acute BE and is common in patients with prosthetic heart valves and intravenous drug users. Acute fever is more likely. Abscess formation and valve destruction is more likely and metastatic infection causing brain abscesses and intracerebral haemorrhage are risks. *S. aureus* and fungi carry the highest mortality.

How would you diagnose endocarditis?

- Acute phase reactants (CRP/ESR) are high
- Blood cultures (multiple, from different sites) are vital for confirmation of diagnosis and institution of appropriate treatment
- Serological assays and polymerase chain reaction testing may aid diagnosis when organisms are difficult to culture
- Transthoracic or transoesophageal echocardiography (TTE/TOE).

List some complications of endocarditis

1. Disseminated sepsis and multiorgan failure.
2. Embolic complications such as cerebral metastatic abscess formation.
3. Valve destruction/heart failure. Changing murmurs are common, indicating change in size of a vegetation or embolisation of part thereof, or worsening valve destruction.
4. Intracardiac abscess formation, e.g. aortic root abscess.
5. Pulmonary emboli (common in intravenous drug users, seeding from tricuspid vegetations).
6. Circulating immune complexes causing glomerulonephritis.

CASE STUDY	5.10 VENTRICULAR SEPTAL DEFECT (VSD)

Instruction: *This man has a heart murmur. Please examine his cardiovascular system and report your findings.*

RECOGNITION

There is a *pansystolic murmur* and often a *thrill* at the *left sternal edge*. This is due to blood flow from the high pressure left ventricle to the low pressure right ventricle. There may be a mid-diastolic flow murmur at the apex and a right ventricular heave due to right ventricular volume overload.

INTERPRETATION

Look for/consider causes

● Usually congenital ● Occasionally post myocardial infarction (coronary heart disease risk factors).

Evidence of decompensation

● Infective endocarditis
● Aortic regurgitation due to prolapse of the right coronary cusp
● Right sided heart failure
● Eisenmenger's syndrome.

DISCUSSION

What investigations would you consider?

● ECG (may show signs of right or left ventricular hypertrophy)
● Chest X-ray (may show enlarged pulmonary arteries)
● Echocardiography and cardiac catheterisation for pressures and oxygen saturations.

What treatments are available?

Small defects often close spontaneously in childhood. Otherwise VSDs should be assessed for complications regularly and closed before the onset of Eisenmenger's syndrome. Indications for surgery include:
● Recurrent endocarditis ● Volume overload ● Acute septal rupture ● Aortic regurgitation.

What is Eisenmenger's syndrome?

Longstanding right sided heart overload leads to pulmonary hypertension and reversal of the left to right shunt (Eisenmenger's syndrome). It leads to *clubbing* and *central cyanosis* and the progressive backward pressure consequences of *pulmonary hypertension* (page 229).

Eisenmenger's syndrome may occur as a consequence of a:
● VSD ● Atrial septal defect (ASD) ● Patent ductus arteriosus (PDA).

What types of congenital heart disease do you know of?

At birth, pulmonary vascular resistance falls as the lungs inflate and more blood flows through them. Left atrial blood flow increases causing closure of the foramen ovale (connection between atria). The ductus arteriosus usually closes < 24 hours after birth. Congenital heart disease is common and often multiple abnormalities occur.

Acyanotic

The majority of congenital heart disease is acyanotic, usually involving a *left to right shunt*, and causes include:

● VSD ● ASD ● PDA ● Aortic coarctation.

Congenital aortic stenosis and congenital pulmonary stenosis are less common causes of acyanotic congenital heart disease.

Cyanotic

Cyanotic heart disease involves a right to left shunt, and causes include:
● Fallot's tetralogy ● Transposition of the great arteries (TGA), which presents at birth ● Eisenmenger's syndrome.

What is Fallot's tetralogy?

The complete syndrome comprises:

● VSD with right to left shunt ● Pulmonary stenosis ● Right ventricular hypertrophy ● Aorta overriding septal defect.

There is cyanosis, clubbing, a right ventricular heave and an intense pulmonary ejection systolic murmur over the left sternal edge with an associated thrill.

Treatments include total correction or Blalock–Taussig shunting in which the left subclavian artery is anastomosed to the left pulmonary artery to increase pulmonary blood flow.

CASE STUDY	5.11 ATRIAL SEPTAL DEFECT

Instruction: *This man has a congenital heart murmur. Please examine his cardiovascular system and report your findings.*

RECOGNITION	

Ostium secundum atrial septal defects (OS ASDs) are the commonest, presenting in childhood or adulthood. Left to right shunting causes increased flow across the pulmonary valve and results in an *ejection systolic murmur* in the left second/third intercostal space (pulmonary area).

ASDs are often large and under low pressure with little turbulence, and it is a common misconception that the murmur is due to the ASD itself. There may also be a mid-diastolic flow murmur across the tricuspid valve and a *right ventricular heave*. *S2 (A2–P2) is widely split* because of delayed pulmonary valve closure, and fixed. *Ostium primum ASDs (OP ASDs)* are less common and usually present in childhood with associated mitral regurgitaiton.

INTERPRETATION

Evidence of decompensation

- Eisenmenger's syndrome (cyanosis)   ● Atrial fibrillation.

DISCUSSION

What might the ECG show?

- OS ASDs cause RBBB and RAD
- OP ASDs cause RBBB and LAD.

Do you know of any syndromes involving ASDs?

- Holt–Oram syndrome: OS ASD + hypoplastic thumbs
- Lutembacher's syndrome: ASD + rheumatic mitral stenosis.

When should surgery be contemplated?

OS ASDs have traditionally been closed in or before the third decade, but recent thinking is that there may be little gained from surgery in asymptomatic adults.

CASE STUDY   5.12 PATENT DUCTUS ARTERIOSUS (PDA)

Instruction: *This woman has a heart murmur. Please examine her cardiovascular system and report your findings.*

RECOGNITION

Small defects cause a loud continuous 'machinery' murmur. This is due to increased blood flow through the lungs (pulmonary arteriovenous fistulae also sound like this). The continuous murmur is *pansystolic/early diastolic* and is heard best over the *left upper sternal edge and clavicle*. There may be an associated *thrill*.

Large defects cause a *collapsing pulse* (aortic diastolic run off), and a *mid-diastolic tricuspid flow murmur* due to right sided heart overload.

Evidence of decompensation

1. Untreated pulmonary hypertension leads sequentially to:
   (i) Attentuation of the early diastolic murmur
   (ii) Attentuation of the systolic murmur
   (iii) Development of a loud P2.
2. Eisenmenger's syndrome (*cyanosis*).

What is PDA?

PDA is an aorto-pulmonary shunt (high to low pressure).

CASE STUDY   **5.13 AORTIC COARCTATION**

Instruction: *This man has a heart murmur. Please examine his cardiovascular system and report your findings.*

The following signs may be present:

There are *large volume radial pulses* (left may be weaker) and there is *vigorous carotid pulsation* (although aortic regurgitation is a much more common cause). Blood pressure would be lower in the legs than in the arms and there is *radiofemoral delay* – the femoral pulse is delayed and of small volume. There is an *ejection systolic murmur* (which may be loud posteriorly but not audible anteriorly). There are *bruits* over the scapulae, anterior axillary areas and left sternal edge (internal mammary artery). *Collateral* blood vessels may be visible when the patient sits forward.

Evidence of decompensation

Tell the examiners that you would be concerned about the following complications/associations:

● Hypertension and its consequences (hypertension may persist post surgery) ● Bicuspid aortic valve ● Cerebral aneurysms ● Infective endocarditis.

What is aortic coarcation?

Narrowing just below left subclavian artery (LSCA) origin. It may be associated with Turner's syndrome or may be a rare complication of vasculitis, but is usually idiopathic. It is more common in males. It commonly results in acyanotic heart failure in neonates, but may be asymptomatic until adulthood, presenting in the third decade with hypertension.

What might the ECG and chest X-ray show?

1. The ECG may show left ventricular hypertrophy.
2. The chest X-ray may show rib notching on the inferior surfaces of ribs due to tortuous arterial collaterals and there may be a 'figure 3' pattern resulting from:
   (i)   an upper bulge (the left subclavian artery)
   (ii) a notch (representing coarctation)
   (iii) a lower bulge (poststenotic dilatation).

CASE STUDY | ## 5.14 HYPERTROPHIC (OBSTRUCTIVE) CARDIOMYOPATHY (HCM)

Instruction: *Please examine this 32-year-old lady's cardiovascular system. She has had presyncopal episodes.*

RECOGNITION

The carotid pulse is *jerky*. A sharp early rise of rapid ejection is followed by a jerky late systolic phase as the dynamic obstruction supervenes. Contrast this with the slow rising pulse of aortic stenosis (page 233), in which there is obstruction from the outset of systole. There may be an *'a'* wave in the JVP reflecting forceful atrial contraction of a hypertrophied atrium. There is a *double impulse at the apex* due to presystolic ventricular expansion from forceful atrial systole followed by a systolic left ventricular heave.

There may be a *fourth heart sound* due to atrial systole. A *late systolic ejection murmur at the left sternal edge* is due to dynamic obstruction. This may be associated with a *left sternal edge systolic thrill* from turbulence. There may also be a *pansystolic murmur at the apex* because mitral regurgitation is commonly associated. Valsalva (strain phase) and standing accentuate the murmur by increasing dynamic obstruction, whilst Valsalva (release) and squatting attenuate it (pages 227–228).

These findings suggest classic hypertrophic (obstructive) cardiomyopathy.

INTERPRETATION

Confirm the diagnosis

Tell the examiners that you would like to ask about presenting symptoms, which may include:

● Dyspnoea ● Syncope or near syncopal episodes ('greying-out' spells) ● Angina ● Palpitations ● A family history of syncope or sudden death.

Assess severity

Neither the severity of symptoms, nor the left ventricular outflow gradient, appear to correlate with prognosis but various features have been shown to be helpful in stratifying risk. Share these with the examiners:

- Young age at diagnosis
- Syncope or family history of syncope or sudden death
- Episodes of non-sustained ventricular tachycardia (NSVT) or previous ventricular fibrillation
- Loss of normal exercise variation in blood pressure
- 'High risk' genetic mutations
- Marked ventricular hypertrophy (defined as > 35 mm in adults) or left atrial enlargement.

DISCUSSION

What do you know about the pathophysiology of HCM?

The myocardium is hypertrophied. Septal hypertrophy usually dominates and is asymmetrical (ASH), although the region of myocardium most affected may vary between different populations—in Japan, apical hypertrophy is common. There may, in addition to hypertrophy, be obstruction to the left ventricular outflow tract, which is dynamic, appearing in late systole (Fig. 5.4):

Fig. 5.4   *Asymmetrical septal hypertrophy (ASH) and systolic anterior motion (SAM) during systole*

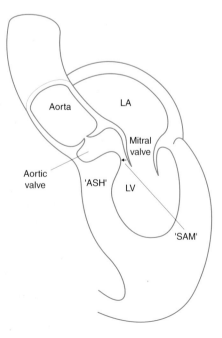

1. The hypertrophied septum distorts systolic movement of the left ventricle.
2. The most significant effect of this is systolic anterior movement (SAM) of the anterior leaflet of the mitral valve.
3. This results in mid–late systolic subaortic obstruction.

HCM also results in diastolic dysfunction. There is increased stiffness of the hypertrophied muscle.

What causes HCM?

The genetic basis of HCM is a mutation in one the genes coding for one of the myocardial contractile proteins—β myosin heavy chain, troponin T, myosin binding protein, α tropomyosin.

An increasing number of different mutations are being described, many with autosomal dominant inheritance, which share the basic histopathological consequence of myocardial fibre disarray.

Increasingly appreciated is the large population of individuals with myocardial fibre disarray without obstruction, sometimes even without echocardiographically detectable HCM. Some of these people—depending upon the underlying genetic aberration—seem to be at risk of sudden death, most likely from conduction abnormalities. HCM may be the commonest cause of sudden cardiac death in young adults. The implications for screening remain unresolved.

What might the ECG and echocardiogram show?

● ECG may show LVH, deep Q waves and conduction defects.
● Echocardiography confirms ASH and SAM in classic HCM, and there may be almost complete obliteration of the LV cavity with a large outflow tract pressure drop or gradient.

What treatments options are there?

● Beta blockers ● Calcium channel blockers ● Amiodarone (first choice antiarrhythmic) ● Dual chamber pacing ● An implantable cardiac defibrillator ● Surgical myomectomy ● Therapeutic septal myocardial infarction ● Endocarditis prophylaxis.

Nitrates and diuretics, which reduce cardiac preload, should be avoided.

What do you know about dilated cardiomyopathy (DCM)?

Causes of DCM include:

● Alcohol ● Genetic (e.g. Duchenne muscular dystrophy, myotonic dystrophy, familial idiopathic DCM) ● Nutritional (e.g. thiamine deficiency) ● Inflammatory (e.g. infection, toxic, eosoinophilic infiltration) ● Drugs (e.g. anthracyclines).

DCM is defined by the presence of a dilated ventricle in the absence of ischaemic heart disease or abnormal loading (hypertension or valvular heart disease), and leads to *systolic dysfunction*.

What do you know about restrictive cardiomyopathy (RCM)

Myocardial infiltration generally results in a degree of RCM. Amyloid and sarcoid are important causes. Haemochromatosis may give rise to RCM or DCM. They may lead to conduction disturbances and *diastolic dysfunction*.

Endomyocardial fibrosis (EMF) affects young Africans and is a chronic non-eosinophilic condition which is difficult to treat. It should be contrasted with Loeffler's endocarditis which occurs in temperate climates and is an aggressive, eosinophilic cause of RCM. RCM may give rise to breathlessness with a positive Kussmaul's sign (page 222) and should be considered in patients with heart failure but a normal cardiac size on chest X-ray. The main differential diagnosis is constrictive pericarditis. Treatment of RCM is unsatisfactory.

What do you know about myocarditis

Myocarditis is uncommon. Causes include:

- Viruses especially *Coxsackie* ● Radiation ● Drugs
- Chemicals (e.g. lead) ● Chagas' disease.

Myocarditis results in a dilated heart and heart failure, often in young adults. The underlying cause should be identified where possible and patients should not overexert themselves until they are better as exertional sudden death is well recognised. One-third of patients return to a normal life, one third have residual symptoms and one third die or proceed to cardiac transplantation.

CASE STUDY   5.15 PERICARDIAL DISEASE

Instruction: *This patient is thought to have pericardial disease. Please examine her and discuss your diagnosis.*

RECOGNITION

Pericarditis

There may be a *pericardial rub*.

Constrictive pericarditis

The signs of a constricted pericardium are similar to restrictive cardiomyopathy (RCM) in that both result in a *raised JVP with prominent x and y descents*, and *non-pulsatile hepatomegaly*. There may be a *pericardial knock*, representing an abrupt halt to rapid ventricular filling.

INTERPRETATION

Look for/consider causes

Look for signs of SLE and tell the examiners that you would ask about recent flu-like illness, other evidence of autoimmune disease (joint symptoms, rashes) and weight loss (for TB or malignancy). All causes

TABLE 5.7   Signs differentiating constrictive pericarditis from cardiac tamponade

Constrictive pericarditis	Tamponade
Prominent x and y descents	Prominent x descent
Kussmaul's sign +ve	Kussmaul's sign –ve
Pulsus paradoxus in one third	Pulsus paradoxus present
Pericardial knock	No pericardial knock

may lead to a pericardial effusion. The causes of constrictive pericarditis are similar.

Assess severity

Pericarditis may lead to pericardial effusion and even tamponade (small volume pulse, hypotension, raised JVP). An ECG might show small complexes. Echocardiography is essential to estimate the volume of fluid accumulated, assess cardiac contractility and guide diagnostic or therapeutic pericardiocentesis.

DISCUSSION

What are the causes of pericarditis?

● Viruses (e.g. *Coxsackie*) ● TB ● Autoimmune/connective tissue disease associated serositis ● Malignancy ● Dressler's syndrome (post myocardial infarction with fever) ● Renal failure.

Which signs might differentiate constrictive pericarditis from cardiac tamponade?

See Table 5.7.

CASE STUDY   5.16   XANTHOMATA AND XANTHELASMATA

Instruction: *What are these skin lesions?*

RECOGNITION

Xanthomata are present (state distribution) (Fig. 5.5). There may also be *xanthelasmata*.

INTERPRETATION

Look for/consider causes

The examiners may wish to discuss the various forms of primary and secondary dyslipidaemia:

Polygenic hypertriglyceridaemia

This gives rise to elevated very low density lipoprotein (VDRL) but its pathophysiology is unclear. Signs of hypertrigyceridaemia include:

Fig. 5.5 *Xanthomata. Reproduced with permission from M.A. Mir (1995) Atlas of Clinical Diagnosis. W.B. Saunders, London*

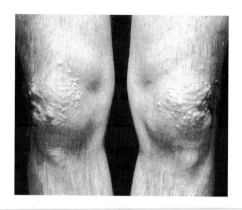

- *Eruptive xanthomata*, yellow nodules especially on the extensor surfaces (elbows, knees, buttocks and back)
- *Lipaemia retinalis.*

Pancreatitis and retinal vein thrombosis are complications.

Familial hypercholesterolaemia

This is an autosomal dominant monogenic disorder of low density lipoprotein (LDL) receptor deficiency/dysfunction, occurring in approximately 1 in 500 in the heterozygous form. Signs of hypercholesterolaemia include:

- *Tendon xanthomata*, common over the extensor surfaces of the hands and the Achilles tendons
- *Tuberous xanthomata*, common over the extensor surfaces of knees and elbows
- *Xanthelasmata*, flat yellow nodules on the eyelids, which can also occur in people with normal serum cholesterol levels
- *Corneal arcus.*

Affected individuals typically have cholesterol levels twice the population average for their age and sex. Myocardial infarction often occurs in early middle age in heterozygotes exposed to a Western diet. Childhood coronary artery disease occurs in the 1 in 1 million homozygotes in all populations.

Polygenic hypercholesterolamia

This is much more common, of uncertain cause, and represents those individuals on the right side of the normal distribution curve.

Familial combined hyperlipidaemia

This refers to polygenic elevation of both cholesterol and triglycride levels, with features of both.

Remnant hyperlipidaemia

This is rare mixed hyperlipidaemia with features of

hypertriglyceridaemia and hypercholesterolaemia and may give rise to *palmar xanthomata.*

Secondary dyslipidaemias

These are usually mixed, but causes of predominant hypertriglyceridaemia include alcohol, obesity and diabetes mellitus (with low HDL levels), and causes of predominant hypercholesterolaemia include hypothyroidism, cholestasis (including primary biliary cirrhosis) and nephrotic syndrome.

DISCUSSION

What do you know about the types of lipid and their transport?

Cholesterol and triglycerides (TG), which are insoluble, are bound in the circulation to *lipoprotein (LP)*. Lipoproteins comprise an outer protein (apolipoprotein) shell and a lipid and phospholipid core. There are various types of lipoprotein:

1. *Chylomicrons (CM)* carry dietary lipid (mostly TG) from the gut to the liver. In the portal circulation LP lipases act on CMs to release free fatty acids (FFAs) for energy.
2. *Very low density lipoproteins (VLDL)* carry TG (and to a lesser extent cholesterol) from the liver to the systemic circulation and tissues. The TG core of VLDL is also hydrolysed by LP lipase to release FFAs. VLDL remnants are termed intermediate density lipoproteins (IDL).
3. *Low density lipoproteins (LDL)* are formed from intermediate density lipoproteins (IDLs) by hepatic lipase. The LDL core is increasingly cholesterol rich and decreasingly TG rich. LDL metabolism is regulated by cell cholesterol needs via negative feedback control of the LDL receptor.
4. *High density lipoprotein (HDL)* carries cholesterol from the tissues back to the liver. HDL is formed in the liver and gut and acquires free cholesterol from the intracellular pools. Within HDL, cholesterol is esterified by lecithin-cholesterol acyltransferase (LCAT). Low HDL levels are generally associated with high TG levels and cardiovascular risk.

The LDL receptor takes up circulating LDL. Cells replete in cholesterol reduce their LDL expression. By contrast, inhibition of HMG CoA reductase, the enzyme controlling the rate of de novo cholesterol synthesis, leads to a fall in cellular cholesterol and an increase in LDL receptor expression. Statin drugs inhibit HMG Co A reductase.

What causes familial hypercholesterolaemia?

Variations in the LDL receptor gene (see page 250).

What is apolipoprotein B?

The component of LDL which binds to the LDL receptor.

Numerous variations in the gene for apolipoprotein B have been described, some of which result in raised cholesterol concentrations.

What is apolipoprotein E?

A ligand for the LDL receptor, which has an important role in clearing cholesterol-rich lipoproteins from plasma.

E3 is the most common allele. The E4 allele of the apolipoprotein E gene occurs in about 30% of the general population. Heterozygotes possessing alleles E3/E4 have slightly higher cholesterol concentrations than E3/E3 homozygotes. A third version of the gene, the E2 allele, occurs in its homozygous form in 1% of the UK population. When combined with a secondary dyslipidaemic risk factor such as diabetes or hypothyroidism, the E2/E2 genotype results in type 3 dysbetalipoproteinaemia, and is associated with high coronary risk.

CASE STUDY | **5.17 HYPERTENSION**

Instruction: *This 46-year-old gentleman has hypertension. Please check his blood pressure and examine his cardiovascular system.*

RECOGNITION

The blood pressure in the right/left arm is (quote reading) in the sitting and standing positions. The diastolic reading is for the fifth Korotkoff sound. The *apex may be displaced.* There may be *hypertensive retinopathy* (Case study 10.2). There may be *other evidence of target organ damage (see below).*

INTERPRETATION

Look for/consider causes

Consider secondary causes of hypertension. In particular, note any:

- *Renal bruit/s* (listen over the renal angles and the epigastrium)
- Signs of *Cushing's syndrome* (Case study 11.6)
- *Radiofemoral delay (aortic coarctation).*

Evidence of decompensation

Tell the examiners that you would consider target organ damage or associated vascular conditions:

- Left ventricular hypertrophy (ECG or echocardiogram)
- Renal disease (proteinuria or raised creatinine)
- Cardiovascular disease (angina, myocardial infarction, heart failure)

- Cerebrovascular disease (transient ischaemic attacks, ischaemic or haemorrhagic stroke, vascular dementia)
- Peripheral vascular disease
- Aortic aneurysm
- Hypertensive retinopathy (Case study 10.2)
- Evidence of atherosclerotic plaques on X-ray or ultrasound (carotid, iliac, femoral, aorta)

Serum TC : HDL ratio and blood glucose should also be obtained in assessing overall risk from hypertension.

DISCUSSION

List some secondary causes of hypertension

- *Renal*, e.g. renal artery stenosis, most renal diseases
- *Endocrine*, e.g. Cushing's syndrome, Conn's syndrome, phaeochromocytoma
- Aortic coarctation
- *Genetic*, e.g. Liddle's syndrome, glucocorticoid remediable aldosteronism, apparent mineralocorticoid excess (Box 5.8)
- *Drugs*, e.g. steroids, alcohol, ciclosporin, NSAIDs.

How may the renin-angiotensin-aldosterone system (RAAS) contribute to the pathophysiology of hypertension?

Hypertension can result from raised peripheral resistance, excessive activation of the RAAS, excessive activity of the sympathetic nervous system, and alteration in the balance of vasoactive molecules derived from the endothelium. A range of genetic factors contribute to these.

Renin is released from the juxtaglomerular apparatus (JGA) of the kidney in response to low sodium or reduced renal perfusion. Renin is an enzyme which converts angiotensinogen to angiotensin I (AI). AI is converted in the lung to angiotensin II (AII) by the action of angiotensin converting enzyme (ACE). AII restores circulating volume via release of aldosterone from the adrenal cortex. Aldosterone acts on the distal renal tubule, promoting sodium and water retention in exchange for potassium and hydrogen ions. Aldosterone also promotes vasoconstriction and thirst. Aldosterone secretion is controlled almost exclusively by the RAAS and not by ACTH. Numerous abnormalities of the RAAS can lead to *hyperaldosteronism* (Box 5.8):

How may the British Hypertension Society (BHS) Guidelines contribute to the management of hypertension?

The principal objectives of the BHS guidelines are to promote the primary prevention of hypertension and cardiovascular disease and to increase awareness, detection, treatment rates and blood pressure control in people with hypertension. The Joint British Societies risk

| Box 5.8 | Some Abnormalities of the Renin–Angiotensin–Aldosterone System |

Primary hyperaldosteronism (Conn's syndrome)

This is most often due to an aldosterone secreting adenoma and suppresses renin production.

Secondary hyperaldosteronism

This is hyperreninaemic, usually in response to low sodium or reduced renal perfusion. A classic example is renal artery stenosis, the kidney perceiving a state of low circulating volume and responding by enhancing its renin secretion.

Pseudohyperaldosteronism (Liddle's syndrome)

This occurs when the tubule sodium channel (ENac), normally stimulated by aldosterone, is switched permanently 'on' in the absence of aldosterone by an autosomal dominant mutation in its gene. Renin is suppressed. Hypertension in Liddle's syndrome may respond to amiloride.

Liddle's syndrome is one of a number of genetically determined causes of low renin hypertension. Two other important ones are *glucocorticoid remediable hypertension* and *apparent mineralocorticoid excess*.

Glucocorticoid remediable aldosteronism (GRA)

Normally two closely related enzymes, 11β hydroxylase and aldosterone synthase, coordinate the synthesis of glucocorticoid and mineralocorticoid from the adrenal gland. In GRA a chimeric gene, comprising the aldosterone synthase gene with an upstream ACTH dependent promoter, results in expression of aldosterone synthase under ACTH regulation. It is inherited in an autosomal dominant fashion. Hypertension in GRA may respond to dexamethasone which suppresses ACTH.

Apparent mineralocorticoid excess (AME)

Normally an enzyme called 11 β hydroxysteroid dehydrogenase (11 βOHSD) within the renal tubules converts cortisol, which has a high affinity for the minerocorticoid receptor, to cortisone, which does not. In AME the 11 βOHSD gene is mutated (autosomal recessive), leading to low enzyme activity and high cellular levels of cortisol which can then act as a potent mineralocorticoid. It may be treated with amiloride and may respond to dexamethasone suppression of cortisol synthesis, as dexamethasone is a less potent mineralocorticoid than cortisol.

Primary hypoaldosteronism
This is due either to Addison's disease or other conditions damaging the adrenal gland (Case study 11.7). Renin is elevated.

Pseudohypoaldosteronism
This occurs when ENac does not work. It is a cause of type 4 RTA (page 95).

---

tables (page 142, Box 4.4) for primary prevention are used in these guidelines. Numerous trials contribute to the evidence base of the guidelines, including the HOT trial (page 141), which reported an overall optimal blood pressure of 139/83 mmHg, with optimal diastolic readings of 82.6 for events and 86.5 for mortality and around 80 in diabetes.

The guidelines also focus on at risk groups including those with isolated systolic hypertension (ISH). ISH is common over 60 years of age, often associated with a lowering of diastolic pressure, and is caused by increased arterial stiffness and decreased compliance. ISH carries significant risk and the evidence is compelling that older patients with hypertension (including ISH) have a high absolute benefit from antihypertensive treatment since they are at high risk of sustaining vascular events.

Thresholds for intervention
Thresholds for intervention based on initial blood pressure are shown in Box 5.9:

Box 5.9	Thresholds for Intervention
● $\geq 160/100$	treat
● 140–159/90–99	treat if target organ damage *or* cardiovascular complications *or* diabetes *or* 10 year CHD risk $\geq 15\%$ observe and reassess CHD risk annually if none of the above is present
● < 140/90	reassess annually
● < 135/85	reassess 5 yearly

Evidence is based largely on standard recording devices, and the place of ambulatory blood pressure monitoring has not been established.

Target blood pressures
Targets are < 140/85 (< 140/80 in diabetes, and increasingly < 130/80 suggested). Minimum recommended levels (although not

always achievable) are < 150/90 (140/85 in diabetes). Both systolic *and* diastolic targets should be reached. Targets in renal disease are on page 91.

Targets in the BHS guidelines, whilst clearly delineated for hypertensive and diabetic patients, are still arbitrary. Increasing evidence from more recent clinical trials suggests that the lower the blood pressure the better, and there even appears to be benefit from lowering blood pressure in normotensive individuals for secondary prevention of cardiovascular events (PROGRESS – Case study 6.13; HOPE – page 141 and Case study 6.13).

Lifestyle modification

Lifestyle modification for blood pressure lowering includes:

- Weight loss via reduced fat and calorie intake
- Regular aerobic physical exercise, e.g. 30 minutes of brisk walking on at least 5 days of the week
- Reduced salt intake
- Increased fruit and vegetable intake
- Limiting alcohol consumption to < 21 units/week for men and < 14 units/week for women.

Choice of drug

The evidence is that blood pressure reduction, regardless of the agent responsible, is the pivotal factor in reducing risk. However, the LIFE study demonstrated the superiority of an AII receptor blocker (ARB) over a beta-blocker in reducing cardiovascular events (less morbidity, less mortality – although no difference in the MI end point), albeit in a select group of patients with LVH. Further, since hypertension in younger patients (< 40 years) is generally associated with higher levels of plasma renin activity, there is theoretical advantage in targeting this group with an ACEI or ARB. Most patients will need combination therapy, approximately 70% of patients responding to some extent to one agent.

A low dose thiazide is generally first line for patients without renal impairment. Agents are listed in Table 5.8.

TABLE 5.8   Choice of drugs for patients with hypertension

	Indications	Contraindications
Beta blockers	Ischaemic heart disease	Asthma/COPD/heart block
Calcium antagonists	ISH in elderly, angina	
ACEIs	Heart failure, renal disease, diabetes	Pregnancy, renovascular disease
AII receptor blockers	ACE inhibitor cough	Pregnancy, renovascular disease
Alpha blockers	Prostatism	Urinary incontinence
Thiazides	Elderly including ISH	Gout

Adequate time for assessment of treatment response should be given and dose escalation where necessary. Whilst postural hypotension is an important side effect, early 'dizziness' may represent cerebral autoregulatory adaptation.

For which patients would you consider antiplatelet primary prophylaxis?

Aspirin is recommended by the BHS for hypertensive patients aged ≥ 50 years with satisfactory blood pressure control (< 150/90 mmHg) and target organ damage or diabetes or a 10 year CHD risk ≥ 15%.

REFERENCES AND FURTHER READING

Day INM, Wilson DI. Genetics and cardiovascular risk. Br Med J 2001; 323: 1409–1412.

Joint British recommendations on prevention of coronary heart disease in clinical practice. Heart 1998; 80 (suppl 2): S1–S29.

The LIFE study group. Cardiovascular morbidity and mortality in the Losartan Intervention For Endpoint reduction in hypertension study (LIFE): a randomised trial against atenolol. Lancet 2002; 359: 995–1003 (a subgroup of the LIFE study in patients with diabetes: 1004–1010).

Ramsay LE, Williams B, Johnston G et al. Guidelines for management of hypertension. Report of the third working party of the British Hypertension Society. J Human Hypertens 1999; 13: 569–592.

Ramsay LE, Williams B, Johnston G et al. British Hypertension Society Guidelines for hypertension management 1999: a summary. Br Med J 1999; 319: 630–635.

Scottish Intercollegiate Guidelines Network (SIGN): Hypertension in older people. Edinburgh: SIGN; 2002. Online. Available: www.sign.ac.uk

Special Writing Group of the Committee on rheumatic fever, endocarditis and Kawasaki disease of the Council on Cardiovascular Disease in the Young of the American Heart Association. Guidelines for the diagnosis of rheumatic fever. Jones criteria, 1992 update. JAMA 1992; 268: 2069.

6. NERVOUS SYSTEM

Scientific exploration into the nervous system is casting light into never before seen depths of this intricate specialty. There is now clearer understanding about the molecular mechanisms of many neurological diseases, opening doors to new treatments. The brain, it seems, is a neurochemical sea, destined to be an aquarium when the windows are securely in place.

Yet even when neurochemistry is seemingly 'normal', the range of human thought and emotion is limitless and, as in chess, the chemical players can play limitless games. Where disease ends and normality begins can be difficult to decide. The brain's complexity is such that we may never have windows to it all.

When preparing for neurology in PACES, it is useful to remember that much neurology remains a scientific mystery. Perhaps more than any other speciality, different neurologists have different ways of approaching their specialty. And perhaps more than any other specialty, it carries an aura of difficulty to 'outsiders'. Lists of signs exist somewhere in memory like fragments of jigsaw but form no real picture. 'Absent ankle jerks and extensor plantars' becomes a list learned by rote, and like so much neurology, exonerated to a mythical proportion of perceived difficulty.

Most PACES candidates fear neurology cases, and should first appreciate that many examiners do, too, hoping only to avoid seeming inept to their co-examiner! But with a basic grasp of the way the neurological system is organised and how disease can sprout from the various components of its organisation, you can turn neurology from one of your feared cases to one of your high scoring ones.

What follows is a journey through the nervous system, from brain to periphery, its organisation systematically explained through six sections of cases:

1. Neuro-ophthalmology and lesions of the cranial nerves
2. Lesions of the cerebral hemispheres
3. Lesions of the brainstem
4. Lesions of the extrapyramidal system and the cerebellum
5. Lesions of the spinal cord
6. Lesions of nerve roots, plexi, peripheral nerves and muscles.

EXAMINATION: GENERAL POINTS

● Neurology is a highly *observational* specialty. Much is missed by instantly stepping forward to examine 'hands on'.

● Neurology is contextual. *I have a headache* can be reported in many ways. We infer if a headache is serious not just by the information elicited but by the way that information is communicated. The brain, unlike a computer, can interpret context. It can handle more than facts. It senses every nuance, knows what information to hold onto, what to suspend and what to discard. Use your 'awareness' when examining patients.

● We have a tendency to 'medicalise' ageing. Systems degenerate with age and, as neuronal reserve declines, so vision, hearing, balance, motor function, reflexes and gait decline.

● Diseases often coexist. An unfathomable mixture of upper and lower motor neuron signs in an elderly patient immediately becomes clear when we discover he or she has degenerative bone disease with cer-

vical myelopathy, multilevel radiculopathy and perhaps even coexistent peripheral neuropathy.

● Signs are more likely to represent pathology if there are associated symptoms. If you think 'maybe the left triceps jerk is a little less brisk than the right', it may well be normal.

Section 1 Neuro-ophthalmology and Lesions of the Cranial Nerves

When we examine the limbs we think of upper and lower neuron lesions. Cranial nerves are simply lower (motor, sensory or both) neurons. Examining them in order from 1 to 12 detracts from the important concept that these *peripheral nerves are in continuum with central nerves*. What we should aim to do is *examine the neurology of the head and neck*.

A *functional* approach to the head and neck is more logical than a *numerical* one. You are more likely to be asked to examine 'the eyes', 'visual fields', 'eye movements' or 'pupils' than 'cranial nerves'.

EXAMINATION: CRANIAL NERVES

Visual acuity (VA) (optic nerve–cranial nerve 2)

1. In practice this is seldom required by examiners. Ask your patient to close each eye in turn and read the letters on a *near vision chart at 30 cm*. Vision should be corrected with glasses if the patient wears them, but a pinhole can also be used to correct refractive errors because it filters out angled rays of light entering the eye. A 6 m Snellen wall chart is more accurate. Normal distance VA is 6/6, meaning that the eye sees at 6 m what it should see at 6 m. 6/60 (the letters on the 6/60 line are 10 times

larger) means it sees at 6 m what it should see at 60 m. If letters cannot be seen, enquire about counting fingers, hands movements and perception of light.
2. Test *colour vision* using a red hat pin. Central vision is especially sensitive for the colour red (peripheral vision monochrome), and if normal a lesion in the optic pathway is unlikely.

Visual fields (VFs) (optic nerve)

1. The *confrontation method* is traditional. Sitting opposite your patient, place your hand over one of their eyes at arm's length, close your opposing eye and ask them to look at you. Then slowly introduce a finger or white hat pin in a plane halfway between yourselves from each quadrant (Fig. 6.2). An easy, nonconfrontational method introduces the hat pin from behind the patient's head but is disliked by some examiners.
2. Examine for a *central scotoma* by moving the hat pin slowly at eye level in a temporal to nasal direction and asking the patient to tell you if it disappears or changes colour. In a central scotoma there will be loss of central vision (see also pages 514–515). The *blind spot* 30° into the temporal field can be mapped out in the same way (Fig. 6.2). It corresponds to the optic disc (see also pages 514–515).

Eye movements (oculomotor nerve–cranial nerve 3, trochlear nerve–cranial nerve 4, abducens nerve–cranial nerve 6)

Gently supporting your patient's head with one hand, ask them to follow the index finger of your other hand. Use midline horizontal and vertical movements, not a letter H.

1. Watch slow, smooth *pursuit* movements ('the lioness on the serengeti eyeing a roaming gazelle') looking for *ophthalmoplegia* (Case study 6.2).

2. Then watch faster *saccadic* movements ('the gazelle catches sight of the lioness'), asking your patient to look from side to side. This may elicit an *internuclear ophthalmoplegia* (Case study 6.3).
3. Note any *nystagmus* (Case study 6.4), normal at extremes of gaze.
4. Note any *ptosis* (Case study 6.5).

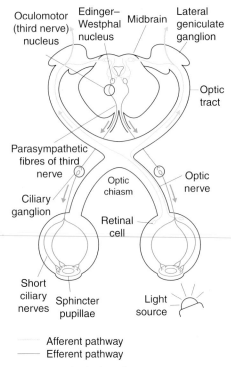

Fig. 6.1   *The light reflex*

Pupils (optic nerve, oculomotor nerve)

1. Check these are of equal *size* (Case studies 6.6, 6.7 and 6.8) and *shape*. *Ptosis* on the side of a *larger pupil* should alert you to a *third nerve palsy*, and on the side of a *smaller pupil* to *Horner's syndrome*.
2. The patient is still looking at your finger. Take it out to a distance (or ask them to look at the ceiling), then quickly close in checking the *accommodation* response. The eyes should constrict as they converge.
3. Check the *direct and consensual light reflexes* by shining the light twice in each eye (Fig. 6.1, Box 6.1).
4. Note any *afferent pupillary defect* by swinging the light (the swinging light test) from eye to eye, dwelling 3–5 seconds

on each eye (Box 6.2). Observe para-doxical dilatation of the pupil of an affected eye, implying a damaged optic nerve with sluggish light impulses.

Fundoscopy

Fundoscopy is discussed on page 513.

Power

1. Assess *facial nerve* (cranial nerve 7) motor function by asking your patient to:
   (i)   Raise their eyebrows
   (ii) Wrinkle their forehead
   (iii) Screw their eyes up tightly
   (iv) Show their teeth
   (v)   Puff out their cheeks.
Note any nasolabial fold flattening, often the first sign of a facial nerve palsy.

Box 6.1　The Light Reflex Mechanism (see also Fig. 6.1)

Light impulses travel along the *optic nerve* and both *optic tracts*. Approximately 10% of the fibres reaching the level of the *lateral geniculate ganglion* subserve the light reflex and connect with both *Edinger–Westphal nuclei* (and adjacent oculomotor/third nerve nuclei) in the periaqueductal matter of the midbrain. Parasympathetic fibres, entwined around both oculomotor nerves are 'excited' by the light impulses, and stimulate the ciliary ganglion, ciliary nerves and ultimately the *pupillary sphincter* muscle of each pupil causing *bilateral pupillary constriction*.

A similar mechanism probably subserves accommodation. The third nerve nuclei also control the action of the medial rectus muscles and convergence. The ciliary nerves also supply the ciliary muscle, altering the lens's shape for focusing. Many more ciliary fibres are dedicated to the ciliary muscle than to the pupillary muscle and the accommodation reflex is often regarded as 'stronger' than the light reflex. This may be the reason why accommodation is preserved in otherwise unreactive Argyll Robertson pupils.

Box 6.2　How the Swinging Light Test Detects an Afferent Pupillary Defect

A. Shining light into the affected eye causes sluggish direct and consensual responses.

B. Shining light into the normal eye stimulates normal direct and consensual responses.

C. When you swing light back into the affected eye, the recovery from B is

faster than the response to A, so the affected eye dilates even though light is shone into it. Because we are referring to A in relation to B, the defect is often referred to as a *relative afferent pupillary defect (RAPD)*. It is also known as the *Marcus Gunn pupil*.

---

2. Assess *trigeminal nerve* (cranial nerve 5) motor function by asking your patient to clench their teeth. Feel for any wasting of the masseters, the muscles of jaw closure.

3. Assess the *glossopharyngeal* (cranial nerve 9) and the *vagus* (cranial nerve 10) *nerves* together by asking your patient to open their mouth and say 'aargh'. Check that the uvula moves upwards and doesn't deviate to one side. It moves to the side contralateral to any lesion. These nerves are complex. They provide sensation to the pharynx and posterior third of the tongue and move the soft palate. Broadly, the glosso-pharyngeal is sensory, the vagus motor; they mediate the gag response and are

vital for normal speech and swallowing. Perhaps the best test that these nerves work is to watch a patient drink a glass of water.

4. Assess the *hypoglossal nerve* (cranial nerve 12). With the tongue at rest inside the mouth observe any wasting or fasciculation. Ask your patient to stick their tongue out and then wiggle it from side to side. The tongue deviates to the side of any lesion.

5. Assess the *accessory nerve* (cranial nerve 11). This innervates the sternomastoid and trapezius muscles. Ask you patient to turn their head against the resistance of your hand (the right sternomastoid turns the head to the left and vice versa)

and then shrug their shoulders against resistance.

Sensation

1. Test the ophthalmic, maxillary and mandibular distributions of both trigeminal nerves.
2. Tell the examiners that you would check the corneal reflex with a wisp of cotton wool (touching the cornea, not the white sclera), its absence often the first sign of a trigeminal nerve lesion.
3. You should not be asked to test *smell* and *hearing* in PACES. Hearing testing is crude without audiometry:

   (i) *Rinne's test* compares sound from a vibrating 512 Hz tuning fork on the mastoid (bone conduction) with the external auditory canal (air conduction). Normally air conduction is better than bone conduction (bone, denser than air, is actually a better conductor of sound but here 'conduction' misleadingly refers to the unimpeded transmission of sound through the air and external canal to the middle ear and inner ear), by convention a Rinne positive test. If bone conduction is better, this implies conductive deafness (everything other than the sensorineural aspect of hearing is conductive), usually due to middle ear disease or wax.

   (ii) In *Weber's* test, sound should be heard in both ears equally when the tuning fork is applied to the central forehead or vertex. In sensorineural deafness (SND) sound is not detected by the affected ear. In conductive deafness sound is louder in the affected ear although neurologists and ENT specialists find this phenomenon difficult to explain. Certainly, when a tuning fork is placed directly on bone, there is no significant sound transmission through the air and all conduction is through bone to the inner ear. Any additional solid material in the ear (causing conductive deafness, e.g. wax, tympanosclerosis, middle ear debris) likely attenuates the normal energy loss at a bone–air interface and enhances sound transmission to the inner ear from the vertex. Whilst this explanation may seem particularly logical for solid occlusive conditions (such as wax or even poking a finger into the ear!), middle ear disease such as effusion, ossicle chain disruption or otosclerosis may also result in a 'denser' middle ear and produce the same effect. (Further, middle ear conditions can lower the inherent resonant frequency, and low frequency sound — such as 512 Hz — tends to be preferentially transmitted to the cochlea; equally, low frequency sound cannot escape from an occluded ear.)

CASE STUDY   6.1 VISUAL FIELD DEFECTS

Instruction: *Examine this patient's eyes/visual fields and comment on your findings.*

RECOGNITION

There is (depending on the site of the lesion):

- A left/right *central scotoma*
- *Tunnel* (more correctly *funnel) vision*
- *Unilateral blindness*
- A *bitemporal hemianopia*

- A *left/right homonymous hemianopia*
- A *left/right homonymous quadrantanopia*
- *Loss of vision in the left/right eye with macular sparing.*

INTERPRETATION

Confirm the diagnosis

What to do next depends upon the visual field defect (Fig. 6.2):

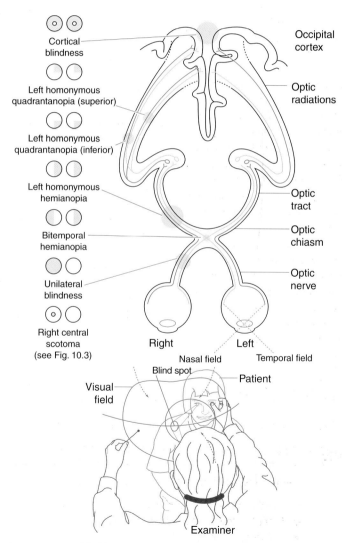

Fig. 6.2   *Visual field testing and visual field defects*

Box 6.3	Five Signs of Optic Nerve Damage

1. Central scotoma
2. Decreased visual acuity
3. Decreased colour vision
4. Relative afferent papillary defect (the most sensitive and specific sign)
5. Optic atrophy

1. Central scotoma

A central scotoma indicates disease of the *central retina (macula)* or of the nerve fibres emanating from the *optic nerve head (optic disc)* which supply it. Candidates get very confused about the macula and the optic disc and why lesions affecting either can cause a central scotoma. This is explained on pages 514–515.

If you elicit a central scotoma, you should *look for evidence of disease at the optic disc and at the macula*, such as optic atrophy or diabetic maculopathy (Case studies 10.4 and 10.1).

Five signs of optic nerve damage (Box 6.3) should be engrained to memory. If you encounter one of them, automatically look for the other four.

2. Funnel vision

Perform fundoscopy to look for *retinitis pigmentosa*. Funnel vision is occasionally due to chorioretinitis or bilateral occipital infarcts. Strictly speaking, *tunnel* vision is psychogenic (page 529).

3. Unilateral blindness

Damage is either in the globe itself, such as a *cataract, retinal detachment* or central retinal artery occlusion, or in the optic nerve. Fundoscopy is essential.

4. Bitemporal hemianopia

This implies a lesion at the optic chiasm. A pituitary tumour may cause compression from below the optic chiasm. Look for signs of *acromegaly* or *hypopituitarism*. Rare causes include craniopharyngiomas, which compress the chiasm from above, meningiomas and aneurysms.

5. Homonymous hemianopia

This usually results from a middle cerebral artery stroke. A right sided lesion cases a left homonymous hemianopia (and left sided upper motor neuron signs). Look for a supranuclear facial palsy and weakness, increased tone and enhanced reflexes in the limbs.

6. Homonymous quadrantanopia

Consider a lesion in the temporal radiations if there is a superior homonymous hemianopia and in the parietal radiations if there is an inferior homonymous quadrantanopia.

7. Cortical blindness

This is classically due to bilateral posterior cerebral artery strokes. The *macula is spared* because the macular cortex is supplied by the middle cerebral artery. Structural lesions destroying a hemioccipital cortex can cause complete contralateral blindness. They can also cause visual hallucinations.

Assess function

Comment on the functional significance of visual loss.

DISCUSSION

Be prepared to discuss the above pathways and causes.

What are the signs of optic nerve damage?

See Box 6.3.

CASE STUDY   **6.2 OCULAR PALSY (THIRD NERVE PALSY, SIXTH NERVE PALSY AND FOURTH NERVE PALSY)**

Instruction: *Examine this patient's eyes/eye movements and discuss your findings.*

RECOGNITION

Third nerve (oculomotor) palsy (Fig. 6.3)

The left/right eye adopts a *'down and out'* deviated position because only the superior oblique and lateral rectus muscles are intact (page 267). There is *ptosis* and the *pupil is dilated* if there is parasympathetic damage.

Because the parasympathetic nerves destined for the pupillary sphincter are entwined around the third nerve, compressive lesions damage them whilst intrinsic (medical) causes like diabetes spare them. Medical causes tend to be painless.

Sixth nerve (abducens) palsy (Fig. 6.3)

There is a gaze palsy, the left/right eye failing to abduct.

Fourth nerve (trochlear) palsy

Isolated fourth nerve palsies are rare. Very slight unopposed external rotation of the affected eye may result in a compensatory head tilt. Trochlear palsies are more commonly part of a *complex (multiple nerve) ophthalmopathy.*

Fig. 6.3   *Ocular palsies*

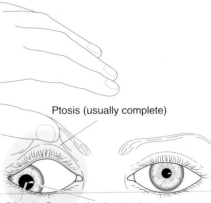

Ptosis (usually complete)

Dilated   Downward and outward
(mydriatic)   deviation of eye
pupil

Right third nerve palsy—neutral gaze

Right sixth nerve palsy—gaze to right

INTERPRETATION

Look for/consider causes

Tell the examiners the possible sites of underlying lesions:

Brainstem

The lesion may be of the nerve or of its nucleus connecting with central pathways. Causes include:

- Vascular lesions. Isolated sixth nerve palsies are often due to diabetes. Look for *diabetic retinopathy*. Tell the examiner that you would check the *urinalysis for glucose*.
- *Demyelination.*
- *Compressive lesions, e.g. pontine glioma.*

Basal area

- Bacterial, fungal or tuberculous infection.
- Carcinomatous meningitis, basal infiltratation from neurosarcoid or lymphoma, or infiltration from the nasopharynx or sinuses. There are often *signs of involvement of multiple lower cranial nerves, including bulbar palsy.*
- A posterior communicating artery aneurysm may compress the third nerve and is often *painful*. The third nerve may occasionally be stretched by a prolapsing temporal lobe (traumatic intracranial

haemorrhage) and the sixth nerve may be stretched over the petrous tip by posterior fossa tumours. Both of these ocular palsies are 'false localising' signs.

Cavernous sinus and orbit

Sepsis, tumours, intracavernous carotid artery aneuryms and infiltrative conditions like Wegener's granulomatosis may damage any of the ocular nerves as they traverse the cavernous sinus.

DISCUSSION

Explain how ophthalmoplegia causes diplopia

When you take a romantic walk with your partner on a sunny day you may catch the sunlight in her or his eyes and you'll see that it falls on exactly the same spot on each eye. Likewise, images from the world around us fall on corresponding spots of each retina. Slight displacement of either eye causes diplopia or double vision.

The direction of gaze in which separation of images and corresponding diplopia is maximal is the direction of action of the paretic muscle. The false image (resulting from the **p**aretic eye) falls progressively away from the macula and is always the outer or **p**eripheral image seen. By covering the paretic eye this false image disappears.

What are the actions of the muscles controlling eye movements (Fig. 6.4)?

1. The actions of the rectus muscles are straightforward. The medial rectus of one eye and the lateral rectus of another work as a conjugate pair for horizontal conjugate gaze.

Fig. 6.4   *Actions of the muscles controlling eye movements (insert: action of superior oblique)*

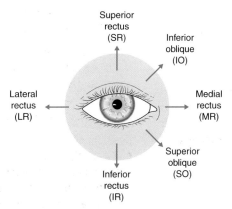

2. The actions of the oblique muscles are more difficult to remember:
   (i) When abducting, superior and inferior rectus dominate vertical gaze.

(ii) When adducting, superior and inferior oblique dominate vertical gaze.

(iii) Superior oblique, unlike superior rectus, depresses the eye whilst inferior oblique, unlike inferior rectus, elevates the eye! This is because the oblique muscles swing through hooks of tissue then double back on the globe to exert traction on it in a line of pull contrary to their nomenclature (Fig. 6.4, insert).

(iv) As the oblique muscles sit slightly medially, they also attempt rotatory movements of the eyes, being unsuccessful in normal circumstances because of the opposing strength of other muscles. Acting alone, superior oblique would cause internal rotation or 'intorsion', and inferior oblique external rotation or 'extorsion'.

By what ocular nerves are these muscles supplied?

The oculomotor nerve supplies: ● Superior rectus ● Inferior rectus ● Medial rectus ● Inferior oblique.

The abducens nerve supplies: ● Lateral rectus.

The trochlear nerve supplies: ● Superior oblique.

What is meant by the term strabismus?

Strabismus or *squint* refers to misalignment—convergence (exotropia) or divergence (esotropia)—in the primary or neutral position (looking straight ahead) which remains constant in all directions of gaze.

What is meant by the term dysconjugate gaze?

Dysconjugate gaze means that the eyes fail to move together in a synchronous fashion. Ocular palsies together with gaze palsies arising from supranuclear pathway disturbances (page 270) and should not be termed 'squints'.

Is diplopia always due to an ocular palsy?

No. Diplopia can arise from nerve, neuromuscular junction or muscle abnormalities. Common causes include:

1. Latent strabismus

The visual axes are misaligned, even in the primary or neutral position, due to an imbalance of muscle tone rather than paresis. We all have a tendency to this, overcome by fusion mechanisms. It manifests in those with a history of a childhood squint, especially when tired. The squint does not settle in either eye. Rather, it is an angle which remains fixed between the eyes in any direction of gaze. The *cover test* may be useful in eliciting a latent squint. To elicit the squint a hand covers one eye. The covered eye moves towards the squinting position, whilst the free eye fixes on an object. When the covered eye is uncovered, the squint is transiently observed.

2. Myasthenia gravis

This causes a *complex ophthalmoplegia* (multiple ocular nerve lesions), and may be *bilateral*. A complex ophthalmopathy may be due to multiple cranial nerve lesions in, for example, vasculitis, but is most commonly due to myasthenia gravis (Case study 6.30). There may also be *ptosis, bulbar involvement* (speech and swallowing impaired) and *limb weakness*. Myasthenic weakness is *fatiguable*. When asking the patient to keep looking at the ceiling, the eyelid will slowly droop.

3. Graves' ophthalmopathy

Eye signs (see also Case study 11.1) can be due to compression from orbital infiltration or thyrotoxic myopathy and include:

- Complex ophthalmoplegia
- *Proptosis* (protrusion of globe)
- *Exophthalmos* (proptosis due to Graves' disease, lower sclera visible between the eyelid and iris)
- *Lid retraction* (upper sclera visible between the eyelid and iris)
- *Lid lag* (upper lid lags behind eye movement on downward gaze).

Other ocular myopathies

Rare ocular myopathies include some mitochondrial cytopathies and oculopharyngeal muscular dystrophy.

CASE STUDY **6.3 INTERNUCLEAR OPHTHALMOPLEGIA (INO)**

Instruction: *Examine this patient's eye movements and then proceed as you think appropriate before discussing your findings.*

RECOGNITION

On horizontal gaze, the abducting eye appears impatient because the *adducting* eye is *slow*. There is *divergent gaze* and the *abducting eye* appears to be coaxing the slow adducting eye, saying to it 'come on, come on!' in the only way it knows—with coarse, jerky *nystagmus* (Fig. 6.5)!

Fig. 6.5   *Internuclear ophthalmoplegia. Abducting eye with nystagmus says 'come on, come on!' to the slower, adducting eye*

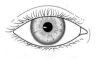
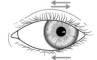

Adducting eye
is slow

Abducting eye
is in a
hurry saying
"come on, come on"

INTERPRETATION

Look for/consider causes

In INO the medial longitudinal fasciculus (MLF) is damaged, most commonly by demyelination in multiple sclerosis. Look for the five signs of optic nerve damage:

Signs of demyelination
- cerebellar signs
- spastic paraparesis
- sensory disturbance
- bladder catheterisation

● Central scotoma ● Decreased, visual acuity ● Decreased colour vision ● Relative afferent pupillary defect ● Optic atrophy.

Tell the examiners that you would look for other signs of demyelination such as cerebellar signs, spastic paraparesis, sensory disturbance or bladder catheterisation.

DISCUSSION

Explain the mechanism of horizontal voluntary conjugate gaze

In neurology we logically think of disease as involving the *upper (supranuclear, or central) neuron* or the *lower (infranuclear, or peripheral) neuron*, the latter referring to root, plexus, peripheral nerve or neuromuscular junction (Fig. 6.6).

We have considered abnormal ocular movements due to *infranuclear* causes. The *supranuclear* or *central* processes governing eye movements are not well established but the following are thought true:

Fig. 6.6   *Supranuclear, nuclear and infranuclear arrangement of the nervous system*

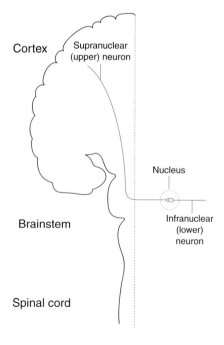

Cortex

Supranuclear (upper) neuron

Nucleus

Brainstem

Infranuclear (lower) neuron

Spinal cord

- Saccadic movements, under voluntary control, are initiated in the frontal cortex.
- Pursuit movements are initiated in the parieto-occipital cortex.
- The eyes must continuously adjust in relation to the position of the head in space, and this requires complex vestibular and proprioceptive inputs mediated through brainstem connections.
- The eyes must move together, requiring synchronous contraction of ocular muscles in one eye and reciprocal muscles in the other. Monkeys relied on the evolution of this binocular vision to judge swinging distances and evade death!

Box 6.4   **Mechanism of Horizontal Voluntary Gaze**

Higher initiating pathways descend from the *frontal cortex* to the level of the contralateral sixth nerve nucleus at the *parapontine reticular formation (PPRF)*. Some neurons from the PPRF stimulate the *adjacent sixth nerve nucleus*. Other neurons from the PPRF travel back upwards and decussate to stimulate the *opposite third nerve nucleus* via a pathway called the *median longitudinal fasciculus (MLF)* (Fig. 6.7). The MLF allows the lateral rectus of one eye and the medial rectus of the other to contract synchronously. Each cerebral hemisphere controls horizontal gaze in the contralateral direction. The *right hemisphere* stimulates the ipsilateral third nerve and the contralateral sixth nerve and the eyes *look to the left*.

Fig. 6.7   *The role of median longitudinal fasciculus in voluntary gaze, looking to the left*

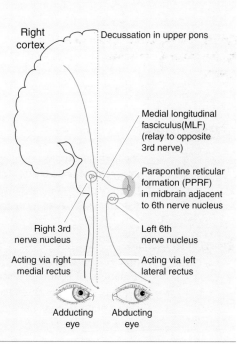

Right cortex

Decussation in upper pons

Medial longitudinal fasciculus(MLF) (relay to opposite 3rd nerve)

Parapontine reticular formation (PPRF) in midbrain adjacent to 6th nerve nucleus

Right 3rd nerve nucleus

Left 6th nerve nucleus

Acting via right medial rectus

Acting via left lateral rectus

Adducting eye

Abducting eye

- Vertical gaze is mediated by the midbrain and not well understood. Skew deviation refers to eyes misaligned at different vertical levels.
- Horizontal gaze is mediated by the pons and the best understood horizontal gaze mechanism is voluntary gaze (Box 6.4).

What causes INO?

Damage to the MLF. Bilateral INOs (BINOs) are common because of the close midline proximity of the right and left MLF.

CASE STUDY 6.4 NYSTAGMUS

Instruction: *Examine this patient's eyes/eye movements and discuss your findings.*

RECOGNITION

There is *difficulty in maintaining conjugate deviation*. The *abducting eye drifts slowly back to the central position (slow, pathological phase)* and *then flicks back to its correct position (fast phase)*. The *direction of nystagmus*, by convention, is the *direction of the fast phase*. This is known as *jerk nystagmus*. Distinguish jerk nystagmus from:

1. *Optokinetic or end point nystagmus.* A few beats of nystagmus at extremes of lateral gaze are normal. This happens when you are a passenger in a car continuously watching the world go by.
2. *Congenital or ocular nystagmus.* Congenital difficulty with fixation leads to a *pendular* nystagmus (no distinct slow and fast phases, the speed and amplitude being equal in all directions) in which the eyes seem to search for a forever elusive resting place.

INTERPRETATION

Nystagmus implies irregular, rhythmic oscillations of one or both eyes, and may be horizontal, vertical or rotatory. Since there is much mystery about the mechanism of conjugate gaze, the pathophysiology of nystagmus is largely obscure.

Assess other systems

Jerk nystagmus occurs in diseases of the peripheral vestibular apparatus or central diseases involving brainstem vestibular connections or the cerebellum. Cerebellar disease is the commonest cause of nystagmus in PACES and you should look for other *cerebellar signs* (Case study 6.16).

DISCUSSION

What are the differences between peripherally and centrally provoked nystagmus?

These are listed in Table 6.1.

In a cerebellar lesion, the fast phase of nystagmus is towards the side of the lesion. In practice, the cerebellum and its brainstem connections are intimately associated and the pathophysiology of these abnormal eye movements likely involves brainstem nuclei. With progressive disease abnormal eye movements may also include *ocular dysmetria*, an overshoot of target directed fast eye 'saccadic' movements resembling limb past pointing and in which the eyes take a few moments to stabilise in the primary position after lateral gaze, *ocular flutter*, in which involuntary horizontal eye movements may occur in the primary position, and *opsoclonus*, in which the eyes continuously oscillate in all directions.

What is vertigo?

Vertigo is an illusion of movement.

Balance depends upon visual, vestibular and proprioceptive inputs to the brainstem and cerebellar connecting pathways. This information is sent to the cortex and also used to mediate ocular movements and postural adjustments.

What are the causes of vertigo?

Peripheral causes include vestibular neuronitis (also known as acute/viral labyrinthitis), benign positional vertigo (BPV), Ménière's disease and local infective causes such as otitis media or a cholesteatoma.

TABLE 6.1   Peripherally and centrally provoked nystagmus

	Peripheral	Central
Causes	Disease of the vestibular system, e.g. vestibular neuronitis	Brainstem or cerebellar demyelination, ischaemia or structural lesion
Direction of fast phase of nystagmus	Away from side of lesion	May be multidirectional. Vertical nystagmus suggests brainstem disease
Associated symptoms	Vertigo ± auditory symptoms common	Vertigo and auditory symptoms rare. May be cerebellar symptoms
Nausea and vomiting	Common	Rare
Effect of lying still	Improves nystagmus and other symptoms	Does not improve symptoms
Recovery	Usually recover quickly (central adaptation)	Slow or no recovery

Box 6.5	Dix-Hallpike Test

1. The patient sits on the couch in such a position that when recumbent their head will hang over the edge.
2. With the head rotated at 45° to one side, lie the patient back rapidly until the head is dependent. This induces self-limiting nystagmus within 30 seconds.
3. The procedure is repeated on the opposite side. The direction of nystagmus (which may be bilateral) indicates the side of the lesion.

- *Vestibular neuronitis* is common in young or middle-aged previously well patients, sometimes following upper respiratory tract infection, and may be due to isolated degeneration of the vestibular nerve. Hearing loss is unusual. The onset of vertigo is frequently on waking, often marked, and associated with nausea and vomiting. There may be horizontal or rotatory nystagmus. Symptoms usually resolve within a few days as vestibular compensation occurs, which precedes regeneration of the nerve. Symptoms may recur but with less severity over subsequent weeks.

- *Benign paroxysmal vertigo* (BPV) refers to recurrent episodes of vertigo provoked by a change in head position, typically turning in bed, bending over/straightening up or extending the neck to look upwards. Nausea may occur but seldom vomiting. There are no associated symptoms such as hearing loss or tinnitus. BPV may be triggered by infection, vasculitis or trauma, but often there is no identifiable cause. Episodes are common in the sixth decade. The Dix–Hallpike test is positive (Box 6.5).

- *Ménière's disease* comprises the triad of vertigo, hearing loss and tinnitus. It tends to affect younger adults and the cause is unknown.

Central causes include ischaemia (the blood supply to the inner ear, brainstem and cerebellum originates from the vertebrobasilar system), demyelination and space occupying lesions affecting brainstem vestibular connections. Vertigo is *not* due to isolated cerebellar disease.

Describe some important distinguishing features between BPV and central vertigo

- In BPV there is a short latent period (of a few seconds) after changing position before vertigo occurs and vertigo is short lived and self-limiting. Central vertigo is immediate, persists and does not recover unless the underlying cause can be treated.
- BPV rapidly fatigues with repeated testing. Central vertigo persists.

- BPV is provoked only by one direction of movement. Central vertigo may occur in all directions.
- BPV usually causes nausea. Central vertigo seldom causes nausea but imbalance is severe.

From what should vertigo be clinically differentiated?

Patients often complain of dizziness or lightheadedness. These terms have no clear definition or associated diagnoses and it is important to differentiate between vertigo and:

1. *Presyncope*, a sensation of impending loss of consciousness. It is caused usually by a decrease in global cerebral blood flow (Case study 4.11).
2. *Disequilibrium*, or *postural unsteadiness*, a sense of imbalance not strictly associated with movement. It is common while standing and is usually worse when walking. It arises if the brain fails to process sufficient information about the body's position in space. Common causes include lower limb weakness, peripheral neuropathy, visual impairment and peripheral vestibular impairment.

CASE STUDY | **6.5 PTOSIS**

Instruction: *Examine this patient's eyes and discuss your findings.*

RECOGNITION

Recognising a *drooping upper eyelid* is easy. Look for signs of the main causes below. Complete unilateral ptosis is highly suggestive of a third nerve palsy.

INTERPRETATION

Look for/consider causes

Determine three things on recognising ptosis:

1. Firstly *check for equal pupils*.
2. Secondly *check the eye movements*.
3. Finally, *note if ptosis is unilateral or bilateral*.

Third nerve palsy

There is a *dilated pupil on the side of the ptosis* and a *'down and out'* *eye. Ptosis is usually complete*, so you would need to retract the lid to see these signs. The degree of ptosis alone should direct you to considering a third nerve palsy.

Horner's syndrome

There is a *small pupil on the side of the ptosis. Ptosis is partial*. Proceed as for Horner's syndrome (Case study 6.8).

Myasthenia gravis

The *pupils are normal*. There is often a *complex ophthalmoplegia* and *fatiguable weakness* of eyelid closure (seventh nerve) and eyelid opening (third nerve). *Ptosis* may be *unilateral or bilateral*.

Myotonic dystrophy

Pupils and eye movements are normal. *Cataracts* may be present. *Ptosis is bilateral*. The face is typically myotonic (Case study 6.32).

Other

Rarer causes, with normal pupils and eye movements, include congenital ptosis, oculopharyngeal muscular dystrophy, and oedema.

DISCUSSION

What other causes of large/small pupils do you know of?

These are discussed below.

CASE STUDY   6.6 LARGE (MYDRIATIC) PUPIL

Instruction: *Examine this patient's pupils and discuss your findings.*

RECOGNITION

There may be difficulty in deciding whether one pupil is *too big* or if the other is too small. Fortunately, knowledge of causes helps you to determine the abnormality.

INTERPRETATION

Look for/consider causes

1. **Third nerve palsy.** Look for *ptosis* on the side of the larger pupil and a *'down and out' eye. Examine eye movements.*
2. **Holmes–Adie (tonic) pupil.** This is of unknown cause, but probably results from damage to the ciliary ganglion, perhaps of viral aetiology. It often affects young women. The dilated pupil may be present long before a patient's attention is drawn to it. Holmes–Adie pupils are often *widely dilated*, and *react slowly to light*, but *react to accommodation*. They are usually *unilateral*, at least at first. Check *ankle and knee reflexes*. Absent *reflexes* suggest *Holmes–Adie syndrome*.
3. **Traumatic iridoplegia.** This may occur unilaterally due to damage to the ciliary pupilloconstrictor mechanism.
4. **Drug causes.** If both pupils are dilated, consider a drug induced cause.

If both eyes are blind for any reason in which light is prevented from reaching both optic nerves and triggering the light reflex response, there will also be bilateral mydriasis.

Which drugs act as mydriatics?

- Tropicamide.
- Cocaine or amphetamines.
- Atropine and other anticholinergics (gardeners may develop mydriasis after contact with an anticholinergically endowed plant, the 'cause–effect' often elusive without a thorough history).

What governs pupil size?

Pupil size is balanced by the effect on the ciliary muscle of constricting parasympathetic fibres acting via the ciliary ganglion and dilating sympathetic fibres acting via the superior cervical ganglion.

CASE STUDY   6.7 SMALL (MIOTIC) PUPIL

Instruction: *Examine this patient's pupils and discuss your findings.*

RECOGNITION

Again, the difficulty may be in determining if one pupil is *too small* or the other too big. If there are *no obvious signs of a third nerve palsy* and the *larger pupil reacts quickly to light*, consider the causes of a small pupil.

INTERPRETATION

Look for/consider causes

1. **Horner's syndrome.** A Horner's syndrome is usually *unilateral* and the *pupil reacts to light.* Look for *partial ptosis.*
2. **Argyll Robertson pupils (ARPs).** These are *bilaterally small, irregularly shaped pupils* which *accommodate but do not react to light.* The site of damage which results in ARPs remains uncertain but the accommodation reflex (page 261) is subserved by more pupilloconstrictor fibres than the light reflex, and this alone may explain the dissociation. ARPs are classically attributed to neurosyphilis.
3. **Anisocoria.** 20% of people normally have pupil asymmetry.
4. **Age related miosis.** Both pupils can become smaller with age, but still react to light and accommodation, and this probably represents autonomic degeneration.

DISCUSSION

Which common drugs cause miosis?

- Pilocarpine ● Opiates.

What causes might you consider in a patient with a depressed conscious level?

● Pontine lesions such as haemorrhage or encephalitis ● Opiate overdose.

What is the cause if the eye is red and painful?

Iritis (pages 184–185).

CASE STUDY	6.8 HORNER'S SYNDROME

Instruction: *Examine this patient's pupils and anything else you think appropriate, then discuss your findings.*

RECOGNITION

1. There is *miosis* (reduced pupillodilator activity) (Fig. 6.8) ipsilateral to the site of the lesion.
2. There is *partial ptosis* (because the levator palpabrae of the upper lid is partially supplied by the sympathetic nervous system as well as the parasympathetic supply that travels with the third nerve) ipsilateral to the site of the lesion.
3. There may be *anhydrosis* or absence of sweating (in preganglionic lesions only because sweat gland outflow is proximal to the superior cervical ganglion).
4. Apparent *enophthalmos* (due to paralysis of the upper and lower eyelid tarsus muscles) is seldom seen.

INTERPRETATION

Horner's syndrome is due to interruption of the sympathetic chain and may originate anywhere along this chain (Fig. 6.9).

Look for/consider causes

It's helpful to consider *three main sites* where lesions can occur and the *lesions at these sites* which may occur:

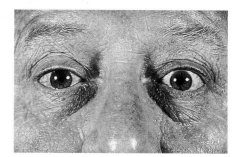

Fig. 6.8   *Horner's syndrome. Reproduced with permission from M.A. Mir (1995) Atlas of Clinical Diagnosis. W.B. Saunders, London*

Fig. 6.9　*Horner's syndrome*

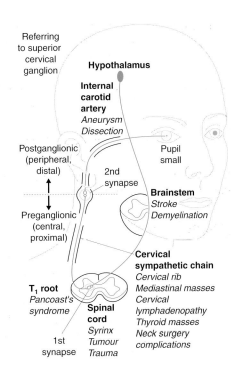

I. The first neuron

The sympathetic pathway starts in the *hypothalamus* and travels through the *brainstem*, terminating in the grey matter of the *spinal cord at C8, T1*. Lesions include:

● **Brainstem strokes** such as lateral medullary syndrome. The sympathetic pathway in the brainstem lies close to the spinothalamic tracts (page 312). *Contralateral body loss of pain and temperature sensation* is therefore a frequent finding in a Horner's syndrome arising from the brainstem.

● **Demyelination** in the brainstem or spinal cord. Other signs of demyelination include the five signs of optic nerve damage (page 264), internuclear ophthalmoplegia, cerebellar signs, spastic paraparesis and sensory disturbance.

● **Syringomyelia/syringobulbia**, resulting in a *'cape' distribution of dissociated sensory loss* (Case study 6.19).

● **Spinal cord tumours or trauma.**

II. The second neuron

Sometimes referred to as the *preganglionic neuron*, referring to the *superior cervical ganglion (SCG)*, the sympathetic pathway travels from C8/T1 via their nerve roots to the SCG. Preganglionic (also known as central or proximal) lesions are the most common causes of Horner's syndrome.

- **Pancoast's syndrome**, in which a tumour of the thoracic inlet may infiltrate and cause pain in the distribution of T1 or C8. *Percuss and auscultate the supraclavicular area for signs of consolidation and look for ipsilateral wasting of the small muscles of the hand.*
- A **cervical rib**, which may be confirmed by chest X-ray.
- A **mediastinal mass** *(look for distended neck veins of superior vena cava obstruction)*.
- **Cervical lymphadenopathy.**
- **Thyroid masses.**
- **Complications of neck surgery** such as endarterectomy disrupting the sympathetic chain. *Look for neck scars.*

III. The third neuron

The *postganglionic* sympathetic pathway travels from the SCG in close proximity to the carotid artery and innervates the pupil (via long ciliary nerves which traverse around the eye), the blood vessels of the eye (via vasomotor fibres in the nasociliary branch of the trigeminal nerve) and the upper and lower lid tarsus muscles (which open the eye and oppose the action of orbicularis).

Postganglionic (otherwise known as peripheral or distal) lesions include *carotid artery aneurysms* and *carotid dissection*.

Evidence of decompensation

A Pancoast's lesion implies invasive disease.

DISCUSSION

How might you determine the site of a Horner's syndrome lesion?

This is usually by identifying the cause. Chemical eye drops methods to determine if a lesion is central or peripheral are historical.

CASE STUDY   6.9 CEREBELLOPONTINE ANGLE SYNDROME

Instruction: *Examine this patient's cranial nerves. Discuss your findings.*

RECOGNITION

Any combination of *cranial neuropathies* involving the *trigeminal, facial* and *vestibulocochlear* nerve may occur. *Corneal reflex loss* is often the first sign, followed by facial sensory loss. Facial weakness can be a late sign. There may be *nystagmus*. There may be *sensorineural deafness*.

INTERPRETATION

Look for/consider causes

Cerebellopontine angle lesions, including *acoustic neuromas* and *meningiomas*, may cause *slowly progressive hearing loss or tinnitus*. Vertigo is a rare and late sign. The next step is neuroimaging.

DISCUSSION

What is the cerebellopontine angle (CPA)?

The CPA is a triangle between the cerebellum, lateral pons and petrous bone (Fig. 6.10). Cranial nerves 5–8 emerge into it from the pons in cranio-caudal sequence. The CPA stops just above nerve 9, which emerges from the medulla.

Tell us about the divisions of the trigeminal nerve

The trigeminal nerve divides into three divisions from the trigeminal ganglion, which lies on the petrous tip. Each division conveys sensation (from many distal branches) from the face:

1. *Ophthalmic.* Runs via the superior orbital fissure and cavernous sinus conveying sensation from the forehead and scalp. The nasociliary branch supplies the nostril and the tip and upper border of the nose, carries sympathetic fibres to the pupil and conveys the sensory limb of the corneal reflex.
2. *Maxillary.* Runs via the inferior orbital fissure and cavernous sinus conveying sensation from the cheek, much of the oral cavity and

Fig. 6.10   *The cerebellopontine angle*

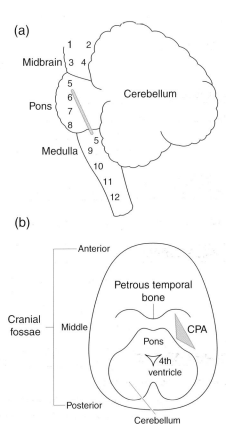

mid-face. One branch thickens into a special ganglion called the pterygopalatine ganglion. This ganglion receives preganglionic parasympathetic fibres which travelled to it with the nervus intermedius (a branch of the facial nerve) and which travel from it to supply the lacrimal gland.

3. *Mandibular.* Exits at foramen ovale and supplies the jaw and lower face. Also carries motor branches to the muscles of mastication, the masseter which is very strong (jaw closure) and the pterygoids which are weak (jaw opening).

What trigeminal neuropathies do you know of?

Trigeminal neuropathies may be part of a wider CPA syndrome, with loss of the corneal reflex often the first clinical sign. Other clinical conditions affecting the trigeminal nerve include *herpes zoster ophthalmicus* and *trigeminal neuralgia.*

What do you understand by the term jugular foramen syndrome?

The final four cranial nerves occupy an area around the jugular foramen. Lesions in this area may be extend from the CPA, or arise as localised or diffuse basal skull lesions (such as chronic tuberculosis or malignancy, including lymphomatous meningitis). Lesions may provoke a bulbar palsy.

CASE STUDY   **6.10 FACIAL NERVE PALSY**

Instruction: *Examine this patient's face. Discuss your differential diagnosis.*

RECOGNITION

There is *paralysis of one side of the face* (Fig. 6.11). In the *upper face*, the *eye does not close fully* (the eyeball may roll up on attempted

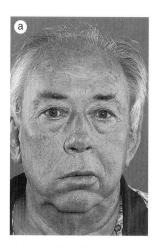 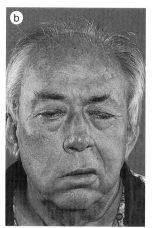 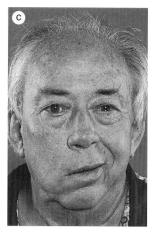

Fig. 6.11   *Facial nerve palsy: (a) at rest; (b) closing eyes; (c) smiling*

closure—Bell's phenomenon). Muscles that do not work include the orbicularis oculi (closes eye), the frontalis (raises eyebrow) and the corrugator superficialis (frowns). In the *lower face*, the *mouth droops* and the *nasolabial fold* is *smooth*.

INTERPRETATION

Look for/consider causes

Tell the examiners that you would consider whether or not *secretomotor function, hearing* and *taste* are affected. These *theoretically* help to localise the lesion, but *in practice* are variable.

Knowing the possible causes of facial nerve palsy enables you to rapidly look for other relevant signs:

1. **Bell's palsy.** This is idiopathic, possibly viral. Usually, but not always, *the only sign is facial weakness*, the presumed site of inflammation or damage distal in the facial canal.
2. **Ramsay Hunt syndrome.** This is due to *herpes zoster* reactivation in the geniculate ganglion. Taste tends to be affected and there may be *vesicles* over the external auditory meatus. Occasionally vesicles hide exclusively within the ear canal.
3. **Parotid swellings.** Look and feel for a swollen parotid gland, which may be due to infection, often secondary to a salivary duct calculus, or a parotid tumour.
4. **Brainstem strokes or demyelination.** These may involve the facial nerve nucleus and precipitate facial weakness.
5. **Cerebellopontine lesions.** These should always be considered, especially if there is *loss of the corneal reflex or hearing.*
6. **Cholesteatoma.** This is a rare cause. Epithelial cells accumulate behind the tympanic membrane, sometimes leading to perforation. Appraisal by an ENT specialist is mandatory.
7. **Bilateral facial nerve weakness.** This is often missed although weakness may not be symmetrical. Causes include bilateral Bell's palsy, acute inflammatory demyelinating polyneuropathy (Guillain–Barré syndrome), neurosarcoid and Lyme disease.

DISCUSSION

Describe the course of the facial nerve. How may knowledge of this help determine the site of a facial nerve lesion?

The facial nerve (Fig. 6.12):

1. Exits the internal auditory canal, where it lies just above the eighth nerve, to *traverse the facial canal within the petrous temporal bone.*
2. Has *two major roots* as it enters the facial canal, a *motor root* and a *sensory root* (*the nervus intermedius*), forming the *geniculate*

Fig. 6.12   *The facial nerve*

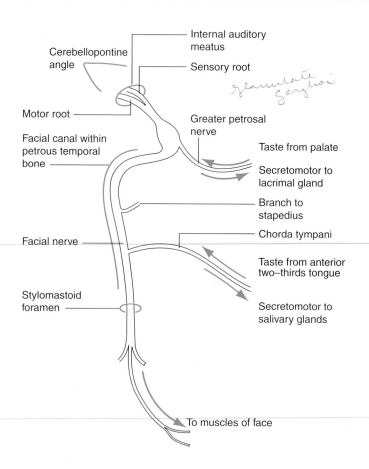

ganglion, in close proximity to the trigeminal ganglion. The *nervus intermedius is an area of convergence of the facial nerve's limited sensory fibres in transit to the brain and also relays secretomotor parasympathetic fibres, which originated in the brainstem, to the submandibular and sublingual salivary glands and (via the otic ganglion) parotid gland.*

3. Gives off an early branch, the *greater petrosal nerve, which carries taste from the palate and secretomotor fibres to the lacrimal gland via the pterygoid canal.* **Lesions distal to or at this site cause, in addition to the signs below, impaired lacrimation.**

4. Further along the facial canal gives off a *branch to stapedius,* which cushions noise. **Lesions distal to or at this site cause, in addition to the signs below, hyperacusis.**

5. Next gives off the *chorda tympani,* which carries *taste from the anterior two-thirds of the tongue* and relays the *parasympathetic submandibular and sublingual fibres* to their final destination. **Lesions distal to or at this site cause, in addition to facial palsy, impaired taste and salivary secretion.**

**Upper motor neuron facial weakness –
left side**

**Lower motor neuron facial weakness –
left side**

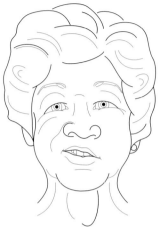
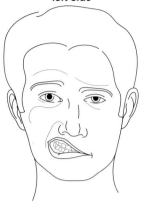

Upper face unaffected.
Slight droop of mouth and flattening of
nasolabial fold

Affects upper and lower face.
Weakness of forehead, eye closure and mouth

Fig. 6.13   *Upper and lower motor neuron facial weakness (patient asked to show teeth)*

6. Finally exits at the *stylomastoid foramen*, sending a branch to the ear muscles and *traverses the parotid gland* dividing into the motor *temporal, zygomatic, buccal, mandibular and cervical branches* which give power to the face. Lesions here cause **facial palsy only.**

How do you distinguish a lower from an upper motor neuron facial weakness?

A facial nerve palsy is just that! There is paralysis of the upper and lower parts of the face due to a lesion in the facial nerve (Fig. 6.13). Candidates often talk of 'lower motor neuron facial nerve weakness.' By definition, facial nerve lesions are lower neuron lesions because the facial nerve is the lower neuron innervating the face! Upper motor neuron facial weakness, due to a lesion in the supranuclear neurons which innervate the facial nerve, spares the upper face and is discussed in Case study 6.13.

Section 2 Lesions of the Cerebral Hemispheres

EXAMINATION: HIGHER CORTICAL FUNCTION, SPEECH AND LOBES OF THE BRAIN

Examining higher cortical function adequately is a complex task which cannot be performed in PACES and should not be requested. A mini-mental state examination (Case study 6.11) is frequently performed on the wards. Detailed examination of higher cortical function requires detailed knowledge of the different functions of the lobes of the brain. In PACES, you could be asked to examine speech or to briefly assess parietal lobe function.

Examining speech and language

You are looking for evidence of one of the problems in Box 6.6.

A scheme for assessing the speech and language problems in Box 6.6 is:

1. **Consider if there is dysphasia:**
   (i) Ask your patient to close their eyes (**?receptive dysphasia**).
   (ii) Ask your patient to tell you their name, address, etc. (**?expressive dysphasia**).
   (iii) If your patient can't perform either, they have a **global dysphasia**.
   (iv) Ask your patient to name exhibited objects (pen, tie, watch) *What is this?* If the patient is unable to tell you, ask *Is it*

a...? (**?nominal dysphasia**). Nominal dysphasia is usually part of a wider dysphasia.
   (v) You could ask your patient to read and write a sentence, but this is not usually expected by examiners in PACES.

2. **Consider if there is dysarthria:**
   (i) **Pseudobulbar palsy.** This refers to supranuclear disease with spastic speech. There is lack of modulation. The tongue appears small and 'tight', and cannot be protruded, lying immobile on the floor of the mouth. Analogies include 'high pitched', 'Donald duck', 'hot potato' or 'strained' speech. Bilateral supranuclear innervation of the lower (bulbar) cranial nerves necessary for speech and swallowing means that bilateral cortical or brainstem lesions are required to induce a pseudobulbar palsy. Causes include bilateral internal capsule strokes or demyelination.

Box 6.6   Speech and Language Problems

Receptive dysphasia
The inability to comprehend, or understand. Receptive dysphasia is due to lesions in Wernicke's area in the dominant temporal lobe.

Expressive dysphasia
The inability to express, despite adequate comprehension. This can cause immense frustration to patients who know 'in their minds' exactly what they want to say but can't formulate the words. Expressive dysphasia is due to lesions in Broca's area in the frontal lobe.

Global dysphasia
Damage to both areas above causes receptive and expressive dysphasia.

Nominal dysphasia
The inability to name objects. When shown a key and asked if it is a pen, a patient may

be able to respond with 'No', and if it is a key, with 'Yes'.

Dyslexia or dysgraphia
The inability to read or write.

Dysarthria
Dysarthria simply means difficulty with articulation or coordinating the structures needed for voice production. It is *not* synonymous with cerebellar disease but may result from supranuclear/upper motor neuron (UMN) lesions (pseudobulbar palsy), cerebellar lesions, extrapyramidal lesions, infranuclear/lower motor neuron (LMN) lesions (bulbar palsy) or local causes such as oral candidiasis.

Dysphonia
Impaired voice production or phonation, as seen in vocal cord disease such as laryngitis or damaged vagal supply.

(ii) **Cerebellar dysarthria.** There is waxing and waning staccato speech. The patient cannot generally say *eee* without undulation. Difficult phrases include *eleven benevolent elephants* and *baby hippopotamus*! Other signs of cerebellar disease are described in Case study 6.16.

(iii) **Extrapyramidal dysarthria.** This is described with Parkinson's disease in Case study 6.15.

(iv) **Bulbar palsy.** This refers to infra-nuclear disease with flaccid speech. Analogies are 'drowning' or 'choking' and a sense that 'everything is in the way'. The tongue seems too big for the mouth and seems to hang out with salivary pooling and nasal escape speech. Unilateral LMN lesions (cranial neuropathies), myasthenia gravis and also myopathies cause bulbar dysarthria.

Note: *ppp* tests lip movements, *ttt* or *lll* tongue movement, *kkk* palatal movement.

3. **Consider if there is dysphonia.** Can the patient cough or produce a sustained 'eee'? Dysphonia with a normal cough implies a local (laryngeal) lesion: a bovine cough (without an explosive start) suggests vocal cord palsy.

Examining the lobes of the brain and recognising lobe syndromes

The cranial nerves, which are merely peripheral nerves, *send sensory information to the brain* and *receive motor information from the brain*. Likewise, the rest of the body, through peripheral nerves and nerve roots sends sensory information to the central nervous system and receives motor information from it. Some of this information does not involve the hemispheres of the cerebral cortex. The corneal reflex, for example, is a rapid involuntary relay between the afferent sensory fibres of the trigeminal nerve and the efferent motor fibres of the facial nerve. It makes evolutionary sense to rapidly protect the eyes from danger. Spinal reflexes are similar. *But for most information, the cerebral cortex prefers to be involved, perceiving everything in our world and initiating almost everything we do. Some of the information to and from the cortex is modified by the cerebellum and extrapyramidal system respectively.* The different lobes of the cortex have specific functions.

The frontal lobe

The frontal lobe is a *motor* lobe. It *plans* and *initiates* tasks. The *precentral gyrus* or *motor strip* is part of the frontal lobe, and puts thoughts into action. It is here that the cascade of messages to move a part of the body begins. Functions subserved by the frontal lobe are shown in Box 6.7.

The posterior parts of the frontal lobe are most important functionally.

Frontal lobe disease may result in those features in Box 6.8:

The frontal lobes not only inhibit undesirable behaviour but also the *primitive reflexes* that are present at birth. These may be disinhibited by frontal lobe disease and include:

- *Grasp*: Stroking the patient's palm induces a grasp
- *Palmomental*: Firmly stroking the patient's thenar eminence induces an ipsilateral grimace
- *Rooting*: Stroking the patient's cheek induces a gnawing mouth movement
- *Sucking*: Touching the patient's lips promotes sucking
- *Snout*: Tapping the patient's upper lip makes it pucker upwards
- *Glabellar*: Tapping the patient's forehead stimulates eye closure.

Box 6.7   Functions Subserved by the Frontal lobe

1. Planning
2. Initiation of movement
3. Speech expression involving Broca's speech area (in the dominant hemisphere)
4. Attention and concentration
5. Voluntary control of micturition
6. Acquired social behaviour.

Box 6.8   Potential Effects of Frontal Lobe Disease

1. *Akinesia* (difficulty with movement)
2. *Apathy* (loss of initiative) and *abulia* (loss of spontaneity)
3. Motor or *expressive dysphasia* (if dominant hemisphere)
4. Distractibility, perseveration
5. Incontinence
6. Mood disturbance and disinhibition

Connections between different parts of the brain explain many neurological signs. Patients with Parkinson's disease may have a positive glabellar tap because of disease in the frontal lobe's extrapyramidal connections.

The parietal lobe

The parietal lobe contains the *sensory cortex* or *precentral gyrus*. Unlike the frontal lobe, the parietal lobe is very much a sensory lobe. It is concerned with appreciating the world around us. It might be considered the lobe for *awareness*.

Both the dominant parietal lobe and the non-dominant parietal lobe are concerned with recognition and awareness of things, and both relay the parietal radiations of the visual pathways (pages 263–264).

Disease in a parietal lobe may manifest itself broadly in one of two ways (Box 6.9).

Lesions in the parietal lobes may cause a specific problem or multiple problems, sometimes grouped into recognised syndromes. The dominant parietal lobe is usually left sided (even in left handed people, whose 'dominant' hemisphere we often assume as being the right). There is much overlap of dominant parietal lobe and non-dominant parietal lobe function.

The occipital lobe

The occipital lobe is the final common endpoint of the visual nerve pathways. Lesions may result in *cortical blindness* (pages 263–264), *visual agnosia* (parieto-occipital connections) or specific visual processing defects such as impaired perception of colour or moving objects.

Box 6.9   Two Important Manifestations of Parietal Lobe Disease

Agnosias

There may be *difficulty in recognising* things, despite intact sensory pathways peripheral to the parietal lobe. These problems with recognition are often termed *agnosias*.

Apraxias

There may be *difficulty in performing tasks*, not because there is any loss of executive function—the frontal lobe and motor pathways (and cerebellum/extrapyramidal system) are all intact—but because the parietal lobe has failed to process information about the environment. It would normally pass on this processed information to the frontal lobe, which in turn would normally initiate a course of action in response to it. These problems with performing tasks are often termed *dyspraxias* or *apraxias*.

The temporal lobe

The temporal lobe subserves memory (hippocampus and other areas), central representation of hearing, taste and smell, speech interpretation, transmission of visual impulses via the temporal visual radiations (pages 263–264), and behaviour via frontal lobe connections. Lesions may result in *memory impairment, auditory agnosia* (via the temporo-parietal connections), *cortical deafness* (if bilateral) and *Wernicke's sensory or receptive dysphasia*.

The limbic system

In summary, the *cerebral hemispheres perceive and initiate*. They are in contact with the outside world through sensory and motor pathways. But what about the inside world? What about thought itself? There is extreme complexity in the visual pathways relaying what we see, but we always see a particular object in the same way. A monkey always looks like a monkey, a giraffe a giraffe and we would never confuse the two. But even visual pathways seem crude compared to mechanisms of recognition, learning, thought and emotion. The limbic system is a part of the brain where science has more questions than answers. It has to do with memory. It is also thought to be a centre for smell. Have you noticed that some smells instantly evoke distant memories?

CASE STUDY	**6.11 MILD COGNITIVE IMPAIRMENT AND DEMENTIA**

Instruction: This 74 year old lady has a history of hypertension. Her husband reports increasing forgetfulness over the past year and some unexplained falls. She has burnt the cooking pot on one occasion. Her minimental state examination (MMSE) score on the ward was 21. Please ask her some questions.

RECOGNITION	

Memory is *impaired for recent events* and she is *disorientated* in time. Memory for distant events is preserved. The *minimental state examination (MMSE)* awards 1 point for each correct of 30 responses and tests:

- *Orientation* (e.g. name season/date/day/month/year/hospital/town/country)
- *Registration* (identify 3 objects by name and ask patient to repeat)
- *Attention and calculation* (patient subtracts serial 7s)
- *Recall* (the 3 objects)
- *Language* (naming objects, repeating a sentence, following a 3 step command, obeying a written command, writing a sentence and copying a design such as intersecting pentagons).

Many objective mental state examination tests evaluate memory, grasp of information, abstract thought, insight, judgement and intellect in more detail. Retentive memory and immediate recall are tested in the MMSE, recent memory can be tested by recall at defined interval, e.g. 5/15 minutes, and remote memory by the patient's ability to provide a coherent chronology of their illness or life events. Proverb interpretation can provide information about judgement and abstract reasoning. Specific higher cortical functions can be tested when clinical circumstances suggest deficits might be present, such as speech assessment and tests of spatial awareness, body perception and praxis (Case study 6.12) such as brushing teeth and combing hair. A full mental state assessment would explore mood and thoughts.

A list of ten questions (*age, time to nearest hour, place, address for recall at end of test, year, recognition of two people, date of birth, dates of Second World War, name of monarch, count backwards from 20 to 1*) should be all that is required in PACES, at least 9/10 normally expected and < 7/10 suggesting established dementia. You should be aware of its limitations and that tests of knowledge should be tailored to a patient's age and background. An MMSE of 21 indicates a mild dementia syndrome.

INTERPRETATION

Look for/consider causes

- Alzheimer's disease (Insidious memory impairment)
- Multi-infarct/vascular dementia (often stepwise periods of deterioration interspersed with periods of stability)
- Prion disease (see below)
- Normal pressure hydrocephalus (NPH)
- A space occupying lesion, especially a chronic subdural haematoma, an important cause of reversible dementia
- B vitamin deficiencies (especially in chronic alcohol misuse)
- Huntington's chorea (family history)

Assess severity

- *Dementia* is a disorder characterised by global impairment of higher mental function (notably memory, cognition, personality and social behaviour) that is not a part of the normal ageing process.
- *Mild cognitive impairment* (MCI) is common. A typical patient might forget to pay bills and collect their pension on the right day, have an MMSE score of 28/30, and not to have a formal diagnosis of dementia at this stage.

Delirium (acute confusion/altered consciousness) and depression can masquerade as dementia.

DISCUSSION

What causes Alzheimer's disease?

Apolipoprotein E (ApoE) is a cholesterol transporter lipoprotein made in the liver with three isomers. The ApoE4 allele in its heterozygous and homozygous form is associated with an increased risk of late onset Alzheimer's disease, whilst rarer early onset Alzheimer's disease may be attributable to rarer mutations in genes for presenilin (1 and 2) and β-amyloid precursor protein. Alzheimer's disease is a neurodegenerative condition with progressive cerebral atrophy characterised histopathologically by neurofibrillary tangles (NFTs) containing the protein tau and beta amyloid plaques.

Acetylcholinesterase inhibitors increase levels of acetylcholine, one of the depleted neurotransmitters in Alzheimer's disease, and are used in early disease. Selected patients with more advanced disease may benefit from N-methyl-D-aspartate blockers.

Do similar changes occur in other neurodegenerative disorders?

The pathogenesis of many neurodegenerative disorders is associated with accumulation of protein deposits in brain parenchyma. A normal soluble cellular protein is converted into an abnormal insoluble toxic aggregated protein rich in beta sheets, as in beta amyloid in Alzheimer's disease. Many neurodegenerative disorders are associated with amyloid accumulation and many are associated with trinucleotide CAG repeat sequences which may cause protein aggregation. Research into treatments which inhibit or breakdown insoluble protein aggregates is ongoing.

What are prions and what do they cause?

The term prion disease is often used interchangeably with Creutzfeldt–Jakob disease (CJD) or transmissible spongiform encephalopathy (TSE). These diseases are caused by proteinaceous infectious agents (which are not organisms) called prions. Prions are proteins derived from simple genes on chromosome 20, coding for the prion protein (PrP). PrP is ubiquitous. We all have Pr, and its natural function is uncertain. When PrP is mutated it causes disease by aggregating into amyloid like plaques.

Prion diseases may be:

- Inherited (familial, autosomal dominant CJD)
- Acquired (iatrogenic CJD, such as that acquired from cadaveric derived growth hormone or from ingestion of brain tissue as in 'kuru')
- Sporadic (more than 85% of all CJD).

How does sporadic CJD present?

- Rapidly progressive dementia ● Myoclonus ● Ataxia.

These result from neuron loss in a spongiform (vacuolated) brain with some gliosis. Most patients have periodic sharp complexes on EEG.

What do you understand by the term new variant CJD (nvCJD)?

nvCJD or bovine spongiform encephalopathy (BSE) tends to affect a younger age group, and presents with early neuropsychiatric symptoms and ataxia. The EEG is not typical.

What is normal pressure hydrocephalus (NPH)?

The arachnoid villi, which absorb CSF, seem to take long tea breaks in NPH! CSF accumulates, giving rise to the following triad:

● Urinary incontinence, due to pressure on the voluntary control micturition centre
● Gait apraxia
● Dementia.

If diagnosed and managed early with a shunt, NPH is fully reversible. Early diagnosis is challenged by frequently normal brain imaging and CSF pressure. NPH should more accurately be called 'intermittently normal pressure hydrocephalus'.

List some causes of acute confusion/altered consciousness

Remember the mnemonic AEIOUTHIPS:

● Alcohol
● Epilepsy/seizure
● Insulin/glucose disturbance
● Oxygenation disturbance
● Urea and electrolyte disturbance
● TIA/stroke/trauma/tumour/temperature disturbance/thrombotic thrombocytopenic purpura
● Heart/cardiac causes
● Infection
● Poisoning
● SLE with cerebral involvement/other connective tissue disorders.

CASE STUDY   6.12 AGNOSIAS, APRAXIAS AND OTHER SIGNS OF PARIETAL LOBE DYSFUNCTION

Instruction: *Please assess this patient's parietal lobe function.*

RECOGNITION

1. There may be *difficulty localising the modalities of peripheral sensation*—light touch, pain, proprioception and temperature, and loss of two-point discrimination. Normally the fingertips are able to distinguish two points a few millimetres apart.
2. There may be a specific **agnosia:**
   (i) *Tactile agnosia (astereognosis).* There is inability to recognise

an object such as a key placed in the hand with the eyes closed. This is despite intact sensory pathways from hand to brain and motor pathways from the brain allowing adequate manipulation of the object. Opening the eyes or rattling the keys may prompt recognition. The lesion is in the contralateral parietal lobe. *Agraphaesthesia* refers to the inability to interpret numbers stroked on the palm of the hand.

(ii) *Visual agnosia.* There is inability to recognise a familiar object by sight, despite intact visual pathways to the occipital lobe. Touching the object may prompt recognition. The lesion is in the contralateral parieto-occipital area. *Prosopagnosia* refers to the inability to recognise a familiar face.

(iii) *Auditory agnosia.* There is inability to recognise familiar sounds such as voices, music or the telephone.

(iv) *Sensory inattention or neglect.* These terms cause confusion for many candidates. *Autotopagnosia* refers to the inability to identify parts of the body. The patient may be *unaware of one side of the body.* The lesion is usually, but not exclusively, in the right non-dominant parietal lobe giving rise to *neglect* of the left side of the body. There may be *anosagnosia* in which a patient is *unaware of any disability* (may move right side if asked to move left).

3. There may be a specific **apraxia.** There may be difficulty in performing tasks such as combing hair, brushing teeth or writing. The key thing to remember is that the sensory pathways, motor pathways and adjustment pathways (cerebellum and extrapyramidal system) all work normally. Common apraxias include:

(i) *Dressing apraxia.* The patient may be unable to put on their pyjama top, especially if turned inside out.

(ii) *Gait apraxia.* The patient is unable to put one foot in front of the other. Sensation of the ground, and the motor mechanisms of walking and balance, are all normal. The problem may be in the parietal lobe itself or in its connections with the frontal lobe or extrapyramidal system. Gait apraxia may be overcome if other parts of the brain assume a greater role than usual. Patients may be able to walk if they look at the ground, especially if 'the cracks between paving slabs' provide assisted visual input.

4. There may be a homonymous quadrantanopia (pages 263–264).

INTERPRETATION

Assess function

The overwhelming difficulties caused by parietal lobe disease are functional.

There is much overlap of dominant parietal lobe (usually left sided) and non-dominant parietal lobe function. Generally, most of the agnosias are due to disease of the non-dominant parietal lobe.

An important specific syndrome of the dominant parietal lobe is
Gerstmann's syndrome, comprising:

AALF

Agrapha

Alexa

fingeragnose

(L)-Ragnose

- Agraphia (inability to write)
- Alexia (inability to read)
- Finger agnosia/acalculia (inability to name and count fingers)
- Right–left agnosia (inability to determine right from left).

Problems with numeracy (such as serial 7s) are more commonly seen
as part of global cortical decline in dementia.

DISCUSSION

Do you know of any other types of apraxia?

- *Topographic apraxia*: patients might not be able to find their way
  back to their bed.
- *Constructional apraxia*: patients are unable to construct shapes or
  patterns using, for example, matchsticks or wooden blocks, and
  are unable to copy shapes such as a 5-pointed star or fill in the
  numbers on a clock face.
- *Ideomotor apraxia*: patients are able to perform a task
  automatically but not on command.
- *Ideational apraxia*: patients are unable to perform a series of tasks.

What are the causes of parietal lobe dysfunction?

Parietal lobe signs may result from structural lesions of one parietal
lobe such as strokes or tumours or from diffuse damage to both
parietal lobes as in hepatic encephalopathy.

CASE STUDY   6.13 ANTERIOR CIRCULATION STROKE SYNDROMES

Instruction: *Examine this patient's face and limbs and discuss your findings.*

RECOGNITION

Each lobe does not have a discrete blood supply. *Stroke syndromes*
are thus different from *lobe syndromes* and there are an infinite
number. It is helpful to briefly revise brain vascular anatomy
(Box 6.10, Fig. 6.14) and cortical representation of body structures
(Fig. 6.15).

Anterior Cerebral Artery (ACA) Syndrome

The anterior communicating artery is a protective anastomosis
between the two ACAs and signs of occlusion are much less common
than for MCA territory. If the anastomosis fails to compensate there is
*contralateral leg weakness and sensory loss. Voluntary control of
micturition may be lost.*

Box 6.10	Blood Vessels of the Brain

The 'Circle of Willis' is a fusion of vessels which supply the anterior and posterior fossae.

Anterior circulation

The *anterior cerebral artery* (*ACA*) supplies the parasagittal cortex including the motor (predominantly frontal lobe) and sensory (predominantly parietal lobe) cortices for the leg. The *middle cerebral artery* (*MCA*) supplies most of the lateral cortex, its main trunk dividing into three major branches. Smaller *lenticulostriate* branches supply the anterior limb of the internal capsule and the basal ganglia. The main vessel terminates as a wisp in the occipital lobe to supply the macular cortex.

Posterior circulation

Bilateral *vertebral arteries* fuse to form a single midline *basilar artery*, and these arteries collectively supply the lower brainstem and cerebellum. The *posterior cerebral arteries* (*PCAs*) are formed from the bifurcation of the basilar artery and supply the upper brainstem, thalamus, posterior limb of the internal capsule and the visual cortex (via the terminal calcarine artery).

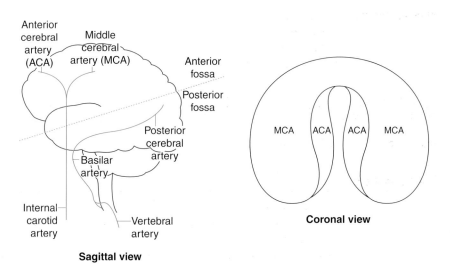

Fig. 6.14   *Blood supply to the anterior and posterior fossae*

Middle Cerebral Artery (MCA) Syndrome

Main trunk occlusion causes devastating infarction of much of one hemisphere. This may be clinically indistinguishable from internal carotid artery occlusion, resulting in a *total anterior circulation syndrome*:

Fig. 6.15   *Cortical representation of body structures*

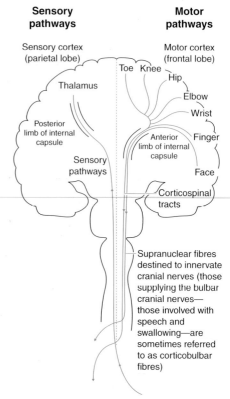

Sensory pathways

Motor pathways

- *Contralateral hemiparesis* — weak face, arm and often leg (leg cortex is spared but fibres running from it may infarct) with *increased tone and reflexes* (limb examination is described in Section 6)
- *Contralateral hemisensory loss*
- *Contralateral homonymous hemianopia* (infarction of optic radiations running through parietal and temporal lobes)
- *Global (expressive and receptive) dysphasia if dominant cortex*
- Severe *agnosias* and *apraxias* (*neglect* if left sided limb signs).

INTERPRETATION

Confirm the diagnosis

In practice, main trunk occlusions are rare and much more likely to occur is occlusion in one of the MCA's branches. *Lenticulostriate* (small penetrating artery) *occlusions* cause the highly prevalent *anterior limb of 'internal capsule' strokes* (see also Box 6.12) seen in dedicated stroke, care of the elderly and medical receiving units. These are motor strokes because the anterior limb of the internal capsule relays only motor fibres. They cause *contralateral limb weakness* due to corticospinal tract infarction and *contralateral lower facial weakness*. Posterior limb internal capsule strokes cause contralateral hemianaesthesia since the posterior limb relays sensory fibres to the thalamus. Small localised infarcts are often due to lipohyalinosis of penetrating arteries and referred to as *lacunar stroke syndromes*, and can affect the anterior or posterior circulation.

The mechanisms of facial weakness caused by a stroke are explained in Box 6.11.

Box 6.11	**Supranuclear Control of the Facial Nerves (and other cranial nerves)**

Twelve cranial nerves (infranuclear) innervate the face ipsilaterally. These receive innervation from supranuclear pathways via brainstem nuclei. Unfortunately, we cannot think of each cranial nerve as being innervated in the same way. Some are innervated only by a contralateral supranuclear pathway from the contralateral hemisphere; some receive bilateral innervation, a supranuclear pathway from each hemisphere:

- The supranuclear control of conjugate eye movements was discussed on pages 270–271.
- The trigeminal nerve's motor nucleus receives bilateral supranuclear innervation. A unilateral supranuclear lesion does not therefore cause masticatory weakness.
- The facial nerve's fibres supplying the upper face are bilaterally innervated from supranuclear pathways (Fig. 6.16). Fibres to the lower face only receive supranuclear innervation from the contralateral hemisphere (Fig. 6.16). A supranuclear lesion therefore causes only contralateral lower facial weakness.
  It makes sense that we have evolved this way, the muscles for eye protection and chewing having a 'spare parachute' supply. However, there is heterogeneity in the way we have evolved, and although some cranial nerve nuclei derive innervation from both hemispheres, the contribution from each hemisphere is rarely 50 : 50. A patient with a left internal capsule stroke and right limb and right lower face weakness may also have subtle weakness of the right upper face, explained if the left hemisphere contributed more than 50% of supranuclear innervation to the right facial nerve.
- If there is a spare parachute for chewing (trigeminal nerve) it makes sense to have one for swallowing. Supranuclear innervation to the nucleus ambiguus (the motor nucleus for the glossopharyngeal, vagus and accessory nerves) and the hypoglossal nerve, motor to tongue, is variable but bilateral in

most people. The palate, vocal cords and tongue may be transiently weak after an internal capsule stroke in some patients, but recover quickly as compensation from the surviving hemisphere kicks in, and any residual speech difficulty is usually attributable to dysphasia rather than pseudobulbar dysarthria. Strictly, supranuclear fibres controlling bulbar function are termed *corticobulbar* fibres.

● The accessory nerve's supranuclear innervation is such that each hemisphere controls the ipsilateral sternomastoid and contralateral trapezius muscles. Contraction of both muscles enables the head to turn away from the hemisphere in question.

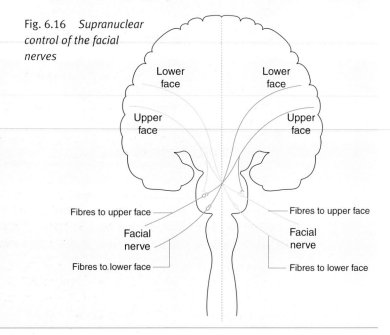

Fig. 6.16   *Supranuclear control of the facial nerves*

Look for/consider causes

Risk factors for strokes and TIAs are discussed in Case study 4.12 and below.

DISCUSSION

Discuss the pathology of stroke

Strokes are characterised by their abrupt (or stepwise) clinical picture.

Many neurological diseases exemplify the eloquence of small parts of the brain. A minor fault often evokes a clinical earthquake. The immune system evolved primarily to fight threats like infection. But evolution takes time, and the contemporary destructive forces of atherosclerosis took evolution by surprise. As it is, the internal capsule, the main thoroughfare for nerve excursion from the cortex, has a disappointing blood supply that is not equipped for breakdown.

Strokes are most commonly occlusive (embolic or atherosclerotic promoting thrombosis) in origin. Small lacunar infarcts are commonly seen on magnetic resonance imaging as deep white matter changes, and illustrate the high prevalence of 'silent' strokes; these may underlie vascular dementia. About 10% of strokes are haemorrhagic (intracerebral, subarachnoid, traumatic) in origin. Arteriovenous malformations are a rare cause of stroke, either through bleeding or through 'stealing' of blood from other territories. Thrombophilic disorders, cerebral vasculitis, dissection of a major artery (trauma may be trivial) and migraine are other causes.

Discuss the principles of stroke management and secondary prevention

Immediate management

1. Patients should be admitted to hospital, preferably to a unit specialising in stroke management.
2. Aspirin should be started within 48 hours. The place of thrombolytic therapy is unresolved.
3. Heparin is not indicated, except where DVT prophylaxis is warranted (appreciable leg weakness).

Investigations

1. Brain imaging is needed to assess the type and size of stroke.
2. Investigations can identify potential embolic sources (ECG for atrial fibrillation, echocardiography for mural thrombus, carotid ultrasound for carotid artery stenosis) or the risk factors below.

Secondary prevention (based on guidelines by the Royal College of Physicians)

1. All patients with ischaemic stroke not anticoagulated should receive an *antiplatelet agent*—aspirin 75–325 mg daily, or clopidogrel, or a combination of low dose aspirin and modified release dipyridamole. Patients intolerant of aspirin should receive an alternative antiplatelet agent, e.g. clopidogrel 75 mg daily.
2. *Anticoagulation* (warfarin):
   (i) should not be used after TIAs or 'minor strokes' unless cardiac embolism is suspected
   (ii) should not be started until brain imaging has excluded haemorrhage and 14 days have passed from the ischaemic event
   (iii) is indicated for patients with atrial fibrillation
   (iv) should be considered for all patients who have ischaemic stroke associated with mitral valve disease, a prosthetic valve or are within 3 months of myocardial infarction.
3. *Antihypertensive therapy* should be considered for all patients (see below).

4. *Statins* should be considered for all patients (Heart Protection Study, page 141).
5. All patients should be assessed for other cardiovascular risk factors and advised/treated appropriately—*smoking cessation, meticulous glycaemic control, low cholesterol/salt diet, exercise.*
6. *Carotid endarterectomy* should be considered if carotid stenosis is > 70%.
7. *Rehabilitation* should not be underestimated since neuronal reserve needs encouragement. Prospects also hinge on how much brain is infarcted and how much ischaemic penumbra with consequent oedema may recover.
8. *Physical activity* is effective in the primary prevention of stroke and may be effective in secondary prevention.
9. Folate supplementation may be protective (page 472).

What do you know about antihypertensive therapy and stroke prevention?

Hypertension is the most important risk factor for stroke. Strict normotensive control should be the aim in *primary* and *secondary* prevention of stroke.

The Heart Outcomes Prevention Evaluation study (HOPE, see also page 141) showed the beneficial effects of the angiotensin converting enzyme inhibitor (ACEI) ramipril on cardiovascular events in patients with vascular disease (previous coronary artery disease, cerebrovascular disease, or peripheral vascular disease) *or* diabetes *plus* an additional risk factor. The impact of prolonged treatment with ramipril was analysed in 9297 patients who were followed for 4.5 years as part of the HOPE study; the analysis showed that ramipril substantially decreased the risk (relative risk reduction 32%) of fatal and non-fatal stroke (and also improved functional and cognitive outcomes) and transient ischaemic attacks in patients with high cardiovascular risk, irrespective of their initial blood pressure and in addition to other preventive treatments such as blood pressure lowering agents or aspirin.

HOPE focused on patients with high cardiovascular risk and controlled blood pressure and was *not a hypertension study*. The underlying mechanisms by which ACEIs prevent vascular events (aside from blood pressure control) are not entirely clear but may include decreased oxidative stress and decreased inflammatory responses with decreased progression of atherosclerotic plaques (pages 143–144), and increased plaque stabilisation.

Whilst blood pressure targets are recommended by the British Hypertension Society (Case study 5.17), the PROGRESS study using perindopril and indapamide (see references) suggested that the lower the BP the better in the secondary prophylaxis of cerebrovascular events and that there may be benefit in treating normotensive patients.

Section 3 Lesions of the Brainstem

CASE STUDY   **6.14 POSTERIOR CIRCULATION AND BRAINSTEM SYNDROMES**

Instruction: *Examine this patient's face and limbs and discuss your findings.*

RECOGNITION

There is a large range of posterior circulation syndromes, many comprising a pot pourri of motor or sensory long tract, cranial nerve and cerebellar signs. Signs include:

- *Bilateral weakness or sensory loss* (if both sides of brainstem involved)
- *Crossed signs* (Box 6.12), e.g. right facial weakness and left limb weakness
- *Cerebellar signs*, e.g. ataxic hemiparesis, a lacunar syndrome caused by an infarct in the base of the pons
- *Diplopia*.

Two classical syndromes caused by infarction in the brainstem are:

Weber's syndrome
~ *ipsilat III nerve palsy & contralat. hemiparesis*

A midbrain lesion causing an *ipsilateral third nerve palsy* (third nerve nucleus/third nerve infarcted) and *contralateral hemiparesis* (the infarcted corticospinal tracts supply the contralateral side of body after decussating in the medulla).

Lateral medullary syndrome   *(Wallenberg's syndrome)*

Also known as Wallenberg's syndrome or posterior inferior cerebellar artery syndrome (although other arteries may be involved) this is due to infarction of the lateral medulla.

It may cause *contralateral loss of pain and temperature sensation* (infarcted spinothalamic tracts, fibres of which have travelled from the contralateral side of the body, pages 311–312), an *ipsilateral Horner's syndrome* (infarcted ipsilateral sympathetic tracts), *bulbar palsy* (slight if there is good bilateral supranuclear bulbar innervation of the bulbar cranial nerves), *ataxia* (infarction of the inferior cerebral peduncle), *vertigo/nystagmus/nausea/vomiting* (infarcted vestibular nuclei) and *ipsilateral loss of facial pain and temperature sensation* (descending tract of trigeminal nucleus invariably infarcted).

The corticospinal tracts are spared in a true Wallenberg's syndrome because infarction is isolated to a specific dorsolateral area of brainstem which in cross section spares these tracts. In practice, most brainstem strokes do not conform to classic syndromes.

Box 6.12	Cortical versus Brainstem Lesions

● A *cortical lesion* such as an internal capsule stroke may cause *contralateral long tract signs* (see below and pages 303–304 and 311–312) and *contralateral supranuclear cranial signs* (Fig. 6.17). Note that some cranial nerves receive bilateral supranuclear innervation (Box 6.11) and function is unaffected.

● A *brainstem lesion* may cause *contralateral long tract signs* (if the lesion is above the medullary decussation of the CSTs and dorsal column — pages 303–304, 311–312; the spinothalamic tracts have already crossed in the spine and any pain and temperature loss is always contralateral to the side of a brainstem lesion) with ipsilateral cranial signs (either because supranuclear cranial pathways are damaged in the brainstem or because the cranial nerve nuclei/cranial nerves themselves are damaged directly) (see Fig. 6.17). This scenario is often referred to as that of *crossed signs*.

● A brainstem lesion may extend bilaterally (e.g. demyelination, space occupying lesion, basilar artery occlusion) causing bilateral motor or sensory signs.

Fig. 6.17 *Cortical versus brainstem lesions*

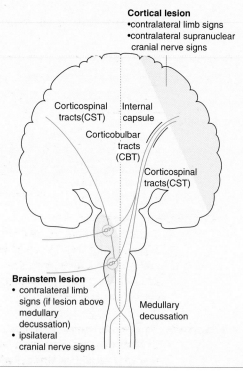

Cortical lesion
•contralateral limb signs
•contralateral supranuclear
 cranial nerve signs

Corticospinal tracts(CST)   Internal capsule

Corticobulbar tracts (CBT)

Corticospinal tracts(CST)

Brainstem lesion
• contralateral limb signs (if lesion above medullary decussation)
• ipsilateral cranial nerve signs

Medullary decussation

Look for/consider causes

Risk factors for strokes and TIAs are discussed in Case studies 4.12 and 6.13.

Which motor pathways traverse the brainstem?

Corticospinal pathways

These descend from the precentral gyrus, through the internal capsule, midbrain cerebral peduncle, and pons, and decussate at the medullary 'pyramids' to supply the contralateral limbs. They are sometimes called pyramidal tracts. Arm fibres lie medial to leg fibres. These long motor tracts synapse at their destined ventral horn exit sites in the spinal cord. Spinal motor pathways are further discussed on pages 303–304, 311–312.

Supranuclear pathways destined to innervate cranial nerves

These descend with the corticospinal fibres as far as the brainstem. Here they synapse with and innervate their respective cranial nerve nuclei and cranial nerves, which may be pure motor, pure sensory, or both. Supranuclear fibres innervating the bulbar cranial nerves are often called corticobulbar fibres.

Which sensory pathways traverse the brainstem?

'Spinocortical' pathways

The dorsal columns (DCs) carrying sensory information for accurate touch, vibration and proprioception synapse and decussate in the medulla and project to the contralateral thalamus and parietal lobe (Fig. 6.18). The spinothalamic tracts (STTs) carrying pain and temperature information have synapsed and crossed already in the spinal cord and also project to thalamus and parietal cortex. Spinal sensory pathways are further discussed on pages 303–304, 311–312.

Supranuclear pathways from cranial nerves

Supranuclear fibres (except those for the corneal reflex) from the trigeminal sensory nucleus project to the contralateral thalamus and parietal cortex. Compare this with the bilateral *supranuclear innervation* of the trigeminal motor nucleus. Chewing persists in the face of hemianaesthesia!

What do you understand by the term cranial nerve nuclei?

Cranial nerve nuclei are the sites where cranial nerves synapse with their supranuclear pathways within the brainstem. The anatomy of the brainstem is complex, made worse by the cerebellar, extrapyramidal and vestibular connecting pathways. Brainstem lesions may, theoretically, be localised in the transverse plane by signs of damage to long motor and sensory tracts (motor being ventral to sensory) and in the vertical plane by cranial nerve lesions. In practice this is unreliable. The twelve nuclei broadly descend from midbrain to medulla (Fig. 6.10a). In reality there are more than twelve nuclei, some nerves have a main nucleus with smaller satellite nuclei.

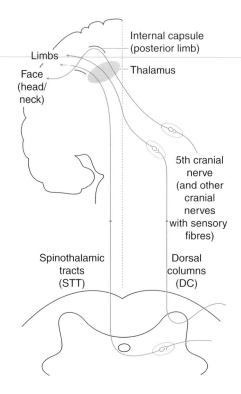

Fig. 6.18   *Sensory pathways from the spinal cord to the parietal lobe via the brainstem*

Section 4 Lesions of the Extrapyramidal System and the Cerebellum: Movement Disorders

EXAMINATION: EXTRAPYRAMIDAL SYSTEM AND CEREBELLUM

Examination points for patients with movement disorders are best devised through the cases below.

The motor cortex exerts voluntary or conscious control of movement via its descending motor pathways to cranial nerves and corticospinal ('pyramidal') pathways and conscious sensory information travels via the ascending dorsal columns and spinothalamic tracts and sensory pathways from cranial nerves to the thalamus and sensory cortex. These spinal pathways or 'long tracts' are discussed in Section 5.

● That conscious motor pathways are not enough to control movement is evident from diseases of the extrapyramidal system. The extrapyramidal system adds unconscious fine-tuning to every move we make.

● That conscious sensory pathways are not enough to appreciate the body's position in space is evident by diseases of the cerebellum. The cerebellum sends unconscious feedback to the cortex about every move we make.

● There is, in essense, a loop (Fig. 6.19). The motor cortex initiates activity, movements are adjusted by the extrapyramidal system, and the cerebellum provides feedback information about the movements made.

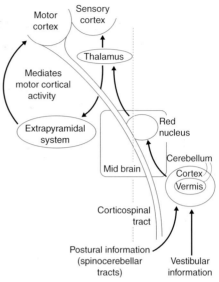

Note that a *left* cerebellar lesion will cause a *left* sided movement disturbance and vice versa (page 309)

Fig. 6.19   *The loop*

Tremor

A tremor is an extra movement whose rhythm is constant but whose amplitude may vary. All tremors are worse with performance, anxiety and tiredness. All tremors may occur at rest or with action but whilst *resting tremors* can be due to many diseases, especially basal ganglia diseases, *action tremors* usually imply cerebellar disease. Red nucleus disease, usually due to demyelination or midbrain vasculopathy, also causes an action tremor which is severe and of wide amplitude, often with head nodding.

CASE STUDY | **6.15 PARKINSON'S DISEASE AND OTHER EXTRAPYRAMIDAL TREMORS**

Instruction: *Examine this patient's movements/limbs/gait OR This patient has Parkinson's disease. Please examine him and discuss your findings.*

RECOGNITION

The classic clinical triad comprises:

1. **Tremor:**
    (i) This is of *low frequency* (4–6 Hz), most conspicuous at rest, and worsens with emotional stress.
    (ii) *'Pill rolling' of the hand* is characteristic (Fig. 6.20).
2. **Rigidity:**
    (i) There is *'cogwheeling'* superimposed on the rigidity. This

Fig. 6.20   *Parkinsonian posture and 'pill rolling'*

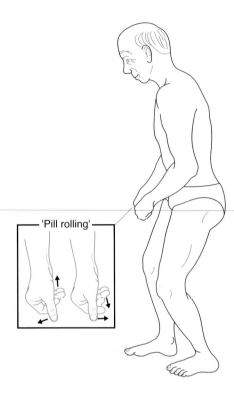

'Pill rolling'

increases with a distracting manoeuvre in the normal limb, for example if the patient taps their knee.

(ii) There may also be *paratonia*, or increased rigidity when the patient tries to relax. This is due to disease in the connections between the extrapyramidal system and the frontal lobe.

3. **Bradykinesia** (slowness and decrease in amplitude of movement):

(i) *Initiating*, rather than sustaining, movement is the biggest problem.

(ii) *Lack of arm swing* whilst walking is an early sign of Parkinson's disease.

(iii) *Diminished gesturing in conversation* is an early sign of Parkinson's disease.

(iv) *Slowing of speech* is an early sign of Parkinson's disease.

(v) There is *blunting of facial expression* (Fig. 6.21).

(vi) There is *difficulty with rhythmic movements* such as stirring tea and cutting food and *rapid alternating movements are poor*. Ask your patient to touch each finger in turn with the thumb of the same hand.

(vii) *'Freezing'* is a later sign. It may take half an hour to do up a shoelace.

These signs may occur in any combination. Early signs are subtle, often predating diagnosis by years.

Fig. 6.21   *Parkinson's disease.*
Reproduced with permission from M.A.
Mir (1995) Atlas of Clinical Diagnosis.
W.B. Saunders, London

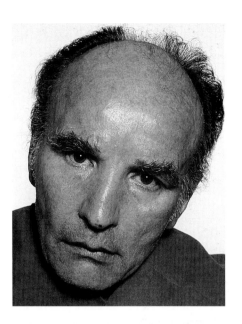

INTERPRETATION

Confirm the diagnosis

- Always check *gait*. Look for *loss of arm swing*, and in later stages *difficulty in starting walking* followed by the *'festinant' gait* with a forward flexed posture (Fig. 6.20) and *shuffling steps*.
- Watch the *difficulty when turning*.
- Check *righting reflexes* by standing behind the patient and gently pushing them forwards and pulling them backwards (it may be best to tell the examiners about this manoeuvre rather than demonstrate it).

Remember the three important characteristics of Parkinson's disease in Box 6.13.

If the features in Box 6.13 are not present, alternative diagnoses should be considered (Box 6.14).

Assess function

- The severity of the clinical triad is important, both functionally and in terms of therapeutic options.

Box 6.13	Three Important Characteristics of Parkinson's Disease

1. Asymmetry
2. Involves the upper body first
3. Fluctuates in severity, 'some days in a wheelchair, some days pushing it!'

| Box 6.14 | Differential Diagnosis of Parkinson's Disease |

1. Vascular 'pseudo-Parkinsonism' (may only be distinguishable at autopsy)
2. Dementia, including the gait apraxia of normal pressure hydrocephalus (pages 292, 293)
3. Drug induced extrapyramidal symptoms
4. Multisystem atrophy (MSA), which may include severe autonomic neuropathy (Shy–Drager syndrome)
5. Progressive supranuclear palsy (PSP), causing impaired upward gaze, and as it progresses over a period of months, extraocular and pseudobulbar palsy
6. Benign essential tremor, a familial tremor usually affecting both hands.

[handwritten margin note: multiple system atrophy]
[handwritten margin note: Progressive supranuclear palsy]

- A history of sudden, unpredictable changes between periods of mobility with disabling levodopa induced dyskinaesias ('*on*') and disabling Parkinsonism ('*off*') is especially important to elicit.
- The neurochemical aberrations in Parkinson's disease may affect *cognitive* and *autonomic pathways*. There is slowing of thought (*depression* may be mimicked or coexist) and even cognitive freezing, and postural instability, especially in late stages.

| DISCUSSION | |

What causes Parkinson's disease?

Parkinson's disease is a slowly progressive neurodegenerative disease associated with degeneration of dopaminergic pathways and neuronal cytoplasmic inclusions called Lewy bodies. Large numbers of cortical Lewy bodies may also be found in patients with dementia (diffuse Lewy body disease), and sometimes coexist with the histopathological features of Alzheimer's disease.

How is Parkinson's disease diagnosed?

Accurate diagnosis remains clinical and can be difficult. Supportive information may be yielded from:

[handwritten margin note: levodopa apomorphine (potent parenteral dopamine agonist)]

- A therapeutic trial of levodopa (a negative short levodopa challenge test may not exclude a positive chronic response)
- An apomorphine (rapidly acting, potent, parenteral dopamine agonist which can cause severe nausea) challenge
- Positron emission tomography (PET)
- Single photon emission computed tomography (SPECT)
- Magnetic resonance imaging (MRI) scanning where other diagnoses warrant exclusion.

Handwritten: Levodopa – nausea, postural LBP, dyskinesia, hypomania

Discuss management principles in Parkinson's disease

1. Levodopa (LD) with a peripheral dopa decarboxylase inhibitor has traditionally been pivotal treatment.
2. LD is less effective for tremor than bradykinesia.
3. Dopamine repletion, once started, is effective for only a limited number of years.
4. LD induces nausea and postural hypotension and dyskinesia affects many patients after 5–10 years of treatment. As the years progress, the fine line between bradykinesia and dystonia is erased and patients may swing unpredictably from one to the other. LD may also trigger hypomania.
5. There is increasing evidence for dopamine agonists such as ropinirole as first line therapy. These carry a much lower risk of dyskinesias. Dopamine agonists are also used as add on therapy to LD. Other dopamine agonists include pergolide, cabergoline and bromocriptine.
6. Other options include anticholinergic drugs (for tremor) and selegiline.

Handwritten: Ropinirole; Dopamine agonists: Ropinirole, pergolide, cabergoline, bromocriptine

CASE STUDY 6.16 CEREBELLAR LESIONS

Instruction: *Examine this patient's coordination and discuss your findings.*

RECOGNITION

To see if the tremor is truly an action tremor, lie the patient on the bed with their arms fully supported to abolish any muscle activation. A cerebellar tremor disappears.

A mnemonic often used by candidates examining for cerebellar signs is *DASHING*:

- **D**ysdiadochokinesis and poor rapid alternating movements
- **A**taxia of limbs
- **S**lurred speech
- **H**eel shin ataxia
- **I**ncoordination with past pointing
- **N**ystagmus (see also page 273)
- **G**ait wide based.

INTERPRETATION

Look for/consider causes

See from Figure 6.19 how unilateral cerebellar disease causes ipsilateral signs. A cerebellar hemisphere feeds information to the contralateral cerebral hemisphere but then that cerebral hemisphere exerts control of movement back on the opposite side.

Midline (vermis) lesions

These cause midline or *truncal* ataxia. Gait is broad based and your patient is unable to tandem-walk or stand like a flamingo!

Cerebellar hemisphere lesions

These cause *appendicular* or limb ataxia, with an action tremor, past pointing and dysdiadochokinesis. Dysmetria—inability to judge distance—also occurs.

These principles may suggest whether cerebellar pathology is unilateral or bilateral, midline, hemispheric or pancerebellar. This should narrow the differential diagnosis to structural lesions and strokes or more generalised insults due to alcohol, drugs, metabolic derangements or one of the neurodegenerative conditions such as a spinocerebellar ataxia. Demyelination in multiple sclerosis is one of the commonest causes of both focal and generalised cerebellar dysfunction.

DISCUSSION

Any abnormal movement is, by definition, a dyskinaesia, but the term has become synonymous with drug-induced abnormal movements.

What is chorea?

Choreiform movements are sudden, rapid, automatic, purposeless jerks. Huntington's chorea is an autosomal dominant disorder which worsens from generation to generation due to trinucleotide repeat sequence expansion. Onset is in early middle age, with choreiform movements and cognitive decline. Other causes include rheumatic fever, pregnancy, phenothiazines, Wilson's disease and carbon monoxide poisoning. Severe chorea looks like hemiballismus.

What is hemiballismus?

Hemiballismus refers to sudden, wild flinging limb movements that are due to a subthalamic nucleus lesion such as an infarct.

What is dystonia?

Dystonia refers to sustained agonist/antagonist muscle contractions and may affect various parts of the body. They are often seen in the 'on' phase of Parkinson's disease due to excess dopamine. Focal dystonias occur as writer's cramp, torticollis and blepharospasm.

What is athetosis?

Athetoid movements are slow, coarse, irregular, unnatural movements and postures. They are often said to be 'writhing' movements. Athetosis can be virtually indistinguishable from dystonia.

What is myoclonus?

Myoclonus refers to brief jerks in a single muscle or a group of muscles. Prion diseases cause myoclonus, but more common causes are hypoxic brain injury and opiate excess. The 'flapping tremors' of liver and renal failure may be considered myoclonic.

Section 5 Lesions of the Spinal Cord

EXAMINATION: LESIONS OF THE SPINAL CORD

The spinal cord extends from behind the C1 vertebral body to the lower end of the L1 vertebra. A cord level is thus above its designated vertebra. (To determine cord levels: C2–7, add 1; T1–6, add 2; T7–9, add 3; T10 = L1, L2; T11 = L3, L4; L1 = sacral and coccygeal segments.) The cord is encased by the pia, subarachnoid space, arachnoid, potential dural space and dura, and supplied by branches of the vertebral arteries.

The long tracts (Fig. 6.22)

1. **Motor (descending) tracts.** The **corticospinal tracts (CSTs)** run downwards and throw off fibres to ventral horn cells. Arm fibres run medial to leg fibres. The CST supplying each side of the body in fact divides into a lateral CST, carrying at least 80% of fibres (decussating in the medulla), and an anterior or ventral CST, carrying less than 20% of fibres (not decussating until lower down, in the spinal cord). For practical purposes, the CST is

Fig. 6.22 *The long tracts. Cross-section of one level of spinal cord, showing the major tracts running up and down it and fibres which connect with a nerve root at that level*

DC=Dorsal columns–carry joint position, vibration and fine touch sense up spinal cord from same side of body eventually synapsing and decussating in the medulla

STT=spinothalamic tracts–carry pain and temperature sense up spinal cord from opposite side of body

CST=corticospinal tracts-carry motor fibres down spinal cord, from contralateral cortex, having decussated in the medulla

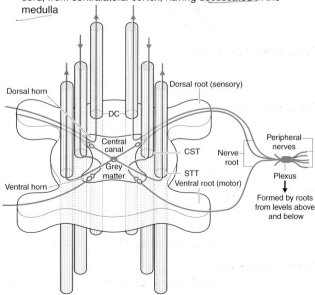

Grey=Right sided tracts and fibres
Blue=Left sided tracts and fibres

considered as one lateral tract in the discussion which follows.

2. **Sensory (ascending) tracts:**
(i) The **dorsal columns (DCs)** (also known as posterior columns) relay *proprioception* (joint position sense), *vibration* sense and *fine two point discrimination* sense from peripheral nerves, roots and dorsal horns, along their gracile (arm) and cuneate (leg) fibres. These fibres synapse in the brainstem then cross, or *decussate*, from the brainstem to the contralateral thalamus and sensory cortex. As you run your finger up the arm of your loved one sequential segments of cortical representation or homunculus (page 296) will be stimulated and each segment will tell them exactly where your finger is.
(ii) The **spinothalamic tracts (STTs)** convey *pain* and *temperature* information to the contralateral sensory cortex but cross early, either immediately or within a few segments in the spinal cord. STTs are fast pathways.

The differential crossing of DCs and STTs accounts for the signs in a Brown–Séquard syndrome (Case study 6.17).

Section 6 describes limb examination and may help with the cases in this section. A detailed description of limb examination was withheld until Section 6 because candidates struggle trying to correlate limb examination with the nerve root and peripheral nerve problems described therein.

Determining the level of a spinal cord lesion: dermatomes, myotomes and reflexes

The level of a lesion can be determined by knowledge of myotomes and dermatomes (Box 6.15).

Dermatomes vary between individuals and overlap in individuals.

Power is most easily assessed in the limbs but sensation can be assessed all over the body.

Box 6.15   Determining the Level of a Spinal Cord Lesion

● In bilateral (rare) **motor cortex lesions** there is global weakness. All muscle movements are affected. In unilateral lesions, contralateral muscle groups are weak (see also Box 6.17). Tone is *spastic* and there is *hyperreflexia*.

● In a **spinal cord lesion** there is *spastic weakness* (see also Box 6.17, page 327) *of all muscle groups below the level of the lesion.* Upper motor neurons normally exert an inhibitory effect on the tone and reflexes in the muscles they supply. In upper motor neuron lesions there is disinhibition of this control, resulting in *spasticity* and *hyperreflexia*. There is *sensory loss in all areas below the level of the lesion* if sensory tracts are also involved. Sometimes only one half

of the cord is damaged (hemisection, or Brown–Séquard syndrome) with ipsilateral weakness, and the sensory loss is said to be dissociated: *ipsilateral loss of sensation carried by the DCs and contralateral loss of sensation carried by the STTs.* Further, there may be detectable *lower motor neuron myotomal weakness at the level of the lesion* if there is damage from the lesion to the ventral horn cell or ventral nerve root at that level.

● **Spinal nerve (or root) lesions** ('radiculopathies') cause discrete *myotomal weakness* and *dermatomal sensory loss.* The term *myotome refers to the muscles supplied by a particular nerve root* (below), no matter how the nerve fibres within that root are

Box 6.15   Determining the Level of a Spinal Cord Lesion

finally distributed via the limb plexuses and peripheral nerves. In root lesions, affected muscles are weak and flaccid, and any reflexes involving that root are lost. The term *dermatome refers to the area of skin supplied by a nerve root* (Fig. 6.23).

Some nerve roots and movements supplied

C5 shoulder abduction, biceps reflex

C6 elbow flexion, supinator reflex

C7 shoulder adduction, elbow extension, wrist flexion and extension, triceps reflex

C8 finger flexion and extension

T1 movements of the small (intrinsic) muscles of the hand

L2 hip flexion, hip adduction

L3 knee extension, knee reflex

L4 hip abduction, ankle inversion, knee reflex

L5 hip extension, knee flexion, ankle dorsiflexion

S1 ankle plantar flexion, ankle eversion

Generally two (and sometimes more) roots contribute to a particular movement, but one (above) usually makes the major contribution. Reference sources vary in ascribing nerve roots to particular movements, and in reality there is considerable biological variation between individuals.

Note on root exit sites

There are 8 cervical roots but 7 vertebrae. Root C1 exits above the C1 vertebra and C8 below the C7 vertebra. All thoracic and lumbar roots exit below their designated vertebra and sacral roots from foramina in the coccyx. Lumbar and sacral roots travel a long distance from their cord segment of origin (page 311) to their exit site (page 325).

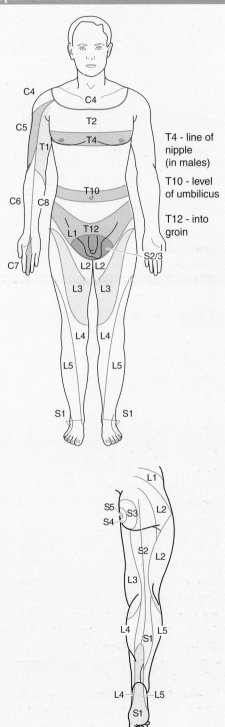

T4 - line of nipple (in males)

T10 - level of umbilicus

T12 - into groin

Fig. 6.23   *Dermatomes*

Lesions of the thoracic cord T2–L1

All muscle groups in the lower limbs are spastic and testing power has no localising value. Seeking where trunk dermatomal sensory loss starts is the most effective way of assessing the level of thoracic spine lesions.

Lumbar, sacral and cervical spinal cord lesions

Seeking dermatomal loss also helps to determine the level of these lesions. Early in disease there may be considerable pain at the level of any spinal cord lesion. When limb dermatomes are painful, spinal cord and root disease is often considered. This is not so for thoracic cord or root disease, when heart, lung and abdominal diagnoses are often considered before dermatomal pain. Thoracic root shingles is a good example.

Abdominal reflexes

Candidates get confused by abdominal reflexes and yet most people know what a 'tummy tickle' feels like. The tickly feeling is due to stimulation of the lower thoracic sensory fibres T8–12 and is lost in lower thoracic lesions.

CASE STUDY	6.17 BROWN–SÉQUARD SYNDROME

Instruction: *Examine this patient's lower limbs and discuss your findings.*

RECOGNITION

There is *spastic weakness* (monoplegia—one limb, or hemiplegia—arm and leg), with *enhanced reflexes* and *loss of proprioception and vibration sense* on one side (ipsilateral to the lesion), and *loss of pain and temperature sensation* on the other (contralateral to the lesion). There may also be ipsilateral root signs at the level of the lesion.

INTERPRETATION

Confirm the diagnosis

True Brown–Séquard syndromes, with 50% hemisection, are rare. Usually lesions are more or less than one wing of the butterfly that is spastic paraparesis. A spastic paraparesis can be markedly asymmetrical. Look for a sensory level (Box 6.15).

Look for/consider causes

Causes are the same as those described for spastic paraparesis (see below). Demyelination and degenerative vertebral disease are the commonest causes. Look for other signs of multiple sclerosis.

Evidence of decompensation

Ask about sphincter disturbance – bladder or bowel symptoms.

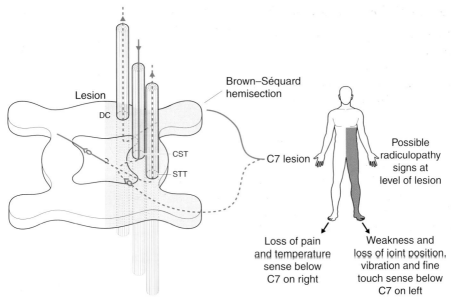

Fig. 6.24   *Brown–Séquard syndrome*

DISCUSSION

Explain the differential dorsal column/spinothalamic tract sensory loss in a Brown–Séquard syndrome?

Refer to Figure 6.24 and pages 311–312.

CASE STUDY   6.18 SPASTIC PARA/TETRAPARESIS AND MULTIPLE SCLEROSIS

Instruction: *Examine this patient's lower limbs and discuss your findings.*

UMN pattern

RECOGNITION

There is *weakness, increased tone and clonus in both legs* with *enhanced reflexes* and *extensor plantar responses*—an upper motor neuron pattern of weakness. There may also be radiculopathy signs at the level of the lesion.

Radiculopathy signs @ level.

INTERPRETATION

Confirm the diagnosis

Check it is spastic paraparesis (lower limbs only) and not tetraparesis (four limbs). Tetraparesis implies a lesion above C4. Try to seek a sensory level (Box 6.15).

✓ **Look for/consider causes**

- Demyelination (commonest)
- Spinal cord compression (trauma, tumours)
- Anterior spinal artery strokes
- Hereditary spastic paraplegia
- Bilateral cortical lesions (bilateral internal capsule strokes)
- Parasagittal meningioma
- Syringomyelia
- The causes of absent ankle jerks and extensor plantar responses (Case study 6.20)
- Cervical spondylosis (page 324)
- Cervical disc prolapse (page 324).

Evidence of decompensation

Tell the examiners that you would ask about sphincter disturbance (bladder or bowel symptoms, ?urinary catheter) and initially wish to exclude acute cord compression, a neurosurgical emergency.

Assess function

How disabled is your patient?

DISCUSSION

What is the pathology in multiple sclerosis (MS)?

There are focal patches of inflammation, oedema and subsequent demyelination. The resolution of oedema and some remyelination accounts for the relapsing–remitting nature of multiple sclerosis but the degree of remyelination does not adequately compensate myelin loss. There is eventual scarring and axon loss, especially as the disease enters a progressive phase.

How is multiple sclerosis diagnosed?

Multiple sclerosis may cause a mixture of central signs (Box 6.16).
Because multiple sclerosis is common, encountering one of the four groups of signs should automatically provoke a search for the others. Sensory examination, inevitably subjective, may be the least rewarding. Neurology clinics see many patients with isolated sensory symptoms (numbness, tingling) without corroborating signs. The extent to which a patient is investigated often depends upon the extent to which that patient can tolerate uncertainty.
Diagnosis of multiple sclerosis remains clinical. It is characterised by multiple lesions in time and space and there are three patterns of disease:

1. Relapsing–remitting course
2. Primary progressive course

Box 6.16	Signs of Multiple Sclerosis

1. Spastic paraparesis
2. Cerebellar/brainstem (which may involve cranial nerve nuclei) signs, e.g. ataxia, dysarthria, diplopia, trigeminal neuralgia, facial nerve palsy, tonic spasms (brief, focal, painful)
3. The five signs of optic nerve damage (page 264) and internuclear ophthalmoplegia (INO) (Case study 6.3)
4. Sensory alteration. These signs may be minimal. Often hot/cold appreciation is disturbed or there is a history of Lhermitte's phenomenon—electric shock like pain on flexing the neck which shoots down the arms and legs and is caused by disease abutting the dorsal columns

3. Secondary progressive (after relapsing–remitting) course, which most patients will have developed within 25 years of onset of relapsing–remitting disease.

Multiple sclerosis has a higher prevalence in young/middle-aged females in northern Scotland.

Which investigations may help?

MRI
CSF
VEP.

- Magnetic resonance imaging (multiple white matter lesions in time and space)
- Cerebrospinal fluid examination (raised protein concentration with oligoclonal bands)
- Visual evoked potentials (VEPs) (often slow, even where there has been no clinical evidence of optic neuritis, indicating that some neuronal loss has nevertheless been sustained).

What treatments are there?

Multiple sclerosis is widely though to be a T cell mediated autoimmune disease in genetically susceptible individuals exposed to environmental triggers. Over time, there is continual accumulation of disabilities with an adverse prognostic effect. The aim of treatment is to delay such accumulation.

Corticosteroids.

Recovery from relapses

A short course of high dose corticosteroids may speed recovery from acute relapses, e.g. methylprednisolone 1 g daily for 3 days or high dose prednisolone.

Disease modifying treatment

Binterferon.

There is evidence that beta-interferon reduces disease activity and delays progression of disability in both relapsing–remitting and secondary progressive disease. There is no clear agreement as to when to start treatment or the cost effectiveness of treatment. Glatiramer (a synthetic peptide which mimics myelin) may also delay progression.

Symptomatic treatment

- Spasticity may respond to baclofen (contraindicated in cardiovascular disease or epilepsy) or tizanidine (requires liver function testing) or diazepam.
- Neuropathic pain may respond to amitriptyline, carbamazepine or gabapentin.
- Tonic spasms may respond to carbamazepine.
- Bladder dysfunction may require oxybutinin, intermittent self-catheterisation, indwelling catheterisation or ureteric diversion with urostomy.
- Constipation may respond to increased fluid intake, diet change, stimulants and softeners.
- Erectile dysfunction may respond to sildenafil.
- Physiotherapy and occupational therapy have pivotal roles.

Are there any factors which confer a loss favourable prognosis in multiple sclerosis?

A less favourable prognosis may be seen with *males*, the *older* the age of onset, a predominantly *motor* rather than sensory picture, a *high number of relapses, incomplete remission* between relapses, and *early disability*. The possibility of various diseases under the broad umbrella of multiple sclerosis has been postulated, since *in many patients multiple sclerosis can run a relatively benign, predominantly sensory, course over many decades.*

What do you know about neurogenic bladder dysfunction?

Bladder control has three main inputs:

1. Parasympathetic, which promotes detrusor contraction and sphincter relaxation and hence promotes micturition.
2. Sympathetic, which does the opposite.
3. Voluntary, causing contraction of a striated muscle sphincter under voluntary control.

Various disorders of bladder control can occur with lesions in these pathways, although incontinence is often multifactorial.

- Commonly in multiple sclerosis, spinal lesions cause regular emptying of a small, contracted bladder without warning, although evacuation is often incomplete.
- Cauda equina lesions, conversely, tend to cause continuous dribbling from a large, atonic bladder whose fullness may not be appreciated.
- These are distinct from detrusor instability and stress incontinence due to alteration in bladder tone or pelvic floor weakness.
- Voluntary control of micturition is sometimes disturbed by cortical lesions.

CASE STUDY	6.19 SYRINGOMYELIA

Instruction: *Examine this patient's arms neurologically. He has a history of altered pain sensation.*

RECOGNITION	

The slowly expanding central canal of syringomyelia results in those signs in Figure 6.25 and described below.

Fig. 6.25   *Syringomyelia*   → Dissociated sensory loss

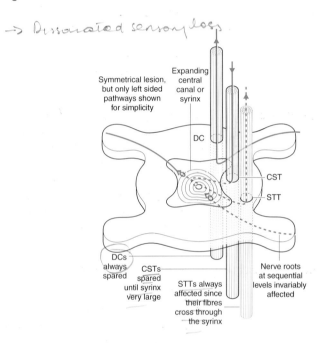

Symmetrical lesion, but only left sided pathways shown for simplicity

Expanding central canal or syrinx

DC

CST

STT

DCs always spared

CSTs spared until syrinx very large

STTs always affected since their fibres cross through the syrinx

Nerve roots at sequential levels invariably affected

- There is bilateral *wasting and weakness of the small muscles of the hands* due to bilateral compression of T1 ventral nerve roots.
- The syrinx generally originates in the cervical cord. Other anterior horn cells and nerve roots are affected as it elongates, resulting in *loss of upper limb reflexes* and *flaccid tone*.
- The spinothalamic tracts (STTs) are always affected because their fibres cross near the centre of the cord and there is *loss of hot/cold discrimination and pain sensation in a 'cape' distribution. This is often the earliest sign.*
- The dorsal columns (DCs) are spared (unlike subacute combined degeneration of cord/tabes/Friedreich's ataxia—Case study 6.20) because they are too far from the site of disease. Because vibration, joint position and fine touch sense are preserved but pain and temperature sense are lost, the sensory loss is referred to as *dissociated sensory loss.*

- The corticospinal tracts (CSTs) may rarely be affected (in late disease) resulting in spastic paraparesis.

INTERPRETATION

Confirm the diagnosis

Diabetes (foot and ankle joints) and tabes dorsalis (knee joints) can also cause Charcot's joints. The clue to syringomyelia should be the dissociated sensory loss.

Assess other systems

- *Horner's syndrome* is common because the syrinx disrupts the sympathetic nerve fibres, especially at C8, T1 (Case study 6.8).
- In longstanding disease loss of pain sensation may cause *Charcot's joints*.
- There may be other skeletal abnormalities such as kyphoscoliosis and cervical ribs. *La main succulemente* is the term given to the cold, swollen, dystrophic hands which may occur in syringomyelia due to autonomic vasomotor disturbance.

Evidence of decompensation

In *syringobulbia* the syrinx originates in the brainstem or extends upwards into it. There may be *facial dissociated sensory loss*, wasting and weakness in the bulbar muscles giving rise to a *bulbar palsy*, *nystagmus* and *cerebellar ataxia*.

DISCUSSION

What is the differential diagnosis of syringomyelia?

Syringomyelia is rare and has an equal sex incidence and an age of onset in early middle age. Intramedullary tumours of the spinal cord may cause a similar clinical picture to syringmyelia.

CASE STUDY   6.20 ABSENT ANKLE JERKS AND EXTENSOR PLANTARS

Instruction: *Examine this patient's legs (you could be asked specifically to examine lower limb reflexes) and discuss your findings.*

RECOGNITION

This implies no more than a combination of lower and upper motor neuron disease, seen classically in:

- Subacute combined degeneration of the cord ● Taboparesis
- Friedreich's ataxia ● Motor neuron disease.

However, it is most commonly encountered when two common conditions occur together, e.g. cervical myelopathy causing extensor plantar responses and diabetes causing peripheral neuropathy with loss of ankle reflexes.

Lesions at the conus medullaris (page 326) may also cause a combination of upper and lower motor neuron signs.

INTERPRETATION

Look for/consider causes

Subacute combined degeneration of cord (SACDC) (Fig. 6.26)

Fig. 6.26   *Subacute combined degeneration of cord*

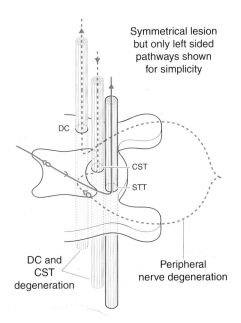

Symmetrical lesion but only left sided pathways shown for simplicity

DC

CST

STT

DC and CST degeneration

Peripheral nerve degeneration

- *Dorsal columns (DC) signs: loss of vibration, joint position and light touch sensation over the feet (± legs and hands) with a positive Romberg's sign.*
- *Corticospinal tract (CST) signs: weakness and extensor plantar responses (and possibly brisk knee reflexes).*
- *Absent ankle jerks* because a full blown upper motor neuron picture is prevented by peripheral nerve damage.
- The spinothalamic tracts (STTs) are spared in SACDC.
- To help to differentiate SACDC from the other conditions, you could look specifically for *optic atrophy* or signs of *dementia*. Both, however, are rare and a *history of malabsorption or autoimmune disease* may be more helpful.

Tabes (Fig. 6.27)

- *DC signs* as above. Without CST involvement the disease is called *tabes dorsalis.*

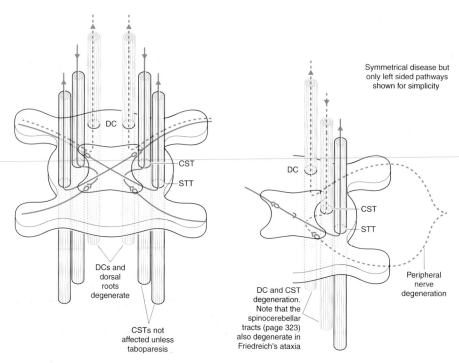

Fig. 6.27   *Tabes dorsalis*   Fig. 6.28   *Friedreich's ataxia*

- *CST signs* as above. This implies *taboparesis*.
- *Absent ankle jerks* as above (taboparesis).
- The STTs are spared in tabes.
- To help differentiate tabes from the other conditions, you could look specifically for *Argyll Robertson pupils*, *Charcot's joints* and *optic atrophy* (rare).

Friedreich's ataxia (Fig. 6.28)

- *DC signs* as above.
- *CST signs* as above.
- *Absent ankle jerks* as above.
- The STTs are spared in Friedreich's ataxia.
- To help differentiate Friedreich's ataxia from the other conditions, look for *pes cavus, kyphoscoliosis* and *bilateral cerebellar signs*, especially ataxia with a wide based gait.

Motor neuron disease (MND)

Anterior (ventral) horn cell degeneration causes a *combination of upper and lower motor signs* with prominent *fasciculation*. There is *never sensory involvement*, and there are never signs of extrapyramidal or cerebellar disturbance, or problems with ocular movements.

DISCUSSION

What causes SACDC?

Vitamin B_{12} deficiency (which is usually detected before it leads to such overt neurodegeneration).

What are the stages of syphylis?

1. Primary chancre
2. Secondary infection (fever, macular rash of hands and feet, condylomata lata)
3. Latent period (years)
4. Late, non-infectious disease which may be asymptomatic or symptomatic comprising:
   (i) Neurosyphylis (tabes dorsalis, generalised paralysis)
   (ii) Cardiovascular syphilis (aortitis).

What do you know about Friedreich's ataxia?

It is an autosomal recessive spinocerebellar degeneration (referring not to spinocerebellar tracts in isolation, but degeneration of multiple tracts within the spinal cord together with cerebellar degeneration) caused by an increased number of GAA trinucleotide repeat sequences at a gene encoding the protein frataxin on chromosome 9. Most patients have hypertrophic cardiomyopathy and skeletal abnormalities. Some have diabetes and visual and hearing problems.

What are spinocerebellar tracts?

These tracts convey unconscious proprioceptive information to the cerebellum. This is in contrast to the dorsal columns which transmit conscious sensation directly to the sensory cortex.

What is a positive Romberg's test?

A positive Romberg's sign (unsteadiness with the eyes closed) is due to dorsal column disease.

What do you know about motor neuron disease?

Motor neuron disease, also called amyotrophic lateral sclerosis, is characterised by degeneration of spinal cord ventral horn motor neurons, cerebral motor pathways and brainstem motor nuclei. The resulting muscle wasting leads to progressive weakness of speech, swallowing, limb movements and ultimately respiratory movements. Presentation is often in an arm or leg, with a mixture of lower motor neuron and upper motor neuron signs. Fasciculation may be an early sign. Progressive bulbar involvement (the predominant feature in some patients) causes drooling (sialorrhoea) because of impaired swallowing, dysarthric speech and occasionally nasal regurgitation of liquids.

Only 5% of motor neuron disease is associated with a family history, a small number of such cases having mutations of the superoxide dismutase (SOD1) gene.

| CASE STUDY | 6.21 CERVICAL MYELOPATHY/MYELORADICULOPATHY |

Instruction: *Examine this patient's arms and legs neurologically. Discuss your findings.*

RECOGNITION

There is *weakness* and *increased tone in the lower limbs* with *enhanced reflexes* and *extensor plantar responses*. There may be sensory impairment (compression of dorsal columns with vibration sense impairment). There may be *inversion of the biceps and reflexes*. In middle aged to elderly patients the most likely diagnosis is cervical spondylosis.

INTERPRETATION

Confirm the diagnosis

The commonest level of cervical spondylosis is C5,6. Always check for *inversion of the biceps and supinator reflexes*. Because these are supplied by C5 and C6 respectively, they are diminished or lost. But upper motor neuron signs are present below the level of the lesion, giving rise to brisk triceps (CT) and finger (C8) reflexes (page 334).

Look for/consider causes

If there is spastic paraparesis or tetraparesis, the numerous differential diagnoses are given in Case study 6.18.

DISCUSSION

What is cervical spondylosis?

Cervical spondylosis is the commonest cause of cervical myeloradiculopathy, and the signs are frequently subtle. It is often painless and may be suspected in an elderly patient with brisk lower limb reflexes but minimal or no other neurological signs. Sometimes it gives rise to Lhermitte's phenomenon (page 317). Commonly C5,6 is affected with signs of radiculopathy at that level and signs of myelopathy below. The lower cervical thoracic spine and roots are less susceptible because their vertebrae undergo less 'wear and tear' over a lifetime. The cervical and lumbar spine is subjected to most movement with greater propensity to degeneration.

What do you know about cervical disc disease?

Cervical disc lesions may provoke cervical myeloradiculopathy. Disc prolapse is more common in young to middle aged adults, and especially affects vertebral levels C5/C6 and C6/C7, with marked radicular pain. Lumbosacral disc prolapse is much more common and causes radiculopathy but not myelopathy because the spinal cord has terminated at the lower level of the L1 vertebra.

Spinal cord ends @ L1.

CASE STUDY	6.22 CAUDA EQUINA SYNDROME

Instruction: *Examine this patient's legs. Discuss your findings.*

- No UMN signs.

RECOGNITION

There is *flaccid weakness* in the lower limbs with *loss of the knee and ankle reflexes* and *normal flexor plantar responses.* There is *dermatomal sensory loss below L1.* These findings suggest a complete cauda equina lesion.

INTERPRETATION

Look for/consider causes

Causes of cauda equina syndrome include compressive lesions such as neurofibromas, expanding conus lesions (which slowly compress roots in an outward fashion, starting from S5) and lumbosacral disc lesions. Any L1–S5 radiculopathy combination may result. If starting at the low sacral roots, perineal pain low or saddle anaesthesia may be most prominent and the anal reflex may be lost. L3 and L4 root involvement may cause quadriceps wasting, anterior thigh pain and an absent knee reflex. Findings may be unilateral or bilateral.

Lumbar disc prolapse causing isolated radiculopathies is very common. For example, the highly prevalent L4/5 and L5/S1 disc prolapses commonly cause compression of the L5 or S1 roots at their foramina exit sites (although these roots originated from their cord level adjacent to a much higher vertebral segment—page 311). However, the term cauda equina syndrome is usually reserved for more widespread damage arising within the canal and involving multiple nerve roots. Note:

1. Pain in the distribution of L4, L5 or S1 may reasonably be attributed to lumbosacral disc disease, but higher lumbar disc disease or lower sacral root damage is unusual and should ring alarm bells to other causes.
2. Because the spinal cord ends at the L1 vertebral level, lumbar disc disease should never cause upper motor neuron signs.

DISCUSSION

What is the cauda equina?

The cauda equina (horsetail) comprises the lower spinal roots.

Because the spinal cord ends at the lower end of the L1 vertebra, the lumbar and sacral roots pursue a long course (unlike cervical roots) within the lumbar canal and can be injured anywhere from the upper lumbar spine to their intervertebral foramina exit sites (page 313). The terminal portion of the spinal cord, at L1, is called the conus medullaris, and from it emerge the lower sacral roots.

Section 6 Lesions of Nerve Roots, Plexi, Peripheral Nerves and Muscles (and Integrated Limb Examination)

EXAMINATION: LIMBS: RAPID SCREEN, POWER AND SENSATION

The examination schemes that follow are appropriate for examining patients with upper or lower motor neuron lesions or both.

In the upper limbs, rapid inspection for wasting then testing for weakness of shoulder abduction, wrist extension and finger extension should detect even subtle upper motor neuron weakness, proximal weakness due to a proximal myopathy and distal weakness due to a lower motor neuron lesion. In the lower limbs hip flexion and ankle dorsiflexion are the most discriminatory tests of power.

Sensation can be left until last when the findings should be predictable from the pattern of weakness.

Testing power

Whilst the above is a useful screen when you don't suspect neurological disease, a more complete examination is required in neurological cases.

The key to examining the limbs is in testing power. There are numerous ways of grading weakness (Table 6.2), but it is more useful to describe weakness in terms of functional loss.

It is useful diagnostically to consider *five patterns of weakness* (Box 6.17). Each pattern has *characteristic signs*. Recognising the pattern will offer you a *clinical correlate* of the pattern of weakness. The clinical correlate connects the site of the lesion, determined from the pattern of weakness, to *multiple pathologies or diagnoses*. Generally, reaching the clinical correlate is by clinical examination and determining the pathology by history and investigations.

When examining limbs, aim to identify the clinical correlate before considering possible diagnoses. This is done by examining power.

TABLE 6.2   **Medical Research Council Grading of Power**

Grade	Definition
5	Normal
4	Active movement against gravity and resistance but not full strength
3	Active movement against gravity but not against resistance
2	Active movement with gravity eliminated
1	Flicker of movement on voluntary contraction
0	No visible or palpable movement

Box 6.17   The Five Patterns of Weakness and their Clinical Correlates

1. **Upper motor neuron (UMN) weakness:**
   (i) The pattern of weakness involves *all muscle groups* in the arm, leg or both. The arm flexors tend to be stronger than the arm extensors and the leg extensors tend to be stronger than the leg flexors
   (ii) Associated signs include *increased tone or spasticity, enhanced reflexes* and an *upgoing/extensor plantar response*
   (iii) The clinical correlate may be a *monoparesis* of one limb, a *hemiparesis* involving the arm and the leg on one side (as in an internal capsule stroke), a *quadri- or tetraparesis* involving all four limbs (due to high cervical cord disease or bilateral brainstem or cerebral hemisphere disease) or a *paraparesis* involving both legs (spinal cord disease below the level of the arms)
   (iv) Diagnoses include strokes, cervical myelopathy, demyelination and so on.

2. **Lower motor neuron (LMN) weakness— focal and proximal:**
   (i) The weakness may be due to disease in a *spinal nerve root*, a nerve *plexus* (a web of neurons with fibres from different roots) or a specific *peripheral nerve*. The site of weakness depends on which root or nerve is affected. *Specific myotomal patterns of weakness and dermatomal patterns of sensory loss are associated with individual root lesions. Specific weakness and sensory loss also occurs in individual peripheral nerve lesions.*
   (ii) Other signs include wasting with or without fasciculation, *flaccid tone* and *attenuated reflexes* in the affected muscle groups
   (iii) The clinical correlates are *radiculopathy, plexopathy* and *mononeuropathy*

   (iv) Important radiculopathies (see also Box 6.15) and mononeuropathies (Case studies 6.23, 6.24, 6.25, 6.27) are described later in this section.

3. **Lower motor neuron (LMN) weakness— diffuse and distal:**
   (i) The pattern of weakness is *symmetrical, distal* and *affects all muscle groups distally*
   (ii) Multiple nerve tips are involved and *weakness, sensory loss and reflex loss starts at the feet and ankles and ascends up the body.* Often the fingertips are starting to be affected by the time disease reaches the knees
   (iii) The clinical correlate of this pattern of weakness is *peripheral neuropathy*
   (iv) There are many causes, some predominantly motor, others predominantly sensory (Case study 6.29).

4. **Neuromuscular junction (NMJ) weakness:**
   (i) The pattern of weakness is the same as for muscle weakness below
   (ii) The best sign to elicit is *fatiguability*, the muscles affected becoming weaker with activity
   (iii) The clinical correlate is myasthenia.

5. **Muscle weakness:**
   (i) The pattern of weakness is *symmetrical, (usually) proximal* and *affects all muscle groups*
   (ii) There are no other neurological signs
   (iii) The clinical correlate is a *myopathy* or a dystrophy
   (iv) There are many causes (Case study 6.31).

radiculopathy
plexopathy
mononeuropathy

Sometimes multiple patterns of weakness occur, e.g. cervical radiculomyelopathy, cervical myelopathy with peripheral neuropathy, SACDC, diabetic peripheral neuropathy with mononeuritis multiplex.

Testing sensation

Usually, examiners will stop you before you embark on sensory examination. The exceptions are in cases of a *radiculopathy*, a specific *mononeuropathy* or *peripheral neuropathy*.

These are the modalities to test for:

1. *Proprioception or joint position sense* (grasping the sides of the finger or big toe, move It up and down, demonstrating to the patient; then ask the patient to close their eyes and tell you the direction of movement being applied) (Fig. 6.29).
2. *Vibration sense* (a tuning fork may be applied over the first metatarsophalangeal joints, medial malleoli, knee, greater trochanters, anterior superior iliac spines, ribs, sternum, wrists, elbows and shoulders). **Note:** proprioception and vibration testing tests dorsal column integrity.
3. *Temperature sensation* (with a cold tuning fork). This tests the spinothalamic tracts. The tests so far are more reliable than testing light touch or pinprick sensation.

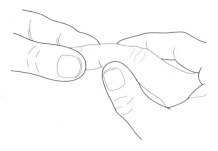

Fig. 6.29   *Testing joint position sense*

4. For *pinprick sensation* you should use a disposable neurological pin, not a venepuncture needle, confirming first on the patient's sternum the difference between sharp and blunt. For *light touch* use a light touch with cotton wool, not a stroking movement.

For all sensory modalities you can test for:

1. *Dermatomal loss* if you suspect a radiculopathy
2. *Specific nerve sensory loss* if you suspect a specific *mononeuropathy*
3. *Peripheral symmetrical loss* if you suspect peripheral neuropathy.

EXAMINATION: UPPER LIMBS

When asked to examine the arms, you are generally being asked to look for a neurological abnormality. Unless there are obvious signs of other pathology (usually rheumatological), proceed as follows:

Inspection

● Note any obvious *wasting, fasciculation, tremor* or *unusual posture* of the limbs.

● The face may reveal asymmetry, wasting, a parkinsonian expression, a Horner's syndrome, nystagmus and so on.

Tone

● The *clasp knife spasticity* of upper motor neuron lesions is best elicited by rapid movements.

● *Extrapyramidal cogwheel rigidity* is best elicited by slow movements.

Power

'Hold your arms out in front of you and close your eyes.'

Look for: — *drift (parietal lesion)*
— *overshoot (cerebellar)*

● Upper motor neuron weakness (the arm falls)

● Drift (the arm wanders in the presence of a parietal lesion)

● Overshoot (when the arm is tapped with eyes closed it fails to rediscover its point of origin) and the action tremor of cerebellar disease.

If there is an obvious UMN weakness it may irk examiners if you laboriously examine every muscle group given below. Use time effectively.

Complete examination of power in the arms would begin by asking the patient to shrug their shoulders whilst adducting the scapulae (C3,4 roots and trapezius muscles), brace back their shoulders (C4,5 roots and rhomboids) and push forward against resistance (C5–7 roots and serratus anterior muscles). To make best use of time test only the following:

Shoulder abduction (Fig. 6.30)

'Hold your arms up like this (chicken wings); stop me pushing them down.'

Root: C5
Nerve: suprascapular (to supraspinatus), axillary (to deltoid)
Muscle: supraspinatus for first 90°, deltoid thereafter.
Hence, by way of example, a C5 root lesion weakens all 180° of shoulder abduction whereas an axillary nerve lesion only weakens the second 90°.

Shoulder adduction (Fig. 6.30)

This generally yields little clinical information because adduction involves multiple roots (but mostly C7), nerves and muscles including pectoralis major and latissimus dorsi.

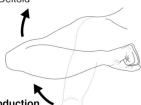

Shoulder abduction(second 90°)
• C5
• Axillary nerve
• Deltoid

Shoulder abduction (first 90°)
• C5
• Suprascapular nerve
• Supraspinatus

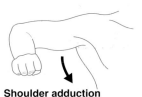

Shoulder adduction
• C7
• Multiple nerves
• Pectoralis major and latissimus dorsi

Shoulder external rotation
• C5
• Suprascapular nerve
• Infraspinatus

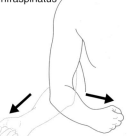

Shoulder internal rotation
• C5
• Subscapular nerve
• Subscapularis and teres minor

Fig. 6.30   *Shoulder movements*

External and internal rotation (Fig. 6.30)

These movements involve the infraspinatus via the suprascapular nerve and the subscapularis via the subscapular nerve respectively. Since both movements are controlled by C5 which has been tested by shoulder abduction, it is unlikely these movements would reveal new information.

Elbow flexion with supinated forearm (Fig. 6.31)

'Bend your elbows, don't let me straighten them.'

Root: C5,6 (mostly C6)
Nerve: musculocutaneous
Muscle: biceps.

Elbow flexion with elbow half pronated (Fig. 6.31)

Root: C5,6 (mostly C6)
Nerve: radial
Muscle: brachioradialis.

Elbow extension (Fig. 6.31)

'Now (against resistance) *straighten them out.*'

Root: C7
Nerve: radial
Muscle: triceps.

Elbow supination and pronation (Fig. 6.31)

Note that brachioradialis flexes the half pronated elbow. It and the supinator muscle are supplied by the radial nerve. The pronator opposing the supinator's action is pronator teres, supplied by the median nerve. The information provided by elbow supination and pronation (*Fig. 6.31*) may also be limited because:

● Elbow flexion has tested the roots (mostly C6) exerting control of these movements

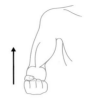

Elbow flexion (supinated)
• C(5), 6
• Musculocutaneous nerve
• Biceps

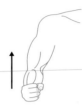

Elbow flexion (half pronated)
• C(5), 6
• Radial nerve
• Brachioradialis

Elbow extension
• C7
• Radial nerve
• Triceps

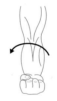

Elbow supination
• C6
• Radial nerve
• Supinator

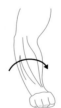

Elbow pronation
• C6
• Median nerve
• Pronator teres

Fig. 6.31   *Elbow movements*

● The radial and median nerves are better tested by examining elbow and wrist extension, and the hand, respectively.

Wrist flexion (Fig. 6.32)

'Bend your wrist; don't let me straighten it.'

Root: C7,8 (mostly C7)

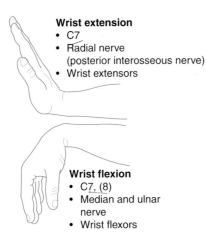

Wrist extension
- C7
- Radial nerve
  (posterior interosseous nerve)
- Wrist extensors

Wrist flexion
- C7, (8)
- Median and ulnar nerve
- Wrist flexors

Fig. 6.32   *Wrist movements*

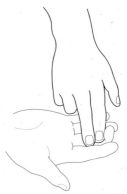

FDP flexes the DIP

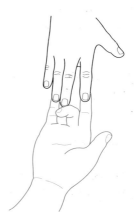

FDS flexes the PIP

Fig. 6.33   *Actions of flexor digitorum profundus and flexor digitorum superficialis*

Nerve: median and ulnar
Muscle: Wrist flexors—flexor carpi radialis (FCR) suppied by median nerve; flexor carpi ulnaris (FCU) supplied by ulnar nerve.

Wrist extension (Fig. 6.32)
'Cock your wrist up; don't let me bend it.'

Root: C7
Nerve: radial (the radial nerve becomes the posterior interosseous nerve as it enters the forearm)
Muscle: forearm extensors—extensor carpi radialis longus (ECR); extensor carpi ulnaris (ECU).

Finger flexion (Fig. 6.33)
'Squeeze my fingers.'

Root: C8
Nerve: median (and ulnar only where stated below)
Muscle: long flexors and short flexors.

● *Flexor digitorum profundus* (FDP) is a long flexor which flexes the distal interphalangeal (DIP) joint of the finger. Only the FDPs to the index and middle fingers are supplied by the median nerve; the FDPs to the ring and little fingers are supplied

by the ulnar nerve. *Flexor pollicis longus* (FPL) does exactly the same at the thumb's interphalangeal (IP) joint.

● *Flexor digitorum superficialis* (also known as sublimis) (FDS) flexes the proximal interphalangeal (PIP) joint of the finger.

● The *lumbricals* flex the metacarpophalangeal (MCP) joints of the fingers when the PIP and IP joints of the fingers are held in extension. The lumbricals for the index and middle fingers (lateral two lumbricals) are supplied by the median nerve; the lumbricals for the ring and little fingers are supplied by the ulnar nerve. Lumbricals are small (intrinsic) muscles of the hand.

● *Flexor pollicis brevis* (FPB) flexes the thumb at the MCP joint. It is also one of the small muscles of the hand.

Finger extension (Fig. 6.34)
'Now hold them straight out.'

Root: C8
Nerve: radial (posterior interosseous nerve)
Muscle: long and short extensors.

● *Extensor digitorum* extends the fingers at the MCP joints

● *Extensor pollicis longus* (EPL) extends the thumb at the IP joint

Finger flexion
• C8
• Median and ulnar nerve
• Flexor digitorum profundus,
 flexor digitorum superficialis,
 flexor pollicis longus, flexor pollicis brevis
 lumbricals

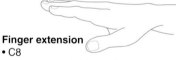

Finger extension
• C8
• Radial nerve (posterior interosseous nerve)
• All extensors

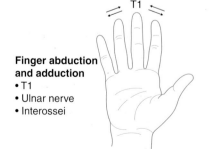

Finger abduction and adduction
• T1
• Ulnar nerve
• Interossei

Fig. 6.34   *Finger movements*

● *Extensor pollicis brevis* (EPB) extends the thumb at the MCP joint.

Finger abduction and adduction (Fig. 6.34)
'Spread your fingers apart; put them together.'
Root: T1
Nerve: ulnar
Muscle: interossei (see below).
Abductor pollicis longus (APL) is also supplied by the ulnar nerve and T1.

Small (intrinsic) muscles of the hand

These muscles all originate within the hand and are supplied from the T1 nerve roots via the median and ulnar nerves.

Median nerve
The median nerve supplies just four small muscles ('LOAF', which are the thenar muscles) in the hand:

1. **L**ateral two lumbricals (lumbricals of index finger and middle finger)
2. **O**pponens pollicis—*'Touch the tips of your little fingers with your thumbs; don't let me pull them apart'*
3. **A**bductor pollicis brevis—*'Let your palms face the ceiling; now point your thumbs up towards the ceiling; don't let me push them down'*
4. **F**lexor pollicis brevis—*'Touch your palms with your thumbs'* (when abducting or spreading fingers apart, the thumb is actually being extended, and on making a fist it is flexed).

Opposition, in which the thumb should normally be able to touch the tip of the little finger, involves abduction at right angles to the palm, flexion and rotation (Fig. 6.35).

Ulnar nerve
The ulnar nerve supplies all other small muscles in the hand. The important ones

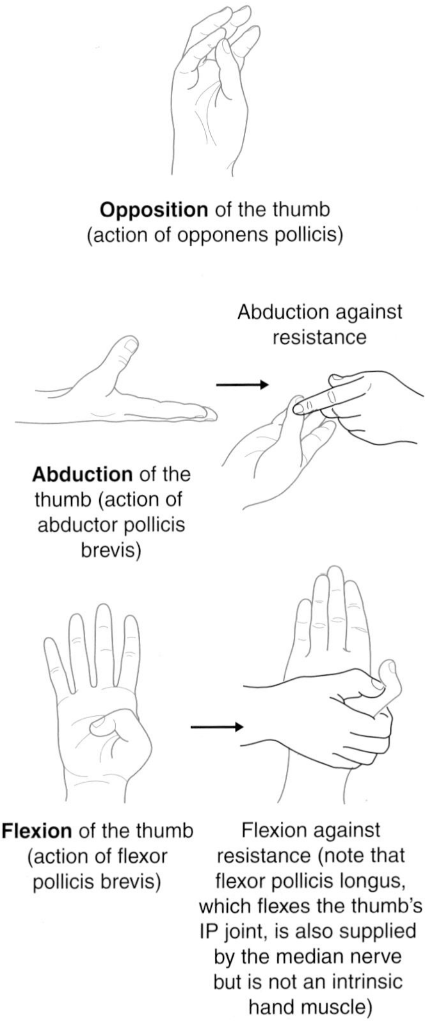

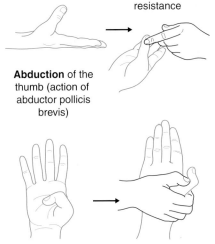

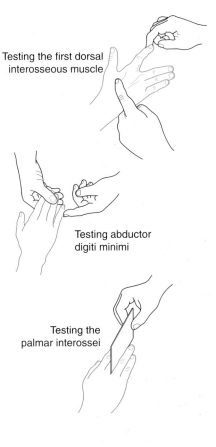

Testing the first dorsal interosseous muscle

Testing abductor digiti minimi

Testing the palmar interossei

Opposition of the thumb
(action of opponens pollicis)

Abduction against resistance

Abduction of the thumb (action of abductor pollicis brevis)

Flexion of the thumb (action of flexor pollicis brevis)

Flexion against resistance (note that flexor pollicis longus, which flexes the thumb's IP joint, is also supplied by the median nerve but is not an intrinsic hand muscle)

Fig. 6.35 *Opposition, abduction and flexion of the thumb*

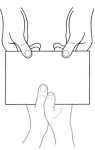

Testing adductor pollicis. Ask the patient to grasp a sheet of paper between the thumbs and sides of the index fingers while you attempt to withdraw it. If the adductor of the thumb is paralysed, the thumb flexes at the interphalangeal joint (Froment's sign)–see Case study 6.24

to remember are the hypothenar muscles, medial two lumbricals described above, the interossei which abduct and adduct the fingers, and adductor pollicis (Fig. 6.36).

1. The **d**orsal interosseoi **ab**duct (DAB)— 'Push your index finger out against my hand' (first dorsal interosseous); 'Push your little finger out against my hand' (abductor digiti minimi)

Fig. 6.36 *Ulnar nerve movements in the hand*

handwritten notes:
Ulnar nerve — hypothenar.
— medial 2 lumbricals.
— DAB
— PAD. — adductor pollicis

2. The **p**almar interossei **ad**duct (PAD)—
  'Grip this piece of paper between your fingers, don't let me pull it away.'

Reflexes

Reflexes are monosynaptic responses to the stretch of muscle fibres, mediated in the spinal cord. Reflexes have a further inhibitory input from higher neurons. In lower motor neuron lesions, reflexes are reduced or absent. In upper motor neuron lesions there is disinhibition from higher neurons and reflexes are increased/ enhanced.

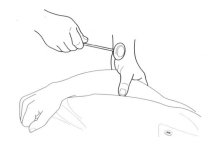

Eliciting the biceps reflex C5 (6)

  Always use a long tendon hammer, and let it fall with its own weight onto the muscle (Fig 6.37). With the patient's arms relaxed and lightly folded, test:

● The biceps reflex C5,6 (mostly C5)— biceps contracts ● The triceps reflex C7—triceps contracts ● The supinator reflex C5, 6 (mostly C6)—involves slight finger flexion and elbow flexion as brachioradialis contracts.

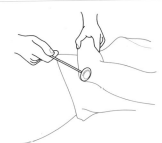

Eliciting the triceps reflex C7

The term inversion of reflexes (page 324) merely implies the absence of a reflex at one, or sometimes more, levels (e.g. C5 and C6) and brisk reflexes below and indicates a spinal cord lesion at the level of the absent reflexes.

Coordination

A rapid finger–nose test should tell you whether or not to pursue cerebellar examination.

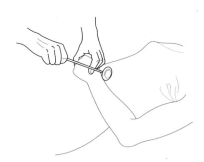

Eliciting the supinator reflex C(5), 6

Fig. 6.37   *Testing upper limb reflexes*

Sensation

Remember that:

● *Global limb sensory loss* suggests a *central lesion*

● *Dermatomal sensory loss* suggests a *root lesion* (page 313)

● *Sensory loss in mononeuropathies* (median, ulnar and radial nerve palsy) is discussed in Case studies 6.23, 6.24 and 6.25.

● *Peripheral symmetrical sensory loss* suggests a *peripheral neuropathy*

CASE STUDY	6.23 CARPAL TUNNEL SYNDROME (CTS)

Instruction: *Examine this patient's hands and discuss your findings.*

RECOGNITION

The patient may be a middle-aged female. There is *thenar wasting*. There is *weakness of opposition, abduction and flexion of the thumb* and weakness of the index and middle finger lumbricals. *Sensation* is *impaired* over the *palmar aspect* of the *lateral side* of the *hand, thumb, index finger, middle finger* and *lateral (radial) border* of the *ring finger* (Fig. 6.38).

INTERPRETATION

Confirm the diagnosis

Tell the examiners that you would ask about symptoms, particularly nocturnal pain or tingling, which often radiates up the forearm. Percussing over the median nerve at the wrist may reproduce the tingling (Tinel's sign). Flexing the wrist for 1 minute may do the same (Phalen's sign). Both of these eponymous signs are unreliable.

Fig. 6.38   *Thenar wasting and sensory loss in median nerve palsy*

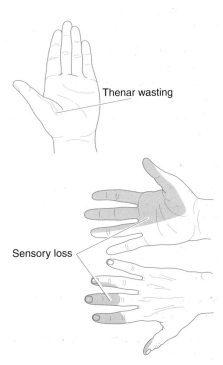

Thenar wasting

Sensory loss

Look for/consider causes

- Often idiopathic.
- Signs of *rheumatoid arthritis* in the hands should be obvious. If the hands seem unusually large, look at the face for other signs of *acromegaly*. Whilst looking at the face, consider if your patient may have *hypothyroidism*. If any of these diagnoses seem possible, pursue them further. If not, let the examiner know that you considered them and mention a few other causes.
- Pregnancy.
- Osteoarthritis.
- Amyloid.
- Sometimes there may be a family history of small carpal tunnels.

DISCUSSION

What is the nerve root supply to the median nerve?

C6–T1.

Which muscles are supplied by the median nerve?

- C6: pronators in forearm (page 330)
- C7: lateral wrist flexors—flexor carpi radialis (page 331)
- C8: long finger flexors (via anterior interosseous branch of median nerve)—FDPs to index and middle fingers (page 331), FDSs to index and middle fingers (page 331) and flexor pollicis longus (page 331). An isolated lesion of the anterior interosseous nerve, albeit rare, causes isolated weakness of pincer grasp.
- T1: 'LOAF' intrinsic muscles of the hand (page 332).

Which common sites are affected in a median nerve palsy?

- Carpal tunnel (CTS) ● Wrist (lacerations, trauma) ● Forearm (fractures) ● Elbow (fractures/dislocations).

In lesions at or above the elbow, there may be lateral forearm wasting and the index (+/– middle) finger is held in extension (Benediction attitude).

What is the investigation of choice?

A nerve conduction study, imperative before surgical decompression is contemplated.

CASE STUDY   6.24 ULNAR NERVE LESION

Instruction: *Examine this patient's hands and discuss your findings.*

RECOGNITION

There is *generalised wasting* of the hand muscles (Fig. 6.39), *sparing only the thenar eminence*. Look especially for *dorsal guttering*. The

Fig. 6.39   *Wasting in ulnar nerve lesion*

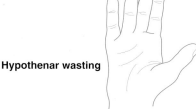

Hypothenar wasting

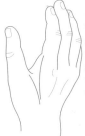

Dorsal guttering
The first dorsal interosseous
muscle is almost always the
first to become noticeably
affected, and hollowing on
the dorsal aspect of the first
web space is often striking

DAB , PAD

first dorsal interosseus is invariably the first muscle noticeably
affected, causing hollowing of the first web space. In a low ulnar
nerve lesion the hand is *claw shaped—the metacarpophalangeal
(MCP) joints of the ring and little fingers are hyperextended* and the
interphalangeal (IP) joints remain flexed. There is *weakness in
abduction and adduction of the fingers and thumb. Sensation is
impaired over the medial side of the hand, little finger and medial
(ulnar) border of the ring finger* (Fig. 6.40).

Check for *Froment's sign*—ask your patient to grip a piece of paper
or a book between the index finger and thumb (Fig. 6.41). Because
adduction of the thumb is weak, the IP joint must flex to perform this
task. This is possible because flexor pollicis longus (page 331 and
Fig. 6.35) is supplied by the median nerve.

INTERPRETATION

Confirm the diagnosis

Consider other causes of wasting of the intrinsic muscles of the hand
(Case study 6.26).

Look for/consider causes

Be sure that you can differentiate between a low and a high ulnar
nerve lesion:

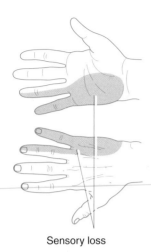

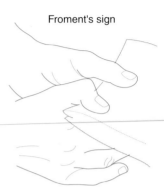

Froment's sign

Sensory loss

Fig. 6.40   *Sensory loss in ulnar nerve lesion*

Fig. 6.41   *Normal and paralysed adductor pollicis giving rise to Froment's sign*

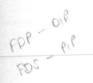

FDP - DIP
PIP
FDS

- **Low lesion**. In a low lesion, the hand is clawed (Fig. 6.42). The lumbricals (page 331) of the ring and little fingers are paralysed causing hyperextension of the MCPs but the FDP muscles (page 331) are intact and flex the DIPs. The paralysed interossei also make a contribution to PIP flexion. Low lesions occur at the wrist.

- **High lesion**. In a high lesion the FDPs are also paralysed. The DIPs are not flexed and so clawing is less obvious (Fig. 6.42). This has been termed the *ulnar paradox*. High lesions occur commonly at the elbow and include osteoarthritis and fractures/dislocations. The ulnar nerve is particularly vulnerable in the cubital tunnel (or ulnar groove). Some people are particularly prone to pressure palsy of the ulnar nerves, which may be provoked by prolonged leaning on desks.

clawing less
obvious

As for all mononeuropathies, consider diabetes, connective tissue disorders and vasculitides.

Assess function

Tell the examiners how you think the palsy might affect your patient's life — at work, around the house, driving and so on.

DISCUSSION

What is the nerve root supply to the ulnar nerve?

C8–T1.

Fig. 6.42　*Claw hand*

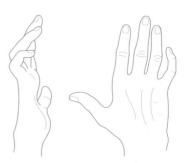

Low ulnar nerve lesion
claw hand

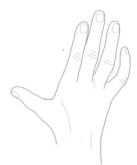

High ulnar nerve lesion
clawing less marked

Which muscles are supplied by the ulnar nerve?

- C8: medial wrist flexors—flexor carpi ulnaris (page 331), long finger flexors—FDPs to ring and little fingers (page 331), FDSs to ring and little fingers (page 331)
- T1: intrinsic muscles of the hand other than the 'LOAF' muscles (page 332).

Which common sites are affected in an ulnar nerve palsy?

- The ulnar tunnel, where the nerve passes between the pisiform and hamate bones (trauma, ganglions)
- Wrist (lacerations, trauma, ganglions)
- Medial epicondyle (friction, pressure, stretching—often in osteoarthritis—or trauma)
- Brachial plexus.

What is the differential diagnosis of a 'claw hand'?

- Volkmann's ishaemic contracture, usually a consequence of brachial artery damage by a supracondylar fracture.
- Diabetic cheiropathy, a complication of longstanding type 1 diabetes mellitus, in which there is skin tightening, joint restriction and sclerosis of tendon sheaths.

CASE STUDY	6.25 RADIAL NERVE LESION

Instruction: *Examine this patient's hands and discuss your findings.*

RECOGNITION	

There is a *wrist drop* and the patient is *unable to straighten their fingers*. There is *sensory impairment over the first dorsal interosseous* (considerable sensory overlap with the other nerves means that the area of sensory loss is small).

Straightening of the fingers at the IP joints is made possible if the wrist is passively straightened because the intrinsic muscles of the hand supplied by the ulnar nerve (interossei and lumbricals) permit some extension. No extension is possible at the MCPs.

Grip strength is impaired in radial nerve lesions, not because any of the flexors are weak but because a degree of wrist extension facilitates good grip. Likewise, abduction and adduction of the fingers are both unaffected in a radial nerve palsy but may appear to be with a flexed wrist. Ask your patient to place their palm flat on a table and test these movements to convince yourself that they are intact (Fig. 6.43).

[handwritten margin note: Grip strength impaired]

Fig. 6.43   *Radial nerve lesion*

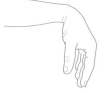

Wrist drop
With the wrist flexed by a wrist drop,
the dorsal intrinsic muscles can easily be
overcome and simulate intrinsic
muscle weakness

**Confirming intact intrinsic
muscles of the hand
in radial nerve palsy**

With the hand placed flat
the interossei can use
their attachments to the long
extensor tendons effectively
to abduct and adduct

Confirm the diagnosis

Check elbow extension, and check the triceps reflex. An intact triceps reflex indicates a lesion below the spiral groove. Triceps wasting and an absent reflex implies a high (axillary) radial nerve lesion or a C7 radiculopathy.

A C7 root lesion causes weakness of shoulder adduction, elbow extension, wrist flexion and wrist extension (Box 6.15, page 313) because it makes a significant contribution to both the median and radial nerves (pages 329–331). A radial nerve lesion cannot affect shoulder adduction or wrist flexion.

DISCUSSION

What is the nerve root supply to the radial nerve?

C6–8.

Which muscles are supplied by the radial nerve?

- C6: supinator (page 330), brachioradialis (page 330)
- C7: elbow extensors – triceps (page 330), wrist extensors (page 331)
- C8: long finger extensors (page 332) – extensor digitorum, extensor pollicis longus, extensor pollicis brevis.

Which common sites are affected in a radial nerve palsy?

- At or below the elbow (fractures, dislocations, ganglions)
- Shaft of humerus (fractures)
- Axilla (crutches, overnight 'stupor' paralysis because a patient has slept with their arm slumped over a chair).

CASE STUDY 6.26 WASTING OF THE SMALL (INTRINSIC) MUSCLES OF THE HAND (WSMH)

Instruction: *Examine this patient's hands. Discuss your findings.*

RECOGNITION

There *is wasting and weakness of all the small (intrinsic) (pages 332–334) muscles of the hand*. The signs are similar to those of an ulnar nerve lesion but with thenar wasting and weakness in addition.

INTERPRETATION

Look for/consider causes

Causes can be considered under the following headings:

● T1 radiculopathy or plexopathy involving T1
● Concurrent median **and** ulnar nerve lesions
● Peripheral neuropathy (if bilateral and with motor predominance)
● Disuse atrophy (bilateral/asymmetrical), e.g. longstanding rheumatoid athritis.

If wasting is unilateral it can be difficult to know in the heat of the exam whether you are looking at a radiculopathy, an ulnar nerve lesion or even a median nerve lesion. A quick way of tackling this is to concentrate on testing the two muscles in Box 6.18. Note that the little finger may be tested (abductor digiti minimi) instead of the index finger (1st DI) to assess ulnar nerve integrity.

Box 6.18   Testing Just Two Muscles Can Yield Much Information!

Abductor pollicis brevis (APB)
'Let your palm face the ceiling; now point your thumb up towards the ceiling; don't let me push it down' (pages 332–334)

First dorsal interosseous (1st DI)
'Push your index finger out against my hand' (could also test little finger—abductor digitorum minimi) (pages 332–334)
- APB weak + 1st DI weak = radiculopathy
  APB weak + 1st DI spared = median nerve lesion
  APB spared + 1st DI weak = ulnar nerve lesion

DISCUSSION

What are the causes of a C8/T1 root lesion?

● Cervical spondylosis (cervical myelo-radiculopathy is discussed in Case study 6.21) ● Syringomyelia (may be bilateral) ● Motor neuron disease ● Pancoast's tumour ● Cervical rib.

EXAMINATION: LOWER LIMBS

As with examining the upper limbs, you could be looking at a non-neurological case such as Paget's disease or a skin lesion. Otherwise, proceed as follows.

Inspection

● Note any *deformity* or *positional abnormality*

● Look for *wasting* and *fasciculation*.

Tone

● Roll the legs, externally and internally rotating the hips.

● Flick them up from behind the knees—the heel will 'fly' if there is spasticity and remain in contact with the bed at all times if the leg is flaccid. Normally there is only minimal departure of the heel from the bed.

● You could flex and extend the knee unpredictably but many patients cannot

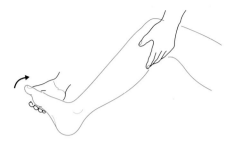

Fig. 6.44   *Testing for ankle clonus*

resist 'helping' you. Tone can only be assessed properly in passive muscles.

Check for ankle clonus. With the knee semiflexed and the foot relaxed, suddenly pull the foot dorsally and hold it, looking for sustained contractions at the ankle joint (Fig. 6.44).

Power

Your patient should be lying supine.

Hip flexion (Fig. 6.45)
'*Lift your leg up towards the ceiling*' (straight leg raising SLR to 90° is automatically assessed doing this; SLR is also achieved if the patient is able to sit down); '*now don't let me push it down*'.

Root: L1, 2 (mostly L2)
Nerve: femoral
Muscle: iliopsoas.

Hip extension (Fig. 6.45)
'*Now push your thighs down in to the bed*' (against resistance)

Root: L5, S1
Nerve: inferior gluteal nerve
Muscle: gluteus maximus.

Full extension is best tested if the patient lies prone but this will most likely complicate your examination sequence without providing additional information.

Fig. 6.45   *Hip movements*

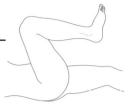

Hip flexion
• L(1), 2
• Femoral nerve
• Iliopsoas

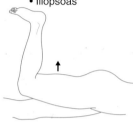

Hip extension
• L5, S1
• Inferior gluteal nerve
• Gluteus maximus

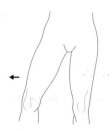

Hip abduction
• L4, 5
• Superior gluteal nerve
• Glutei

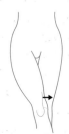

Hip adduction
• L2, (3)
• Obturator nerve
• Adductors

Hip abduction (Fig. 6.45)

This movement adds little useful information (internal rotation at the hip also involves these muscles)

Root: L4,5
Nerve: superior gluteal nerve
Muscle: gluteus medius/minimus.

Hip adduction (Fig. 6.45)

'Push your thighs outwards against my hands.'

Root: L2, 3 (mostly L2)
Nerve: obturator
Muscle: adductors.

Knee flexion (Fig. 6.46)

'Pull your heel in towards your bottom' (against resistance).

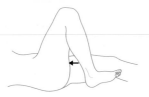

Knee flexion
• L5, S1
• Sciatic nerve
• Hamstrings

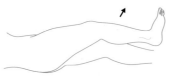

Knee extension
• L3, (4)
• Femoral nerve
• Quadriceps femoris

Fig. 6.46   Knee movements

Root: L5, S1
Nerve: sciatic
Muscle: hamstrings.

Sartorius, from roots L2, L3 via the femoral nerve, flexes the knee if the hip is in external rotation.

Knee extension (Fig. 6.46)

'Now push your shin out against my hand and try to straighten your leg.'

Root: L3,4 (mostly L3)
Nerve: femoral
Muscle: quadriceps femoris.

Ankle dorsiflexion (Fig. 6.47)

'Cock your foot back against my hand/point your toes at the ceiling.'

Root: L4,5 (mostly L5)
Nerve: sciatic—via its common peroneal nerve (the deep peroneal nerve is the division of the common peroneal nerve largely responsible for dorsiflexion) – see footnote to Fig. 6.47.
Muscle: anterior tibial (tibialis anterior).

Ankle plantar flexion (Fig. 6.47)

'Now push your foot down against my hand.'

Root: S1
Nerve: sciatic—via its tibial nerve – see footnote to Fig. 6.47
Muscle: calf muscles—gastrocnemius/soleus.

Ankle inversion (Fig. 6.47)

This adds little information.

Root: L4,5 (mostly L4)
Nerve: sciatic—via its tibial nerve
Muscle: posterior tibial (tibialis posterior).

Ankle eversion (Fig. 6.47)

This adds little information.

Ankle dorsiflexion
- L(4), 5

L4|5.

- Common peroneal nerve (deep peroneal branch)
- Tibialis anterior

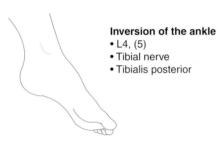

Ankle plantar flexion
- S1
- Tibial nerve
- Calf muscles

Inversion of the ankle
- L4, (5)
- Tibial nerve
- Tibialis posterior

Eversion of the ankle
- L5, S1
- Common peroneal nerve (superficial peroneal branch)
- Peroneus longus/brevis

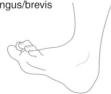

Note: The *sciatic nerve* has *two divisions*—the *common peroneal nerve* (or lateral popliteal) and the *tibial nerve* (or medial popliteal).
The common peroneal nerve has two divisions — the *deep peroneal* nerve and the *superficial peroneal* nerve

Fig. 6.47   *Ankle/foot movements*

Root: L5, S1
Nerve: sciatic—via its common peroneal nerve (the superficial peroneal nerve is a division of the common peroneal nerve which supplies the anterolateral aspect of the lower leg and is largely responsible for eversion) – see footnote to Fig. 6.47.
Muscle: peroneus longus/brevis.

Toe flexion
'*Curl up your toes.*'

Root: S1,2 (S1 mostly)
Nerve: sciatic
Muscle: small muscles of foot and flexor digitorum longus (flexes toe).

Toe extension
'*Now straighten them out.*'

Root: L5, S1 (L5 mostly)
Nerve: sciatic
Muscle: extensor digitorum longus extends toes, extensor hallucis longus extends big toe, extensor hallucis brevis (the main muscle of the foot) dorsiflexes the foot.

Knee reflex L3.4.

Reflexes (Fig. 6.48)

● *Knee reflex* L3,4: support your patient's knees at about 15°. Make sure the heels are in contact with the bed and that the quadriceps are relaxed. Strike each patella tendon just below the patella and watch the quadriceps muscle contract and the knee extend (Fig. 6.48). *Ankle reflex L5 S1*

● *Ankle reflex* L5,S1 (mostly S1): '*Bend your knee slightly and let it flop to the side.*' Holding the forefoot, strike the Achilles tendon, having induced relaxed tone in the calf muscle by adjusting the amount of ankle flexion. Watch for plantar flexion and calf muscle contraction (Fig. 6.48). A method favoured by many neurologists is

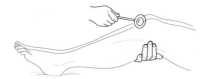

Eliciting the knee reflex L3, 4

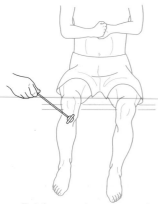

Reinforcement may be used
to enhance reflexes which
are difficult to elicit
(ask patient to clasp hands
slightly as shown or clench teeth)

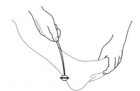

Eliciting the ankle reflex of recumbent
patient S1

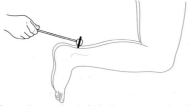

Alternative method of eliciting ankle reflex S1

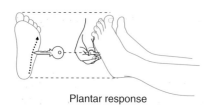

Plantar response

Fig. 6.48   *Testing lower limb reflexes*

to strike the sole of the foot to stimulate sudden Achilles stretch (not illustrated).

● *Plantar response*: scrape the outer border of the foot from heel to toe and then across sole of the forefoot. Watch the toes plantarflex (normal) or dorsiflex (upper motor neuron lesion) (see Fig. 6.48).

Coordination

Ask your patient to run their heel smoothly up and down the shin and watch for any tremor or difficulty coordinating this movement.

Sensation

● *Global limb sensory loss* suggests a *central lesion*

● *Dermatomal sensory loss* suggests a *root lesion* (page 313)

● *Sensory loss in a specific mononeuropathy* (common peroneal nerve palsy) is discussed in Case study 6.27.

● *Peripheral symmetrical sensory loss* suggests a *peripheral neuropathy*.

EXAMINATION: GAIT

Observing gait is an essential part of lower limb examination. Proceed to do this, but your examiners will likely stop you. You are more likely to be asked to examine gait as a separate instruction.

1. Watch your patient walk.
2. Watch your patient turn and note if there is loss of arm swing (*parkinsonian*).
3. Watch your patient stand (and then walk) on their heels and toes (*?foot drop*).
4. Watch your patient walk heel to toe— 'tandem walking' (*?cerebellar disease*).
5. Check Romberg's test (*?sensory ataxia*). This is only positive if your patient is

more unsteady with their eyes closed than with the eyes open. Positive 'pseudo-Rombergism' is common— without vision, unsteadiness is always a little worse. With a truly positive Romberg test there will be associated proprioceptive and vibration sense impairment.

6. Ask your patient to squat (*?proximal myopathy*); if unable, ask them to raise their arms above their head as further evidence.

CASE STUDY   **6.27 COMMON PERONEAL NERVE (CPN) PALSY**

Instruction: *Examine this patient's lower limbs and discuss your findings.*

RECOGNITION

There is wasting of the lateral muscles of the lower leg, and weakness of dorsiflexion and eversion (pages 344–345) of the ankle. There may be sensory loss over the anterolateral aspect of the lower leg and dorsum of the foot, but in practice sensory loss tends to be slight.

INTERPRETATION

Confirm the diagnosis

1. Check the ankle reflex. It should be intact. The sciatic nerve has two branches—the peroneal and tibial nerves (page 345, Fig. 6.47). The ankle reflex is conveyed through the S1 root via the tibial branch of the sciatic nerve, and is therefore spared in a peroneal nerve lesion. An absent ankle reflex indicates one of three possibilities:
   (i) a tibial nerve lesion (much rarer than lesions of the common peroneal nerve or its deep/superficial divisions)
   (ii) a complete sciatic nerve lesion
   (iii) an S1 radiculopathy (by far the commonest cause in practice).
2. Observe gait. A CPN palsy causes a foot drop, resulting in a high stepping gait. Correcting callipers may be at the bedside.

Look for/consider causes

- Compression (plaster casts) or trauma at the fibula neck. The CPN traverses around this.
- Diabetes mellitus.
- Vasculitis.
- Leprosy is perhaps the commonest cause worldwide (but not in PACES). It causes thickening of peripheral nerves which become palpable, notably the greater auricular nerve.

DISCUSSION

Give some other causes of foot drop:

- Peripheral neuropathy, especially hereditary sensory and motor neuropathy (HSMN) type 1 (Case study 6.29)
- Sciatic nerve palsy (see Fig. 6.47)
- L4,5 radiculopathy (see Fig. 6.47), a prolapsed lumbar disc being the commonest cause.

CASE STUDY | 6.28 ABNORMAL GAITS

Instruction: *Examine this patient's gait. Tell us your impression. You may briefly examine anything else you feel relevant.*

RECOGNITION

Spastic

The *foot is turned inwards*. It may be part of hemiplegia or paraplegia. In hemiplegia the pelvis on the affected side is tilted upwards to raise the spastic leg off the floor. The arm may be held in flexion, the leg in extension (Fig. 6.49). In paraplegia the gait is said to be *scissoring*, as if the legs are trying to cross over each other. The gait is *awkward and slow, as if wading through mud*.

Spastic

hemiplegia — raise spastic leg off floor.
Paraplegia — scissoring — trying to x over.
awkward
slow

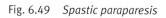

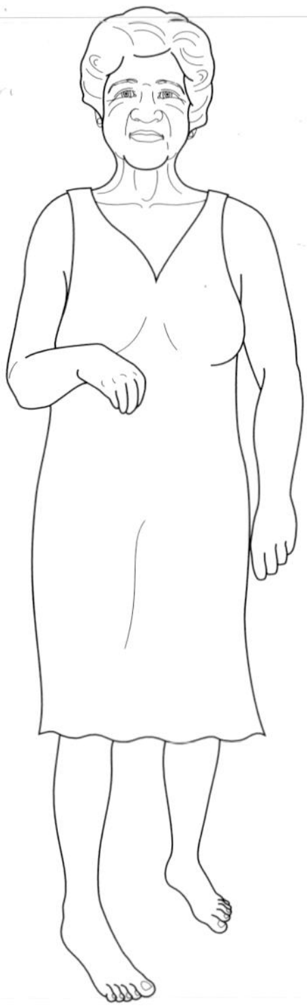

Fig. 6.49   *Spastic paraparesis*

Cerebellar

This is a *wide based*, unsteady gait. The patient lurches from side to side (or towards the side of the lesion) as if on the deck of a ship. The *foot is turned outwards*.

Parkinsonian

festinant gait

There are *short, shuffling steps* and the patient *watches the floor* as he or she walks. There is a distinct *lack of arm swing*. The body leans forwards and it is as though these short, shuffling steps are hurrying to keep up with it—the so called *festinant* gait.

Sensory ataxic

stamping gait

The foot seems to stamp down onto the floor—the so-called *stamping* gait. The gait is *wide based*, the *movements of the leg(s) bear(s) no relation to its/their position in space*, and the patient *must look at the floor* to aid their unsure steps. This should not be confused with an apraxic gait (pages 292, 293).

High stepping (foot drop)

There is a *foot drop* and the patient must *lift the leg/bend the knee* to avoid the forefoot maintaining continuous contact with the ground.

Waddling

The gait is *wide* and *weight is shifted from side to side* as the patient waddles forward.

INTERPRETATION

Assess other systems

Spastic

Examine power, tone and reflexes for evidence of hemiplegia and include a search for a sensory level if paraplegia (most likely a myelopathy).

Cerebellar

Look for other cerebellar signs (Case study 6.16).

Parkinsonian

Look for other signs of Parkinson's disease (Case study 6.15)

Sensory ataxic

impaired proprioception + vibration

Check for a positive Romberg's sign and impaired proprioception and vibration sense.

High stepping (foot drop)

Check for signs of a CPN palsy (Case study 6.27).

common peroneal nerve

Waddling

> Assess power and perform a brief inspection for likely causes of proximal myopathy (Case study 6.31), for example Cushing's syndrome.

DISCUSSION

List some causes of a spastic gait?

> ● Stroke (hemiplegia) Note that diffuse cerebrovascular disease may cause marche a petit pas, an upright gait with short steps and marked arm swinging ● Demyelination ● Spinal cord compression (paraplegia).

List some causes of a cerebellar gait?

> ● Alcohol ● Drugs (phenytoin toxicity) ● Cerebellar degeneration.

List some causes of a sensory ataxic gait

> ● SACDC ● Tabes dorsalis ● Friedreich's ataxia ● Cervical myelopathy.

List some causes of a high stepping (foot drop) gait

> ● CPN palsy ● HMSN1 ● Sciatic nerve palsy ● L4,5 radiculopathy.

List some causes of a waddling gait

> ● Cushing's syndrome ● Thyrotoxicosis ● Polymyositis.

CASE STUDY | 6.29 PERIPHERAL NEUROPATHY

Instruction: *Examine this patient's legs and discuss your findings.*

RECOGNITION

> There may be *symmetrical impairment of sensation to all modalities in a stocking (and sometimes also glove) distribution.*
> There may be *distal wasting* and *weakness* and *distal areflexia.*
> A severe, predominantly motor, peripheral neuropathy with marked wasting (causing distal narrowing or *inverted champagne bottle legs)* may be caused by *hereditary sensory and motor neuropathy (HSMN) type 1* (Fig. 6.50). There may also be *clawing of the toes* and *pes cavus* (page 354) with marked weakness of dorsiflexion. Note that HSMN (otherwise known as Charcot–Marie–Tooth disease or peroneal muscle atrophy) is a very rare cause of peripheral neuropathy, but may appear in PACES.

[handwritten margin note: predominantly motor]

INTERPRETATION

Confirm the diagnosis

> Peripheral neuropathies may be predominantly *sensory* (all modalities of sensation are lost, entire peripheral nerves subject to disease in an

Fig. 6.50   *Hereditary sensory and motor neuropathy (HSMN) type 1*

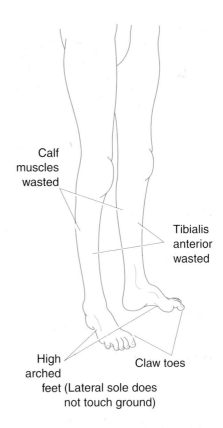

Calf muscles wasted

Tibialis anterior wasted

High arched feet (Lateral sole does not touch ground)

Claw toes

ascending circumferential fashion, so do not talk about spinal levels, roots or dermatomes!) or predominantly *motor*, or *mixed*.

Although the clinical presentation of peripheral neuropathy can widely vary, the classic picture of stocking sensory loss and/or distal wasting, weakness and areflexia is likely in PACES and should be easy to recognise.

Look for/consider causes

1. Look for punched out foot ulcers suggesting diabetic neuropathy. *Diabetes mellitus is the commonest cause of peripheral neuropathy.*
2. Tell the examiners you would like to:
   (i) Take a drug history
   (ii) Take a full medical history (especially for diabetes, connective tissue disease, chronic renal failure, liver disease and thyroid disease)
   (iii) Ask about exposure to potential toxins such as insecticides or solvents
   (iv) Ask about alcohol intake.
3. If you suspect HSMN type 1 (clawing of toes and high arches—pes cavus or marked distal wasting) a marked bilateral high stepping gait due to bilateral foot drop is likely. This is predominantly due

to bilateral common peroneal nerve palsy (Case study 6.27), these nerves being especially vulnerable in this condition and often thickened. The neuropathy often ascends relentlessly to cause wasting of the intrinsic muscles of the hands, whilst sensory impairment is usually minimal. Ask about a family history.

Assess severity

If there is a predominant symmetrical motor neuropathy, tell the examiners that you would wish to exclude Guillain–Barré syndrome, which can cause acute severe ascending paralysis involving arm, chest, neck, facial and bulbar muscles, and respiratory failure.

DISCUSSION

Discuss the causes of peripheral neuropathy?

Three patterns of peripheral neuropathy may be distinguished on the basis of clinical signs, each with a different differential diagnoses.

1. **Acute symmetrical peripheral neuropathy**. This is rare, but most commonly due to *Guillain–Barré syndrome* (motor or mixed neuropathy, see below). Other causes include vasculitis (mixed), diabetes (predominantly sensory), drugs (predominantly sensory, e.g. nitrofurantoin, vincristine, cisplatin), porphyria (motor), diptheria (mixed), paraneoplastic neuropathy (predominantly sensory) and critical illness neuropathy (predominantly motor).
2. **Multiple mononeuropathy.** This is most often due to *vasculitis* (primary systemic vasculitis or vasculitis secondary to connective tissue disease, e.g. rheumatoid arthritis, SLE). This, like Guillain–Barré syndrome, is an acute neurological emergency and requires immunosuppressive therapy. Other causes include sarcoidosis, lymphoma, carcinoma, amyloid, lead toxicity and multiple compression palsies (associated with metabolic or toxic neuropathies or hereditary neuropathy with liability to pressure palsies).
3. **Chronic symmetrical peripheral neuropathy.** This usually evolves over several months, and is the commonest clinical presentation of peripheral neuropathy. There are two types of chronic symmetrical neuropathy, *demyelinating* and *axonal* (Box 6.19).

List some investigations you might consider in assessing the causes of peripheral neuropathy?

Stage 1 investigations

- Urine (glucose, protein)
- Haematology (FBC, ESR, B_{12}, folate)
- Biochemistry (fasting blood glucose, renal function, liver function, TSH).

Box 6.19	Chronic Symmetrical Peripheral Neuropathy

Demyelinating neuropathy

This is usually *motor*, and due to a limited number of causes that include:

- Chronic inflammatory demyelinating polyradiculoneuropathy *(CIDP)*
- HMSN type 1
- Hereditary liability to pressure palsies
- Paraproteinaemic demyelinating neuropathy associated with myeloma or monoclonal gammopathy of undetermined significance (usually sensory)
- Other rare genetic causes.

Axonal neuropathy

This may be *sensory* or *mixed sensory and motor*. Loss of pain and temperature sensation and burning or prickling neuropathic pain can be prominent features. Sometimes no cause is found but there are many important causes, including:

- Diabetes mellitus (the commonest)
- Alcohol
- Metabolic disturbances (chronic renal failure, chronic liver disease, hypothyroidism)
- Vitamin B_{12} deficiency
- Carcinoma, e.g. bronchial, breast
- Vasculitis
- Drugs and toxins.

Stage 2 investigations

- Neurophysiological tests (below)
- Biochemistry (serum protein electrophoresis, serum ACE)
- Immunology (ANA, ENA, ANCA, pages 475 and 85)
- Chest X-ray.

Stage 3 investigations

- Urine (Bence Jones proteins)
- Cerebrospinal fluid (cells, protein, immunoglobulin oligoclonal bands)
- Immunology (anti-HIV antibodies, antineuronal antibodies (HU, Yo), antigliadin antibodies, antimyelin antibodies and other antibodies directed against nerve components)
- Tests for Sjögren's syndrome
- Molecular genetic tests.

How may a nerve conduction study (NCS) aid diagnosis?

A nerve conduction study involves the stimulation of a peripheral nerve and recording, further along that nerve, the latency and amplitude of the action potential. From the latency, a conduction velocity may be calculated. In *demyelinating* neuropathies, the velocity is slowed but the amplitude preserved. The opposite is characteristic of axonal neuropathies.

What is Guillain–Barré syndrome (acute inflammatory demyelinating polyradiculoneuropathy)?

This is a predominantly motor peripheral neuropathy, although it often starts with distal paraesthesia. Areflexia is characteristic but may not occur in the first few hours. Progression is swift and life threatening respiratory muscle paralysis can occur. The pathogenesis usually involves autoimmune demyelination of peripheral nerves, often secondary to respiratory (*Mycoplasma*) or gastrointestinal (*Campylobacter jejuni*) infection some weeks previously. Some cases of Guillain–Barré syndrome are due to axonal neuropathy. Raised CSF protein (higher the longer the evolution of the illness) with a normal white cell count is characteristic. Intravenous immunoglobulin, with or without steroids, hastens recovery and reduces long-term disability.

Miller–Fischer syndrome is a variant of Guillain–Barré syndrome characterised by areflexia, ataxia and ophthalmoplegia.

What is chronic inflammatory demyelinating polyradiculoneuropathy (CIDP)

This is a predominantly motor, relapsing and remitting neuropathy causing proximal as well as distal weakness. The CSF protein concentration is high. The cause is unknown but likely autoimmune, and treatment is with immunosuppressive therapy. There is a variant— multifocal motor neuropathy—in which demyelination is patchy.

What is the genetic basis of hereditary sensory and motor neuropathy (HSMN)?

HMSN type 1 is frequently caused by duplication of a gene encoding myelin protein on chromosome 1. The clinical picture ranges from almost undetectable clawing of the toes to classic pes cavus with severe distal wasting ('inverted champagne bottle legs'). Unlike HSMN type 1, HMSN type 2 is an uncommon axonal neuropathy which may only become detectable in later life.

What is pes cavus?

In pes cavus, the arch of the foot is high, the foot shortened with bunched up toes, and its lateral border does not contact the ground. Foot drop usually develops later.

What is diabetic amyotrophy?

Pain, weakness and wasting in one or both quadriceps muscles in diabetes mellitus, probably caused by microvasculitis in the lumbosacral plexus.

What is meralgia paraesthetica?

Entrapment of the lateral cutaneous nerve of the thigh, which gives rise to lateral mid-thigh pain or tingling. It is usually self limiting.

[handwritten annotations in top margin: Postural drop. Constipation, urinary incontinence, Sexual dysfunction]

How may autonomic neuropathy present?

- Postural hypotension   ● Constipation/change in bowel habit
- Urinary incontinence   ● Sexual dysfunction.

It may occur in many of the peripheral neuropathies, notably diabetes mellitus.

What are the principles of treatment in peripheral neuropathy?

- Removal of any exogenous cause
- Treatment of any underlying medical cause
- Immunosuppressive therapy for certain causes
- Painful peripheral neuropathy is difficult to treat. The most useful agents are anticonvulsants (especially gabapentin and carbamazepine) and tricyclic antidepressants (especially amitriptyline)
- Foot care, ankle supports and physiotherapy.

[handwritten margin notes: gabapentin, Carbamazepine — TCA, i.e. amitriptyline]

CASE STUDY　　**6.30 MYASTHENIA GRAVIS (MG)**

Instruction: *Examine this patient's eye movements/arms and discuss your findings.*

RECOGNITION

There is *weakness* of (order of likelihood):

- The extraocular muscles giving rise to a *complex ophthalmoplegia* (two-thirds of patients)
- The bulbar muscles giving rise to *dysarthria* and *swallowing difficulties* (10% of patients)
- The limbs (10% of patients).

The weakness is induced or worsened by sustained activity— *fatiguability*. Ptosis and diplopia are worsened by 2 minutes of upward gaze. *Ptosis* is present in the majority (two-thirds) of patients, and may be unilateral or bilateral. Rapid lid retraction on re-fixing from downward gaze may occur (*Cogan's sign*). The pupil is never involved.

INTERPRETATION

Confirm the diagnosis

Suggest an edrophonium (Tensilon) test (page 356)

Signs of associated diseases

Look for overt signs of other autoimmune diseases, especially Graves' disease (3% of patients), rheumatoid arthritis and SLE.

DISCUSSION	

What causes myasthenia gravis?

MG is an autoimmune disease of the neuromuscular junction in which autoantibodies mediated against the postsynaptic acetylcholine receptor (AChR) cause functional blockade and destruction of receptors. AChR negative MG is recognised, in which there are autoantibodies against other muscle antigens. Most patients have detectable antibodies althought the titre does not correlate with disease activity or progression. Many patients have thymic hyperplasia especially those with AChR antibodies. The thymus is abnormal in 75% of patients with MG (most of whom have thymic hyperplasia but a smaller proportion will have a thymoma).

Who tends to be affected?

MG tends to have two epidemiological peaks. It often affects females in early adult life or males in later life. Many patients first present with episodic diplopia, worse with tiredness.

Which investigations might aid diagnosis?

- Edrophonium (Tensilon) test (a short acting anticholinesterase which produces rapid improvement in signs which wanes within minutes; unfortunately a negative test does not disprove a diagnosis of MG)
- Electromyography (EMG) in which repetitive stimulation results in a diminishing amplitude of evoked response
- Mediastinal imaging.

What is the treatment?

Treatments include long acting cholinesterase inhibitors (e.g. pyridostigmine slowly titrated up to 60 mg three times daily), thymectomy for thymoma, corticosteroids and more potent immunosuppressive agents. Azathioprine is the steroid sparing agent of choice. Bone densitometry is advisable for patients embarking on long-term corticosteroids.

List some causes of a myasthenic crisis?

- Tiredness ● Infection ● Drugs (many).

What is Eaton–Lambert syndrome (ELS)?

Commonly a paraneoplastic syndrome (such as in small cell lung cancer), ELS similarly has an autoimmune basis and causes fatiguability but does not affect ocular or bulbar muscles. Ptosis is not a feature. Reflexes are absent but return with exercise, unlike MG, and the EMG shows improved amplitude with repetitive stimulation.

CASE STUDY	6.31 PROXIMAL MYOPATHY

Instruction: *Examine this patient's arms and legs and discuss your findings.*

RECOGNITION	

There is *symmetrical weakness* (and possibly wasting) in the *proximal muscles*. The patient is *unable to rise from a squatting position or raise their arms above their head*. There are no other neurological signs.

INTERPRETATION	

Look for/consider causes

There are many potential causes. Two conditions to be especially alert to are *polymyositis* and *muscular dystrophy*. Otherwise, discuss the differential diagnosis, which includes:

Metabolic/endocrine causes

- Cushing's syndrome (usually iatrogenic)
- Thyrotoxicosis
- Acromegaly
- Diabetic amyotrophy (This is a relatively uncommon asymmetrical polyneuropathy causing painful wasting and weakness, often in one thigh)
- Osteomalacia
- Carcinoma/paraneoplastic
- Alcohol
- Periodic paralysis due to ion channelopathies.

Inflammatory causes

Polymyositis/polydermatomyositis.

Genetic causes

- Muscular dystrophy
- Myotonic dystrophy (an exception because the weakness is distal).

DISCUSSION	

What is polymyositis?

Polymyositis is an idiopathic proximal myopathy in which the muscles are painful and tender. It may be associated with skin manifestations (dermatomyositis, Case study 8.8).

What is polymyalgia rheumatica (PMR)?

PMR is characterised by pain and stiffness without weakness or wasting. It is not, therefore, a proximal myopathy. The ESR is often very high but the creatinine kinase, EMG and muscle biopsy are normal. PMR is associated with giant cell arteritis.

What do you know about the muscular dystrophies?

Duchenne muscular dystrophy   (X-linked)

This is X-linked, the gene responsible being on the short arm of the X chromosome. A translocation at the disease locus, Xp21, prevents production of a protein called dystrophin. Patients develop severe proximal myopathy and pseudohypertrophy of the calf muscles in early childhood with difficulty in rising to standing position—the hands 'walk up' the front of the legs to assist standing (Gower's sign). In childhood the gait is waddling but patients are invariably wheelchair bound before their teens. Death is common in the second/third decades due to respiratory infection. Tall R waves may be present on the ECG and cardiac failure is not unusual. Becker's muscular dystrophy is a milder form, with dystrophin produced in smaller quantities than normal. In neither is facial weakness predominant.

Facio-scapulo-humeral dystrophy   (Autosomal Dominant)

This affects the face and shoulder girdle. There is marked *facial* weakness with impaired expression and difficulty smiling, whistling and closing the eyes. The lips at rest are slack, the mouth being open. There is dysarthria due to weakness of the buccal muscles. The neck muscles are weak, as are the shoulder girdle muscles with winging of the scapula. Onset is often in early adult life with a normal life expectancy. It is autosomal dominant.

Limb girdle (Erb's) muscular dystrophy

This involves the upper and the lower limbs, starting proximally in the glutei and hip flexors or the shoulder girdle. In the arms it frequently starts at the biceps and progresses to the wrists. It is autosomal recessive. Onset is in early adult life and life expectancy is normal.

Rarer muscular dystrophies include ocular and oculopharyngeal myopathies.

What is electromyography (EMG)?

EMG involves stimulating motor nerves and recoding the ensuing compound action potential from the muscles it supplies. It is useful for diagnosing myopathies.

CASE STUDY   **6.32 MYOTONIC DYSTROPHY**

Instruction: *Examine this patient's muscle strength and proceed as you think best.*

RECOGNITION

The *face is myopathic* (it looks sad, sleepy and lifeless) with *bilateral ptosis* (Fig. 6.52). There is *wasting of the frontalis and temporalis muscles*, other facial muscles, neck muscles and muscles of the shoulder girdle (Fig. 6.51). There is also *distal weakness and wasting*.

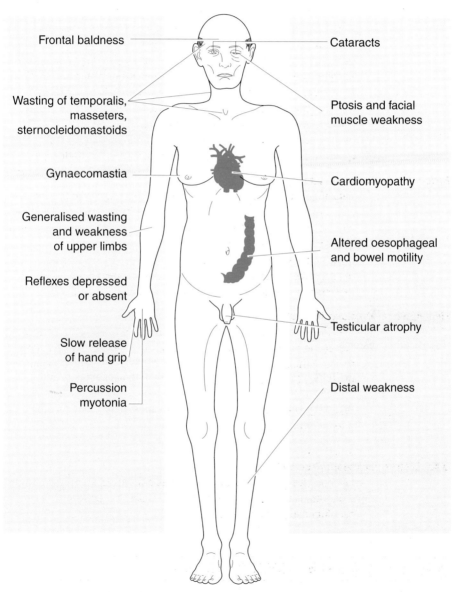

Frontal baldness

Cataracts

Wasting of temporalis, masseters, sternocleidomastoids

Ptosis and facial muscle weakness

Gynaecomastia

Cardiomyopathy

Generalised wasting and weakness of upper limbs

Altered oesophageal and bowel motility

Reflexes depressed or absent

Testicular atrophy

Slow release of hand grip

Distal weakness

Percussion myotonia

Fig. 6.51   *Myotonic dystrophy*

Fig. 6.52   *Myotonic dystrophy.*
Reproduced with permission from M.A.
Mir (1995) Atlas of Clinical Diagnosis.
W.B. Saunders, London

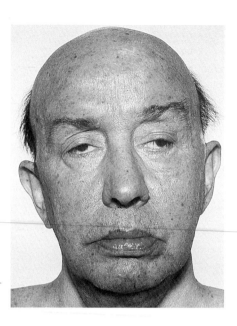

The forehead is smooth. There is *frontal balding*. When you shake
hands with your patient you may notice *slow release of grip*. The
same occurs if they are asked to make a fist (worse if cold or excited).
Percussion myotonia is present on the thenar eminences—when you
percuss, a dimple appears which is slow to resolve. There is also slow
opening of the eyes after firm closure. The deep tendon reflexes may
be attenuated.

INTERPRETATION

Assess other systems

- Look for cataracts or ask about eye surgery.
- Tell the examiners you would check for gynaecomastia and
  testicular atrophy.
- Tell the examiners you would also expect percussion myotonia of
  the tongue.
- Tell the examiners that you would assess for bulbar dysarthria.

Evidence of decompensation

- Diabetes mellitus is common. Tell the examiners that you would
  check for glycosuria.
- Cardiomyopathy is a complication which can cause a variety of
  ECG conduction abnormalities, bradycardia and sudden death.

Assess function

- The muscle wasting and weakness is disabling. Tell the examiners
  you would ask about daily activities and wish to test eyesight.

DISCUSSION

What do you understand by the term myotonia?

Myotonia implies continued contraction of muscles after voluntary contraction with slow, delayed relaxation.

What is the genetic basis of myotonic dystrophy?

Autosomal Dominant chrom 19
Anticipation

An autosomal dominant condition on chromosome 19 which shows genetic anticipation due to increasing trinucleotide repeat sequences with successive generations.

What is myotonia congenita?

There is delayed relaxation after muscle contraction, but no other features of myotonic dystrophy are present.

REFERENCES AND FURTHER READING

Batty GD, Lee I-Min. Physical activity for preventing strokes. Br Med J 2002; 325: 350–351.

Bosch J, Yusuf S, Pogue J et al. Use of ramipril in preventing stroke: double blind randomised trial. Br Med J 2002; 324: 699–702.

Folstein MF, Folstein SE, McHugh PR. 'Mini-mental state.' A practical method for grading the cognitive state of patients for the clinician. J Psychiatr Res 1975; 12: 189–198.

Hughes R. Peripheral neuropathy. Br Med J 2002; 324: 466–469.

Intercollegiate Working Party on Stroke (Royal College of Physicians): National Clinical Guidelines for Stroke. March 2000 (now updated and available at www.rcplondon.ac.uk)

Lucchinetti C, Bruck W, Noseworthy J. Multiple sclerosis: recent developments in neuropathology, pathogenesis, magnetic resonance imaging studies and treatment. Curr Opin Neurol 2001; 14: 259–269.

Lyp GYH, Kamath S, Hart RG. Antithrombotic therapy for cerebrovascular disorders (ABC of antithrombotic therapy) Br Med J 2002; 325: 1161–1163.

National Institute for Clinical Excellence. Full guidance on the use of beta-interferon and glatiramer for the treatment of multiple sclerosis. February 2002. Online: Available: www.nice.org.uk

Patten JP. Neurological differential diagnosis, 2nd edn. Berlin: Springer; 1996.

Petersen RC, Doody R, Kurz A et al. Current concepts in mild cognitive impairment. Arch Neurol 2001; 58: 1985–1992.

PROGRESS Collaborative Group: randomised trial of a perindopril based blood pressure lowering regimen among 6105 individuals with previous stroke or transient ischaemic attack. Lancet 2001; 358: 1033–1041.

Schrader J, Lüders S. Preventing stroke. Br Med J 2002; 324: 687–688.

Weatherall MW. The mysterious Weber's test. Br Med J 2002; 325: 26 (Responses: Mbubaegbu CE. Physics renders Weber's test not so mysterious ... Br Med J 2002; 325: 1117. Kroukamp G. ... and a collaborative group of otorhinolaryngologists reports its findings. Br Med J 2002; 325: 1117.)

COMMUNICATION SKILLS AND ETHICS

7. COMMUNICATION SKILLS AND ETHICS

COMMUNICATION SKILLS

Effective Communication and Problem Solving

Effective communication in medicine means simply that doctor and patient (relative, colleague, etc.) understand each other.

We could, broadly, think of an encounter with a patient in two parts:

1. The first part of the encounter is concerned with information gathering, the principles of which were described in 'History taking skills' in Chapter 4. The aim is to answer the question 'What is the problem or what are the problems?'
2. The second part of the encounter is concerned with developing a management plan, aiming to answer the question 'How do I solve this problem or these problems?' As with history taking, management plans should be developed not just for patients, but with patients. A plan is seldom a case of saying:

D: *You have an overactive thyroid. You will need to take a tablet called carbimazole.*

It is more a case of:

D: *Let's look at how we could treat your overactive thyroid.*

It is a two-way process of information sharing. The doctor does not so much know the solution to the problem (although he or she may know what is clinically best), but reach a solution through communicating with the patient. This method of problem solving is more *patient centred*.

Doctor and patient centred communication

At a glance, allowing patients to be involved in management decisions might seem to be relinquishing medical expertise and merely facilitating what patients want. This would be unprofessional, and we could deservedly question how patients can know what they want without medical knowledge and training.

If you were to say to the thyrotoxic patient:

D: *We could treat your overactive thyroid with tablets called carbimazole or we could use radiotherapy or we could arrange for you to have an operation. Now which will it be?*

she would likely respond:

P: *Well, I don't know what's best. You're the doctor.*

Many doctors are still concerned about patient centred communication. But it does not mean abdicating decision making to patients. It is the process of providing patients with the appropriate knowledge and understanding to enable them to make informed decisions and take appropriate responsibility for their care. Such an approach combines the professional knowledge and opinions of the doctor with respect for the autonomy of the patient.

D = doctor; P = patient.

A better way to approach the thyrotoxic patient would be:

D: *There are a number of ways to treat an overactive thyroid. One would be to take tablets for a few months to see if they settle it down. They are often very effective, although some patients do eventually need to have an operation. Another choice would be to consider surgery at the outset, but in my experience most surgeons prefer to operate if the tablets don't work. A third option would be something called radiotherapy, but this may not be a good idea if you were planning to become pregnant in the near future. I usually prefer patients to take advice from a doctor who specialises in thyroid problems before deciding, but wonder if you have any immediate thoughts about these treatments.*

The degree to which we engage in open discussion depends upon the patient. At one end of the spectrum are patients with seemingly very little interest in decision participation—'I'll go with whatever you think is best, doctor'. At the other extreme there are patients who ruminate over everything that happens to them, and want to know the minutiae of every management option—'How many stitches would the surgeon need to use, doctor?'

Patients vary.

Yet when we look for evidence based management of disease, we find management plans that *focus on disease* and not the permutations of our patients. Traditionally, doctors have been trained to be *disease centred*, but *diseases are wrapped up in packages that are patients* and a fundamental clinical skill is applying evidenced based medicine to the spectrum of different patients. Guidelines might advise against radioactive iodine in pregnancy and the patient might say:

P: I *was thinking about having a family soon.*

But what if she were then to mention her mother?

P: *My mother had a thyroidectomy 30 years ago and had terrible swallowing problems afterwards until the day she died.*

The swallowing problems her mother had may or may not have been associated with the thyroidectomy. One could also say that surgery has moved forward in 30 years. But she may nevertheless have decided that she does not want to contemplate surgery. The point is simply that *the optimal management of a disease is not automatically the optimal management for a patient with that disease.*

Taking into account how a patient feels about their disease and its management is what is meant by *patient centredness*. Because patients have a fundamental ethical right to be involved in decisions about managing their disease, doctors have a duty to be patient centred.

Patient centred physicians do not abandon their focus on disease. The terms

---

Box 7.1   Disease, Doctor and Patient Centred Encounters

Disease centredness focuses on disease and its management.

Pure **doctor centredness** is doctor controlled and tends to be inflexible from patient to patient. Management decisions are made by the doctor and the patient is expected to comply.

The key to **patient centredness** is not to abandon the strengths of disease and doctor centred clinical practice, but to share information so that the diagnosis is put in context and so that decisions about management are shared with and acceptable to the patient.

patient centredness and *doctor centredness* (Box 7.1) are now popular, but it may be inferred (mistakenly) that they are at opposite poles. In reality, they should work together. We could think of *disease centredness* (Box 7.1) as being similar to *doctor centredness*, referring to clinical knowledge of disease and how it should be managed, and we could think of *patient centredness* as a means of harnessing the patient's perspective in order to convert that knowledge into an acceptable management plan.

Clinical knowledge is not disbanded in favour of patient choice. Rather, it is central to helping patients decide what is best for them. Consider that the surgeon of the thyrotoxic patient felt that thyroidectomy was the best course of action. It would certainly be right to explore her understandable concerns about the operation. Negotiating the best course of action for her should address these concerns. A balanced explanation by the surgeon may emphasise the low incidence of serious complications, despite her fears, and include an expectation of what may happen if she does not proceed to surgery now. Despite this process of shared understanding, if the' patient, competent to decide and aware of the risks, declines surgery, she is exercising her autonomy. More likely, she will be reassured and begin to find surgery an acceptable option.

Patients have a right to be involved in decisions that affect them. Practising modern medicine is not just about knowledge, but about having the skills to share that knowledge in ways that encourage patients to make sound informed choices. Patients, in general, value our ability to guide. When they are guided, rather than pushed, they are far more likely to keep going along the treatment path we suggest.

ETHICS

The Importance of Ethical Decision Making

Every day we make ethical decisions in medicine. Some of these decisions are based on documented professional or legal frameworks. Most are less clearly defined. How much information about the side effects of a drug should we tell a patient, for example?

Ethical decision making involves the application of ethical principles. Often, the decisions we reach seem intuitively right. Yet intuition, whilst valuable, may alone be inadequate and even detrimental to a patient's care. For one thing, a purely intuitive approach alone may lead to inconsistent behaviour in the way we care for patients, especially with complex issues. If we aspire to provide the best care, we need to be more analytical.

Ethical principles

Four broad ethical principles underlie ethical decision making:

1. Respect for persons
We have a duty to respect the rights, autonomy and dignity of the person. This duty incorporates concepts such as honesty, truthfulness, sincerity and trust. In medicine, respecting a patient's *autonomy* is a fundamental ethical principle.

Autonomy is the capacity to think and decide, and act on the basis of such thought and decision, freely and independently. This requires health professionals to provide the necessary information to help patients reach decisions for themselves and respect such decisions even if these do not appear to be the best course of action.

2. Justice

Justice refers to our duty of universal fairness or equity. It incorporates our duty to avoid discrimination, abuse or exploitation of people.

3. Beneficence

The duty to do good (in the medical context, to our patients) is a fundamental guiding ethical principle. It entails doing what is best for patients, but raises the question as to who is the judge of what is best.

Beneficence is often seen as being applied in practice when a health professional determines, by objective assessment, what is in a patient's best interests. The patient's views are encapsulated in the principle for autonomy. Usually, that which the health professional determines and the patient's views lead to the same conclusion, because most patients choose what is objectively in their best interests.

4. Non-maleficence

The duty to avoid doing harm runs, in most situations, parallel to the duty to do good. Most treatments carry some risk of doing more harm than good but it does not follow that such treatments should be avoided on grounds that avoiding harm takes priority over doing good.

Applying ethical principles

Specific cases have a vital role in ethical argument. Ethics is not a science where we agree upon a set of principles and then deduce what is right or wrong from these. Rather, the *implications* of the principles in specific cases must be explored.

Ethical reasoning is an interactive process that involves consideration of individual situations and application of general principles. One logical requirement to this process is *consistency*. If what you believe to be right in one situation seems inconsistent with what you believe to be right in another, you must either identify a morally relevant difference between the two situations or change your view.

COMMUNICATION SKILLS AND ETHICS CASES

At the Communication Skills and Ethics Station the examiners are observing many of the communication skills taught in Chapter 4, History Taking Skills. Your case may be biased more towards demonstration of specific communication skills or centred around an important ethical issue. You are expected, where possible, to have agreed a summary and plan of action with your patient/subject before closure and discussion. During the subsequent discussion you are likely to be asked to summarise the problem before being asked wider questions about the case and issues raised by it.

| CASE STUDY | 7.1 EXPLAINING A DIAGNOSIS |

Instruction: *This 40-year-old lady has been diagnosed with systemic lupus erythematosus (SLE). She has a malar rash and the joints in her hands are swollen. Investigations have not shown involvement of other systems. Please explain the diagnosis to her.*

Stronger candidates are guided by their patients when giving explanations, as they are when history taking. They understand that

Case Box 7.1   **Explaining a Diagnosis**

1. Introduction
Introduce yourself and confirm the name/identity of your patient.

2. Identify the diagnosis for discussion
Be clear in your own mind what problem or diagnosis needs to be discussed.

D: *I see that you have been diagnosed with a condition called SLE, sometimes called lupus.*

3. Establish previous experience
Try to establish what your patient knows about their diagnosis before launching into your explanation. Rather than saying:

D: *SLE is a condition which...*

a better approach would be one of:

D: *Have you heard of this condition before?*
D: *I wonder if you know anything about this condition before we start?*
D: *Have you any ideas about this condition?*
D: *What have you been told so far about this condition?*

A specific, uncommon condition like SLE may mean very little to a patient. Other diagnoses such as multiple sclerosis, cancer and rheumatoid arthritis are well known but often poorly understood. Establishing your patient's prior knowledge or preconceptions helps you determine at what level to start your explanation. She may not know that SLE can be a multisystem disease affecting more than skin and joints. Alternatively, she might say:

P: *Well, I was reading about it and learnt that it can affect the kidneys and that some patients end up on dialysis. Is that likely to happen to me in the end, doctor?*

Patients vary not only in their knowledge of the diagnosis but in their desire for knowledge. Trying to clarify how much a patient wants to know can be useful but difficult to ask. Sometimes a patient will tell you:

P: *I want to know if it's bad news; you would tell me, wouldn't you, doctor?*

4. Be alert to beliefs, concerns and expectations
Establishing prior experience can help you understand any specific fears that may relate to it. Throughout your explanation, try to take account of any beliefs, concerns and expectations you elicit.

Examples of concerns that a patient with SLE might have include:
- No longer being able to go on sunny holidays
- An unsightly rash
- Arthritis
- Needing to take dangerous drugs
- Having a disease of the immune system
- Ending up on dialysis.

5. Order

Try to provide a framework for your explanation of the disease itself. You might talk about:
- Why SLE occurs—a 'misdirected' immune system
- Possible clinical problems—focusing especially on those affecting your patient
- The likely natural history, with and without treatment.

6. Keep it short and simple

Keep your explanation as clear and simple as possible. Use language that your patient will understand (without being patronising), avoiding complex medical terminology. Sometimes it helps to use similar phrases to your patient:

P: *How does it look on the whole, doctor?*

D: *It looks alright, on the whole. Most patients with your condition continue to live a very normal life.*

7. Repeat important information

Repeating important information can be a very effective way of emphasising 'take home' messages:

D: *I think I should emphasise to you again that most people with this condition do not end up with kidney problems or need dialysis. Most patients have skin and joint problems very similar to yourself, and these problems do tend to get better with treatment.*

8. Encourage feedback, invite questions and check understanding

D: *I appreciate that we have covered a lot there. Is there anything you would like me to go over again?*

D: *Are there any questions you would like to ask me?*

Although you do not wish to *test* your patient, it can *sometimes* be useful to ask if your patient would mind repeating to you what they feel to be the important points of the discussion you have just had.

9. Be honest in your explanation

Be prepared to admit uncertainty if the patient asks something you can't answer.

diabetes and cancer and arthritis are different things to different people. They operate within a patient-centred framework. Weaker candidates think 'Oh no,! What do I know about SLE?' and proceed to tell their patients very little or far too much, often in a very disorganised fashion. A suitable framework for tackling this instruction is given in Case box 7.1.

What general steps do you take when explaining a diagnosis to a patient?

The examiners know that there is no single correct way to answer this. They merely wish to see that you can give it some logical thought (steps 1–9, Case box 7.1).

CASE STUDY | 7.2 EXPLAINING AN INVESTIGATION

Instruction: *Your consultant has asked you to explain to this 64-year-old lady that she needs a bronchoscopy to investigate her haemoptysis. Her chest X-ray has shown a 2-cm central opacity. Please explain this procedure to her.*

Investigations in medicine generally serve one of three purposes:

1. Furthering a diagnosis
2. Assessing the severity of a diagnosis
3. Monitoring the response to a treatment.

Case Box 7.2   Explaining an Investigation

1. Introduction
Introduce yourself and confirm the name/identity of your patient.

2. Identify the investigation for discussion
Be clear in your own mind what investigation needs to be discussed, and the purpose for which it is being performed.

3. Establish previous experience
Try to establish what your patient knows about their problem before explaining the investigation. Rather than saying:

D: *You need to have a test called a bronchoscopy,*

a better approach might be:

D: *The chest specialist feels that we should look more closely into this problem of coughing up blood. He suggests some further tests. Can I ask you what you've been told about the results of your tests so far?*
P: *I know the X-ray wasn't completely normal. What tests does he suggest?*
D: *He suggests a test called a bronchoscopy. Have you heard of a bronchoscopy before?*

4. Be alert to beliefs, concerns and expectations

Establishing prior experience can help you understand any specific fears that your patient may have relating to the potential diagnosis or to the test itself. These should be addressed before proceeding.

P: *What do you think the X-ray means, doctor? The other doctor said it could be a growth in the lung. I've smoked all my life so I wouldn't be surprised, to be honest with you. Is it bad?*

D: *The X-ray does show that there is a possibility of a growth in the lung. A bronchoscopy is the best way of knowing this for certain. It's very hard to say what it means for you until we know for sure what it is. Once we know, we are in a much better position to know how best to treat it.*

5. Order

Try to provide a framework for your explanation of the investigation. You might talk about:

(i) The purpose of the investigation, if not already covered in the discussion above
(ii) The nature of the proposed investigation
(iii) Any risks that may be involved.

D: *The bronchoscopy involves an anaesthetic and passing a small tube into the airways to examine them. If there is anything seen, such as a growth, then the specialist will take a biopsy, a small piece of tissue, from it and send it to the lab. to be looked at under the microscope. A bronchoscopy is a very common test these days, and generally very safe.*

6. Keep it short and simple

Keep your explanation as clear and simple as possible. Use language that your patient will understand and avoid jargon.

7. Repeat important information

8. Encourage feedback, invite questions and check understanding

9. Seek consent

Remember that you are explaining the reason for an investigation and not telling your patient that they must have it. Following your explanation, you should seek informed consent to proceed. Obtaining consent for an investigation is discussed in Case study 7.19.

The steps in explaining an investigation are very similar to those for explaining a diagnosis and are given in Case box 7.2.

What do the terms reliability and validity mean?

A *reliable* method is one that produces repeatable results.

A *valid* method measures what it sets out to measure.

What criteria would you consider important in determining whether or not to implement a screening test for a disease?

Ideally, the disease should be common, important and diagnosable by an accepted method. There must be a latent interval between disease onset and important manifestations during which effective intervention is possible. The screening test should be simple, cheap and performed on a group deemed by policy to be at high risk. It should have a high sensitivity and a high specificity.

What is meant by the following terms—sensitivity, specificity, positive predictive value (PPV) and negative predictive value (NPV)?

Note: a = disease positive, test positive; b = disease negative, test positive; c = disease positive, test negative; d = disease negative, test negative.

Sensitivity

This refers to the ability of a test to detect a disease. It is the proportion of true positives detected by the test of all those who have the disease.

$$Sensitivity = a/a + c$$

Specificity

This refers to the ability of a test to detect the disease in question and no other; in other words to exclude those who do not have disease. It is the proportion of true negatives of all those who do not have the disease.

$$Specificity = d/d + b$$

Sensitivity and specificity look primarily at disease positives and negatives respectively.

PPV

This refers to the proportion of people with positive test results who have the disease.

$$PPV = a/a + b$$

NPV

This refers to the proportion of people with negative test results who do not have the disease.

$$NPV = d/d + c$$

PPV and NPV look primarily at positive and negative tests respectively.

CASE STUDY	7.3 EXPLAINING A TREATMENT

Instruction: *This gentleman was recently in your ward following a myocardial infarction. 6 weeks later, in clinic, you see that he has not been started on lipid lowering therapy. His total cholesterol is 5.3 mmol/L. You feel he would benefit from a statin. Please discuss this option with him.*

When explaining a treatment try to cover the points in Case box 7.3

Case Box 7.3	Explaining a Treatment

1. Explain the reasons for considering treatment

D: *I'm glad to see that you are recovering from your recent heart attack. Your test results are largely encouraging but your blood cholesterol level is still a little high. When the cholesterol is high and we don't treat it, this can increase the risk of future heart attacks. Fortunately, the risk can be reduced with medication and I think we should discuss starting this medication in your case.*

2. Give your patient a chance to react to the need for treatment

Remember that a lot has happened to him recently. His world has likely been turned upside down by the heart attack. He likely had an enormous fright when he came into hospital, and is still coming to terms with the repercussions of his diagnosis, learning that his life is as vulnerable as anybody else's. He might have been forced to change his job or stop working altogether. He might have new financial worries. He will have received a great deal of advice from doctors, nurses and members of the cardiac rehabilitation team. He will be on a range of tablets, all of them indefinitely.

All this is not meant to sound patronising. It should be obvious. But it is important to recognise that his hopes for the outcome of today's clinic appointment and yours may not immediately be the same. There may be a mismatch of *agendas*. You have heard that he is well and checked his results. You want him to start taking a statin and then you will see your next patient. But he desperately wants to hear some good news. Yet another tablet may not be what he had in mind. Give him a chance to react to what you see as the most important reason for his being here today.

Usually, patients will ask for more information. Sometimes a patient will ask a question such as:

P: *Is more medication really necessary?*

3. Explain the likely benefits of treatment

Explain these as precisely as possible, but beware of overwhelming patients with outcomes of studies. It often helps to reassure patients that others are taking the same drug and that your advice is commensurate with the larger body of current medical opinion.

D: *Most doctors are now keen that patients with high cholesterol are on this drug and it has certainly helped a large number of patients.*

4. Explain what the treatment will mean for your patient
Explain:
(i) The frequency of dosing
(ii) The duration of therapy
(iii) Any special instructions, e.g. the tablet should be taken with meals or at a certain time of day
(iv) Any requirements for blood monitoring, if relevant, and how this would be arranged.

5. Explain the likely side effects of treatment
(i) In general, advise about side effects that are common or serious.
(ii) Try to explain how in your view the side effects weigh up against the benefits.
(iii) Allow your patient to weigh up the pros and cons as they see them.
(iv) Explain what should be done if a side effect occurs. Many patients know that NSAIDs can cause heartburn, but carry on taking them. Patients have not worked in GI units. Do not assume that what is obvious to you is obvious to your patient.

6. Give ample opportunity for questions
Allow your patient time to consider the treatment and seek further information if so wished.

7. Seek consent
Remember that you are explaining the reason for a treatment and not telling your patient they must have it. Following your explanation, you should seek informed consent to proceed. Obtaining consent for a treatment is discussed in Case study 7.20.

What is meant by relative risk (RR) and relative risk reduction (RRR)?

- RR is the ratio between the risk in an intervention group and the risk in the control group. The risk of an event in the intervention group is sometimes called the experimental event rate (EER). The risk of an event in the control group is sometimes called the control event rate (CER). Assume the risk of myocardial infarction (MI) in those treated with lipid lowering therapy is 1 in 100 (EER) and the risk in the control group is 2 in 100 (CER). The relative risk of myocardial infarction with treatment is $(1/100)/(2/100)$ or 0.5.
- RRR refers to the amount by which risk is reduced and may be calculated using the formula $1 - RR$. In our example $1 - 0.5 = 0.5$ or 50%. In our example treatment reduces the risk of MI by 50%. RRR can also be calculated using the formula $(CER - EER)/CER$.

What is meant by absolute risk reduction (ARR)?

ARR is useful in determining if the RRR is important. It is calculated from CER – EER. In our example CER = 2% and EER = 1%. ARR is therefore 1%. In other words, 1 in 100 people benefit from treatment. By contrast, if the CER of a disease is much smaller, say 0.001%, the ARR achieved by the same RRR of 50% is 0.0005%. This ARR would warrant a much higher 'number needed to treat'.

What do understand by the term number needed to treat (NNT)?

NNT = 1/ARR and refers to the number of people needed to be treated in order for 1 person to benefit (1 event to be prevented). In our initial example, the NNT is 100. In our latter example, it is 2000.

CASE STUDY   **7.4 DISCUSSING PROGNOSIS AND POSSIBLE COMPLICATIONS**

Instruction: *This 49-year-old man had a partial gastrectomy for gastric cancer 2 years ago. It was diagnosed very early, and was very likely an incidental finding discovered at endoscopy for investigation of dyspeptic symptoms. After surgery and a course of H. pylori eradication therapy he had no further symptoms. His surgeon told him 6 months ago that unless he had further symptoms he was 'in the clear'. He now has recurrence of dyspepsia and is seeing you urgently in the gastroenterology outpatient clinic. He asks 'What is the outlook, now, doctor?' Please talk with him.*

Discussing prognosis requires that you have all of the facts in front of you. In this case, there is not as yet a diagnosis and clearly a central investigation to obtain more facts will be further endoscopy:

Case Box 7.4   **Discussing Prognosis and Possible Complications**

1. Obtain the facts
It can be easy to be drawn by patients into discussion of likely outcomes when you do not possess all of the facts. As far as possible, try to avoid discussing outcomes of a range of hypothetical diagnoses.

2. Discuss the prognosis of any diagnosis with and without treatment
Discussion should utilise the patient centred approaches outlined in Case study 7.1 for explaining a diagnosis and emphasising the benefits of any treatment.

3. Discuss the complications of any diagnosis and treatment
Complications of both the diagnosis and its treatment should be discussed. As a general rule, those complications that are either common or serious should be discussed.

D: *I think that we should strongly consider having a look down into your stomach by endoscopy. This will tell us quickly whether or not there is anything we need to be worried about. I'm hoping it will show an ulcer which we can treat with tablets. In the unlikely event that it were to show something more serious we would be able to decide how best to deal with it sooner rather than later.*

Discussing prognosis and complications of a diagnosis should broadly follow the steps in Case box 7.4.

How do you break bad news to a patient?
Refer to Case study 7.10.

CASE STUDY	7.5 DISCUSSING DIAGNOSTIC UNCERTAINTY AND RISK

Instruction: *You have been seeing a 24-year-old woman in clinic for follow up of Crohn's disease. She has been asymptomatic for 6 months. At the end of the consultation she mentions that she has had pain in her right calf for the past week. She didn't want 'to bother her GP' and hoped you might take a quick look at it. She started the combined oral contraceptive pill (COCP) 2 months previously whilst touring in Australia with her boyfriend. They returned home 10 days ago. She has no family history of thromboembolic disease. Examination is unremarkable. Please discuss management options with her.*

This patient probably has no concerns about a deep venous thrombosis (DVT). She appears to lead an active lifestyle, has no signs of a DVT, and the absolute risk of thromboembolic disease on the COCP is very low. The pain could well be due to 'muscle strain'. Conversely, you know that signs of a DVT can be 'hit or miss' and that she has two possible risk factors—the COCP and a recent long haul flight. You also know that thromboembolic disease, although rare in this age group, can be life-threatening and is treatable. A symptom may have a low probability of representing serious pathology but a high probability of serious consequences if ignored. Such information should always be shared with a patient.

The management of disease in textbooks is often clear cut: investigation A for suspected disease B; treatment Y for disease Z. But outside textbooks, whether or not to embark on an investigation in the face of limited evidence is a complex decision, which should involve sharing your knowledge, concerns and expectations.

Three important steps in discussing diagnostic uncertainty are given in Case box 7.5.

Case Box 7.5   **Discussing Diagnostic Uncertainty**

1. Outline the possibilities, including the most serious

D: *This is most likely a harmless muscle pain. There is a small possibility that your pain is due to a clot of blood in one of the deeper veins of the leg. It is difficult to exclude this without further tests. Although I don't think a blood clot is likely, there is a risk that a blood clot that isn't treated can travel to the lungs and this can be dangerous. We could arrange a scan of the leg just to be on the safe side, if you wished.*

This sounds straightforward, but in practice there can be a problem with sharing information in this way. Patients frequently don't warm to the idea of being asked to make a decision and saying *if you wished* may be too open-ended to actually help a patient decide. This patient might well respond:

P: *Well, you're the doctor, I'll take your advice,* or *Do you think it's really necessary?*

placing you back at square one. Sharing information is more than showing patients the menu!

2. Give an honest professional opinion

If these decisions are difficult for us, with years of medical training, then they can be enormously difficult for patients, given only snippets of the distilled medical wisdom. Since there is no clear history of muscle strain, the potential seriousness of a DVT may persuade you to say:

D: *I'd advise a test called an ultrasound...but if you'd prefer not to have tests then...(in which case you should cast a safety net).*

3. Use a 'safety net'

Always have a follow up plan, such as suggesting follow up by the patient's GP or to seek medical advice if the pain gets worse rather than better or if swelling develops.

Any decision that involves waiting for something else to happen before acting should be 'safety netted' and patients should be clear about which symptoms should prompt reassessment.

A 48-year-old non-smoker is being discharged from your ward today following investigation for chronic diarrhoea. No sinister cause has been found. He tells you that a few weeks ago he had a single episode of 'coughing up a teaspoonful of blood' which he'd forgotten to mention until now and says 'but that's not anything to worry about, is it, doctor?' Your further questions confirm that it was most likely an episode of small haemoptysis and reveal no other symptoms of note. He is a non-smoker and you know that his chest X-ray was normal. What are the important issues here?

The nature of the problem is clear—one episode of unexplained haemoptysis. There may be no sinister cause at all. It has not recurred and he is a non-smoker with a normal chest X-ray. Nevertheless, the symptom remains unexplained. There is a small chance of something serious—a small endobronchial tumour, a laryngeal tumour, or even the first manifestation of systemic vasculitis.

There are numerous potential approaches to this problem. At one dangerous extreme he might be reassured and told 'No, it doesn't sound like anything worrying'. At the other safer extreme he could be advised that urgent investigations are needed to exclude a tumour. Each doctor has his or her own 'risk threshold' for undertaking investigations, but the problem with each of these extremes is that they do not involve the patient.

It would certainly be important to share with him that a small lesion may not show up on chest X-ray and that the only way to be certain of excluding this would be with further tests.

How would you manage this particular patient?
- Sharing of information
- Urinalysis for haematuria (if positive, microscopy for dysmorphic red cells and casts)
- Blood tests including renal function, and, if haematuria, vasculitis screen
- Discussion with respiratory specialist and/or referral for bronchoscopy.

Teamwork is integral to good clinical care and when you feel out of your depth in making a decision then you should seek advice. Patients (and PACES examiners) are more impressed by your ability to know your limitations than your proceeding without all the information you need.

CASE STUDY | **7.6 NEGOTIATING A MANAGEMENT PLAN**

Instruction: *This 60-year-old man is soon to leave hospital, 7 days after an uncomplicated myocardial infarction. He has some concerns about his return to a normal life. What advice would you give him on the further management of his condition?*

The key word in this question is that this man has some *concerns*. It is very easy to assume what a patient's concerns are, and then address our assumptions without actually tackling the concerns of the patient. A suitable approach to this case is given in Case box 7.6.

Do you think that guidelines have an important role in clinical decision making?

Guidelines clearly have an important role in presenting evidenced based medicine in an easily accessible form for guiding decision

Case Box 7.6   Negotiating a Management Plan

1. Clarify the task
Introduce yourself and establish the facts. Confirm that he is recovering from a recent heart attack and that you hope to reassure and guide him on his road back to health.

2. Explore concerns and expectations
A patient's specific concerns can be overlooked when giving advice after a myocardial infarction, because there are standard areas that are usually discussed. Patients do not always voice their concerns. Often they think that 'the doctor has too many important things to think about' or 'is busy' or they are afraid to mention them or simply don't know how. It is important to ask about specific concerns. You could say:

D: *We usually have a list of things we go through before our patients go home, but before we start is there anything worrying you in particular?*

Or you could invite your patient to mention anything that you do not cover at the end.

3. Keep to a doctor's framework
Patient centredness means shepherding patients rather than abdicating all responsibility for decisions to them. A framework of points you need to discuss or management options you wish to consider keeps the consultation 'on track'. Patients prefer doctors who are open, informative and considerate to their wishes, but with one proviso—that their doctor appears to be *actively in control of the problem*. A good analogy is with active and passive listening. A doctor who sits forward, makes good eye contact and appears attentive is more likely to inspire a patient than one who sits back and appears uninterested. Equally, a doctor who is actively trying to reach the best management strategy through careful, well controlled discussion, is more likely to achieve a better outcome than one who seems happy to let patients 'do what they like'.

4. Share management options
Management options may include further investigations and pharmacological or non-pharmacological treatments. Patients vary in the extent to which they wish to be involved in management decisions, but most want to be informed about possible options.

For each option it is often worth stating your position, particularly where there appears to be a strongly 'right' option clinically. If there is a range of clinically acceptable options, you could deploy 'thinking aloud' skills:

D: *I wonder...*
D: *It might help if...*
D: *I often find that this is helpful...*
D: *I expect that if we...* (but never say what will happen, only what seems likely)

Throughout, ask what your patient thinks, encouraging good ideas whilst gently countering bad ones.

5. Confirm understanding and acceptance

D: *Does all of that make sense?*
D: *Are there any questions you'd like to ask?*
D: *We've covered a lot there...is there anything you'd like to go over again?*

---

making. The problem with guidelines is that they are created primarily for disease management and cannot be explicitly applied to every patient with the disease.

CASE STUDY | **7.7 ENCOURAGING PATIENT CONCORDANCE**

Instruction: *This 49-year-old gentleman was in hospital 6 weeks ago following a stroke with minimal right-sided weakness. Brain imaging confirmed a small left sided infarct. He has made a complete recovery and you are seeing him for follow up in the medical outpatient clinic. His ECG, echocardiogram and carotid Doppler study are normal. Blood tests have been unremarkable and you may assume that there was no underlying cause for his stroke other than hypertension. His hypertension was discovered 2 years ago, and is sustained, but his compliance with treatment has been poor. His blood pressure today is 180/100. Please discuss future management with him.*

Compliance (the term concordance is often preferred since it suggests agreement between patient and doctor) should always be checked before evaluating the effectiveness of a treatment.

Non-compliance with antihypertensives is a common dilemma, and it is important not to apportion blame—either to the patient or to the patient's general practitioner (GP). Patients don't take medications for many reasons and GPs struggle tirelessly to persuade patients to follow the best advice. Your discussion should begin with this premise and not by highlighting this patient's 'failure'.

Before you attempt to influence him in taking his medications, consider the following three questions:

1. *Are you dealing with poor compliance?*

Often the importance of taking medications has not been carefully explained or sufficiently emphasised. Even when explained, patients may still not fully understand or may forget the importance of medication.

2. Is poor compliance due to iatrogenic symptoms?

Always consider drug side effects or drug–drug interactions as a reason for a patient not taking prescribed medication.

3. Is the poor compliance due to another reason that needs to be explored?

Very often, poor compliance is the result of a discordance between what the doctor sees as important and what the patient sees as important.

If the above questions have been explored, the skills for *influencing* him in taking his medications are similar to those of negotiating a management plan, but particularly important elements of each skill are shown in Case box 7.7.

Case Box 7.7   **Encouraging Patient Concordance**

1. Clarify the task

Make it clear that shared understanding of the importance of hypertension treatment is the goal of this discussion.

2. Explore any concerns

D: *I know how difficult it can be to take medicines sometimes, but it would help me to know if there are any particular reasons you find your tablets difficult to take.*

3. Keep to a doctor's framework

We have seen (page 380) that a framework inspires patient confidence. In particular, frame your discussion around advantages that are likely to be important to your patient—the reduction in risk of stroke, reducing the need for future hospital admissions and so on. This sort of *giftwrapping* of treatments can be highly effective. Sometimes illustrating your point by reference to a similar case can help.

4. Share management options

Keep management options simple and keep your patient involved in decision making. Explicit categorisation can help, telling your patient that there are three things, for example, you want him or her to know, and that you will now explain 1, 2 and 3 in turn.

5. Confirm understanding

And offer to write down the key points of your management strategy for your patient's future reference.

A 34-year-old man was being treated for a high-grade non-Hodgkin's lymphoma on your haematology ward. He is 3 days into a chemotherapy regimen involving high-dose steroids but this morning, according to your junior house officer (JHO), was in a strange mood. He was apparently tearful but also declared that he believed himself now to be cured. He left the ward in his pyjamas and an overcoat and has not returned. Your JHO asks what, if anything, should be done. What should be done?

Patients have the right to decide how they are going to be treated and indeed whether they are going to be treated. Such autonomy should be respected. But in a case such as this, where declining further treatment is likely to have serious consequences, it is imperative to explore the patient's reasoning. In this example, iatrogenic mood disturbance from high-dose steroids must be the first consideration, and this patient's 'choice' should be held circumspect until further assessment has been made. Informing the ward staff, consultant, the patient's GP, relatives, and, on discussion with the consultant, involving hospital security and the police (restraint under the Mental Health Act is generally a last resort but may need to be instituted), are steps which may be needed to ensure this patient's safety.

CASE STUDY	7.8 DISCUSSING SMOKING CESSATION

Instruction: *This man wants to stop smoking. Can you help him?*

As well as the serious cardiac, respiratory and neoplastic risks of smoking, smoking carries considerable social harms and promotes premature ageing. Stopping smoking carries immediate benefits, including mortality reduction.

Nicotine addiction is now acknowledged as a treatable condition and there is substantial evidence of the effectiveness and cost effectiveness of behavioural and pharmacological interventions.

Some key approaches to helping a patient stop smoking are given in Case box 7.8.

Smoking cessation reduces the risk of many diseases. List some

- Stroke
- Coronary heart disease
- Peripheral vascular disease
- COPD
- Cancer of lung, mouth, throat, larynx, oesophagus, pancreas, bladder, cervix
- Peptic ulcer disease
- Pregnancy complications.

Do you know of any contraindications to treatment with amfebutamone?

- History of seizures
- Drugs which lower seizure threshold
- Pregnancy
- History of certain psychiatric disorders.

Case Box 7.8   Discussing Smoking Cessation

1. Ask about current smoking status
This includes asking about whether other household members smoke.

2. Advise about the benefits of smoking cessation
These include physical (see disease list, page 384), social and cosmetic. Emphasise the health benefits of stopping smoking rather than the risks of continuing to smoke. Reinforce the patient's own motivation for wanting to stop.

3. Ask about reasons for wanting to stop and assess motivation
(i) Ask your patient if they really want to stop smoking and if they would be prepared to stop now or within the next few weeks
(ii) Find out about previous attempts to stop and what measures helped or hindered
(iii) Ask whether other household members are willing to stop, too.

4. Discuss ways of assisting
These could include:
(i) Setting a date and stopping completely
(ii) Enlisting the help of family and friends. It helps many patients to consider themselves 'non-smokers' rather than 'ex-smokers'.
(iii) Enlisting the help of health promotion services and the patient's GP
(iv) Nicotine replacement therapy (best avoided in severe cardiovascular disorders)
(v) Amfebutamone.

CASE STUDY   7.9 CROSS-CULTURAL COMMUNICATION

Instruction: *You are seeing this 54-year-old Asian man in the diabetes clinic. He has some concerns about his treatment. Please explore these.*

Cultural factors can have large influences on disease management. Further, patients from different cultures may have differing beliefs about causes of their disease and effects of treatment.

During Ramadan, for example, Muslim patients may not eat anything, including tablets, during daylight hours, and often eat a large meal after dark. Type 2 diabetes is especially common in many Asian populations and Muslim beliefs may have important repercussions on the style of management chosen.

As a general rule, the same principles of good communication and explaining skills described earlier in this chapter apply when consulting with patients from different cultures. In other words, you should try to do more of the same, rather than treat such patients differently. In particular, it is important to adhere to the points in Case box 7.9.

Case Box 7.9   **Cross-cultural Communication**

- Allow plenty of time
- Show interest and concern and give non-verbal reassurance
- Keep explanations clear and simple
- Avoid jargon
- Check understanding.

Be aware of prejudice. We all tend to stereotype people—to assume people have characteristics because they appear to belong to a certain group. When stereotyped, people can become victims of prejudice—opinions, often unfavourable, formed without good reason. This can jeopardise good care.

What potential problems may arise when using interpreters?

- Failure to check that interpreter and patient speak the same language
- Assuming the patient can't understand any of what is being said— beware of assumptions and seek to find out what a patient can and can't understand
- Failure to address both the patient and the interpreter
- Failure to communicate simply and in small chunks
- Incorrect understanding or transmission of information
- Avoidance of delicate topics
- Domination of the patient by the interpreter
- Failure to allow sufficient time (at least a doubling of time is required).

CASE STUDY   **7.10 BREAKING BAD NEWS AND TALKING ABOUT DEATH AND DYING**

Instruction: *This is a previously well 48-year-old patient on your ward with a history of recent night sweats and abdominal pain. He has been under stress at work and had attributed his symptoms to this. He has splenomegaly and his full blood picture suggests chronic myeloid leukaemia. The haematology team plan to perform a bone marrow examination but he wants to know what diagnosis you suspect. 'Please tell me what you're thinking, doctor. Is it bad?' Please tell him.*

The skills for breaking bad news build on the skills of explaining a diagnosis, but with 'added ingredients' (Case box 7.10).

Examiners may ask you about how you would handle sensitive questions about death and dying.

Talking with patients about death and dying can be one of the most difficult areas of communication. Frequently, patients have specific

Case Box 7.10	**Breaking Bad News**

1. Scene setting

Many candidates are naturally adept at creating rapport and building a feeling of trust with their patients. Important components include:

(i) Ensuring that your patient does not sense that you are pressured for time. Ideally, this means setting aside time when you are not going to be interrupted. Happily, this is the case for 15 minutes in PACES!

(ii) Sitting close enough to your patient to allow good eye contact and observe non-verbal cues. Sitting at the same level, rather than above (or worse, standing), is less threatening to an already frightened patient.

(iii) Opening with a neutral statement:

D: *I believe you have had these sweats at night for a couple of months, and some pain in the tummy.*

(iv) Active listening. This means being attentive to what your patient tells you, showing your interest and concern through eye contact, head nodding and other natural body language.

In a nutshell, your patient should be made to feel that his or her problem is the most important problem in the world to you for the duration of the interview.

2. Establish previous experience

The golden rule is to *ask before telling*:

D: *I believe you put your symptoms down to stresses at work. Did any other possibilities cross your mind?*

Such a question both explores his beliefs and concerns, and prepares him for more serious news. The skill now is to encourage him to respond and elaborate. This might be with non-verbal skills such as silence, active listening and with simple words such as *hmm, yes*, and *and then?* Repeating and reflecting back important information he tells you can be effective:

D: *So you had been worried about something like that?*

3. Discover how much your patient wants to know

This can be a very helpful step if handled well, because it allows you to know what to tell. It can be handled poorly. Possible questions include:

D: *You said you wanted me to be honest and open with you. Are you the sort of person who likes to know everything about his condition?*

D: *We can't be certain of what is wrong from the test results so far. But are you the sort of person who likes to know all the possibilities?*

D: *Do you know why we did the biopsy?*

D: *Have you thought about what might be causing your symptoms?*

Many patients indicate immediately that they think they know what's wrong:

P: *I'm worried about cancer.*

It can be useful to clarify this:

D: *Are there any reasons why you think that?*

You are then in a position to confirm rather than break bad news.

When your patient appears not to be aware of potential bad news, the skill is in conveying the bad news without provoking overwhelming distress or pushing your patient into denial:

D: *I'm afraid it doesn't look like a straightforward ulcer.*

Your patient can then signal that no more information is wanted:

P: *Just tell me what we have to do next.*

or may indicate that they are ready for more information:

P: *What do you mean by not straightforward?*
D: *When the pathologist looked at the biopsy he found some abnormal cells.*

Again your patient can signal 'enough' or 'more':

P: *What do you need to do next?*

or:

P: *What do you mean by abnormal cells? I need to know if it's what I think it is.*
D: *They are cancerous.*

4. Break the bad news

The bad news may have been communicated by this time. Important principles for communicating bad news include:
(i) Ordering the information, building up the news layer by layer
(ii) Giving information in clear, simple, small pieces
(iii) Repeating important information
(iv) Encouraging feedback and giving your patient plenty of opportunity to respond
(v) Checking understanding
(vi) Being realistic and honest, but leaving room for hope.

One way to do all of this can be to recount previous events as a narrative, building up to the results of tests and explaining what can be done:

D: *We were worried about these night sweats and the lump in your tummy. The blood count you had is not completely normal. It shows some abnormal looking cells in your blood. We would need to do further tests before knowing why you have these cells. There are a number of possible reasons, but one of the possibilities would be a serious blood disorder, a type of leukaemia.*

The word leukaemia is the key word likely to register with your patient and provoke a response. It is best to reserve the use of such a 'fear-word' for when you have established that the patient does want to know the worst and that the diagnosis is either a strong possibility awaiting confirmation or one that has been established beyond doubt.

5. Acknowledge and respond to your patient's concerns/distress

You can do this non-verbally, practically (e.g. by offering tissues) or by putting emotions into words and acknowledging that such emotions are understandable (legitimising).

When bad news has been confirmed, it is tempting to rush in and offer immediate reassurance (but this is strongly discouraged):

D: *I'm sorry to have told you it's cancer, but the good news is...*
D: *Let me tell you what we can do...*

Unfortunately, patients at this point are usually too preoccupied to assimilate further information, and doctors can help far more by actively acknowledging distress:

D: *I can see this news has really upset you. Can you bear to tell me what distresses you most about all of this?*

It is particularly important to elicit specific concerns before giving more advice or information:

D: *How does this news make you feel?*
D: *It obviously hurts a lot to ask how long you might live if this is a type of leukaemia. It would help me understand how you are feeling if you could explain why you asked that question. I will give you the most honest answer I can.*

When asked about their fears, some patients say: *Am I going to die?* Assuming this to be an obvious question is natural, but it may be important to find out why your patient is asking.

6. Summarise, emphasising what can be done

Your patient may now have a number of questions, and it is time to give some positive news. Never remove all hope. However bad things may seem, always find a reason to be optimistic.
Talking with patients about death and dying

concerns and it is very important to discover what questions they have. Common questions include:

1. Questions about death

> P: *Am I going to die?*
> D: *I can answer that. But could I firstly ask you why you've asked me?*
> P: *Well, you've talked about more treatments, doctor. Chemotherapy and so on. But this problem with my liver doesn't sound good. I know that secondaries are a bad sign.*
> D: *I'm afraid it does look like your cancer is getting worse*
> P: *I just don't want to go through any more treatment if it's not going to make me better*
> D: *Are you thinking that chemotherapy is maybe not the best thing for us to consider?*
> P: *It won't cure me, will it?*
> D: *Well, it might buy us some more time.*
> P: *Could we do anything else?*
> D: *We could make sure that you were as comfortable as possible and try to let you spend as much time at home as possible.*
> P: *I think that might be best.*

2. Questions about how much time is left

> P: *How long have I got, doctor?*
> D: *The problem is, I don't know for certain.*
> P: *Can you guess?*
> D: *Well, the way things have been going, it could only be a few months.*
> P: *Will I be here for Christmas?*
> D: *I would hope so. Is there any particular reason you mention Christmas?*
> P: *I'd hate to die just before Christmas. My sister died just before Christmas. Christmas is always a terrible time of the year. I know it sounds stupid, doctor. I don't want my children to think about me dying at Christmastime.*
> D: *Is there anything else worrying about how much time you might have left?*

3. Questions about the impact on others

Frequently, the impact on others rather than dying is feared most:
> P: *I realise there's no cure now.*
> D: *Are there any specific concerns that you would like us to discuss?*

P: *Well, I know my time is up. I just feel a burden now.*

D: *A burden?*

P: *I can't do things for myself. The nurses are doing a lot. My daughter comes in each day but she's got a lot of problems of her own.*

D: *(Silence or acknowledging Mmn.)*

P: *I feel so sad for her. I look terrible now. I know it hurts her so much to see me like this.*

CASE STUDY   7.11 REQUESTING AN AUTOPSY (POST-MORTEM)

Instruction: *This lady's 86-year-old mother has died on your ward. She had a CT scan recently which showed bilateral adrenal masses, thought to be malignant, but had been awaiting further investigation. Your consultant has asked if you might seek permission from the family for an autopsy. Please discuss the possibility with her.*

Asking for permission to carry out an autopsy at a time when relatives are distressed is not an easy task and one which should not be delegated to the more junior member of the team. Most hospital trusts have guidelines for autopsy requests.

Most autopsies in hospital will be hospital requested and not at the request of the Coroner (Procurator Fiscal in Scotland), and for this relatives must grant permission. Before approaching relatives, it is important to establish if the patient had made any prior wishes (Case box 7.11).

Can relatives request a limited autopsy?

Yes. Most autopsy request forms allow relatives to choose a limited autopsy.

Is permission required for organ retention?

Yes. The autopsy request form should contain a question seeking separate permission for this. The usual organs retained are brain or lungs. Disposal of such organs can either be by the pathology department or they may be returned to the funeral director at the family's request.

Is permission needed for information from the autopsy to be used for educational purposes?

Most autopsy request forms contain a clause informing relatives that information may be used for such purposes unless they disagree.

Is permission needed for the use of retained tissue for research purposes?

Most autopsy request forms contain a clause asking relatives if they agree that research studies may be carried out on small samples of tissue removed at autopsy. Relatives may be assured that research projects need to be approved by the Local Research Ethics Committee.

Case Box 7.11   Requesting an Autopsy

1. Acknowledge that it is a difficult time

2. Explain the reasons for asking for an autopsy
Reasons might be:
(i) That the cause of death was not clear
(ii) That whilst the cause of death was clear, some features of the disease remained unusual or puzzling
(iii) That the disease was rare and an autopsy could shed new light on the disease
(iv) That information from the autopsy might help the management of other patients (or even family members) who suffer from the condition.
Additional benefits of an autopsy are that it can assist medical education, audit and research.

3. Explain the autopsy request form
If relatives seem happy to grant permission for an autopsy, the request form may need to be explained. Most autopsy request forms seek separate permission for organ retention and contain questions about information being used for medical education and small tissue samples being used for research.

4. Be prepared to discuss arrangements about the body
(i) Explain that an autopsy will not (usually) delay funeral arrangements.
(ii) Relatives may ask if the body can be viewed after autopsy. They should be assured that in the hospital autopsy standard incisions are used which are not visible when the body is gowned and that the body can be viewed after the autopsy.

Does a coroner requested autopsy require the consent of a relative?

No. Relatives do not have the right to either grant or refuse permission for an autopsy requested by the Coroner, nor any organ retention. Relatives may choose how they wish retained organs to be disposed of.

CASE STUDY   7.12 TALKING WITH ANGRY, UPSET AND DISTRESSED PATIENTS

Instruction: Please talk to this patient. He is very unhappy that your team seem to have lost the results of his blood tests. He thinks 'doctors and the NHS are useless'.

Two simple communication skills underlie dealing with angry, upset and distressed patients:

1. Try to calm emotions before dealing with the facts

2. Ask what is concerning the patient and listen to these concerns before you try to give any explanations or information.

Anger is usually secondary to another emotion such as fear, guilt or uncertainty. Discovering the underlying emotion is far more likely to achieve a resolution than taking anger at face value. Since minor disagreement can explode unpredictably into more serious confrontation, dialogue should, from the start, work towards de-escalation and resolution. Three general steps are helpful (Case box 7.12).

Case Box 7.12   Talking with Angry, Upset and Distressed Patients

1. Acknowledge (legitimise) your patient's emotions

D: *So you feel angry about the way you've been treated.*
D: *You feel that the treatment has been messed up.*
D: *Obviously you are very upset about this.*
D: *I think it's understandable that you should feel that way given what has happened to you.*
D: *It sounds as though you're feeling really upset/bad about this.*
D: *What bit of this has upset you most of all?*

2. Explore the emotions and concerns

D: *I agree that we must sort this out as quickly as possible. I will do everything I can, but it will help me if I know which aspects of how you have been treated concern you most of all.*

3. Work towards resolution

How might you work towards resolution?

(i) By steering away from areas of conflict (the fact that result was lost)

(ii) By avoiding comments which might incriminate colleagues

(iii) By identifying constructive actions

(iv) By giving clear advice and information or undertaking to seek it

(v) By finding realistic grounds for optimism in the face of anxiety or uncertainty

(vi) By finding common ground

(vii) By remaining polite and avoiding confrontation at all costs. The nature of medical training often equips doctors well with the skills of negotiation. Some patients simply do not have these skills. People are capable of acting out of character and appearing aggressive when upset. The primary motivation is more likely to be upset, distress or fear than desire to harm. It is essential to show willingness to listen and help.

CASE STUDY | **7.13 LEGAL POINTS IN CONFIDENTIALITY**

Instruction: *This 27-year-old Thai woman, who speaks good English, was admitted to your infection unit with jaundice, now confirmed to be a result of hepatitis B infection. She also has inguinal lymphadenopathy and you have asked for her consent for an HIV test. She has lived in the UK for 6 months with her English husband whom she met and married a year ago. She refuses the test. She also tells you not to tell her husband her diagnosis. They have a child 2 months old. Please talk with her (Case box 7.13).*

Case Box 7.13 | **Legal Points in Confidentiality**

1. There is potential conflict between the right of this patient to confidentiality and the right of contacts (her husband and the baby) to information and possible treatment. From the outset, you may be balancing her right to confidentiality against potential risks to others. But you should avoid giving her 'ultimatums' at this stage. It is vital not to 'rush in'. Your first duty is to her, analysing her problems and how you may best help her. Your first concern is that she may be infected with HIV in addition to hepatitis B. You should explain this to her, and assure her that you are there to help.

2. Try to explore her concerns. Is she scared about being diagnosed with HIV? If so, why? Is she scared for herself, or for the effect it will have on her family or marriage? Perhaps she knows that she has been exposed to HIV in the past and has always feared this sort of predicament. Is it possible that she that has been diagnosed with HIV in the past but has been living in denial?

3. Try to let her see the importance of excluding or confirming the diagnosis. A supportive approach is essential, letting her see the potential advantages—that the HIV test may be negative; were the test positive, it would allow earlier institution of treatment and testing of contacts (who could well be negative). Denial will not make the problem go away. She will know this, and her decision to avoid testing and telling is almost certainly motivated by fear.

4. Allow her time to think about what has been discussed and to ask questions.

She may have initially decided that the worst outcome would be for her husband to know that she has hepatitis or HIV. Your task is to identify other outcomes for her to consider.

Why is confidentiality important?

> Confidentiality is central to the trust that exists in the relationship between a doctor and a patient. This has been enshrined in doctors' codes of professional conduct including the Hippocratic Oath and the General Medical Council's (GMC) Guidelines.
>
> Information that a doctor learns from a patient 'belongs' to that patient. From a legal point of view a patient's case records do not belong to that patient, but from an ethical point of view patients should have the right to determine in general who has access to the information that they provide.
>
> Respect for patient autonomy supports confidentiality and opposes paternalistic attitudes, common in the past, in which doctors 'knew what was in a patient's best interests'.

What do you know about your legal commitment to confidentiality?

1. The general obligation is for doctors to keep information about patients confidential.
2. This obligation is not absolute—the law may allow or obligate breach of confidentiality, but any breach should only be to the relevant person or authority.
3. The issue of whether or not breach of confidentiality is lawful is often a question of balancing harm to the individual patient if confidentiality is breached, against harm to others if it is not breached. However, the equation of balancing public interests is seldom simple and the law sees a strong public interest in individual doctor–patient confidentiality being maintained.
4. The GMC's guidelines do not have the force of law but are taken seriously by the Courts.
5. Breach of confidentiality does not occur if a patient is not identifiable or if a patient has consented to the disclosure of information.
6. Sharing information about patients with other members of the health care team is not generally viewed by the law as breaching confidentiality.
7. Doctors have a duty to take reasonable precautions to prevent confidential information from falling into the wrong hands.

Under what circumstances may confidential information be disclosed?

Confidential information *must* be disclosed:

1. When legally required by a Court Order.
2. When a statutory duty, as in communicable disease notification and the reporting of births, deaths, abortions and work related accidents.
3. In cases of national security such as terrorism or in major crime prevention or in assisting in the solving of a major crime.

Confidential information *may*, at a doctor's discretion, be disclosed:

1. When a third party is deemed to be at risk of harm, for example at risk of contracting a serious infectious disease.
2. When it is in the public interest, for example informing the medical officer at the DVLA in the case of a patient with seizures who is known to be continuing to drive illegally.
3. Through sharing information with the health care team. When disclosure of relevant information between health care team members is clearly required for investigation or treatment to which a patient has agreed, the patient's explicit consent may not be required. Examples include passing information to medical secretaries for typing and writing information on request forms for laboratory or radiological investigations.

Breach of confidentiality should usually be the 'last resort' and a patient whose confidential information is intended to be breached should be given an explanation as to why. A doctor breaching confidentiality must be able to justify that decision. Before deciding to breach confidentiality, a doctor might sensibly seek advice from colleagues, professional bodies such as the BMA, and their medical defence organisation.

What are the possible consequences of breach of confidentiality?

- Loss of trust and breakdown in the doctor–patient relationship
- Disciplinary action by the GMC
- Investigation of serious professional misconduct by the GMC
- Civil legal action.

Does information remain confidential after death?

Yes, and information cannot be released without the consent of the patient's executor or a close relative who is fully informed of the consequences of disclosure.

What type of consent is needed when disclosing information to third parties such as employers and insurance companies?

Express consent (see Case study 7.19) is always needed from a patient, except where breach is necessary under the circumstances outlined above. Express consent may be *verbal* or *written* and is needed for disclosure of information to any third party, including a nearest relative.

Verbal consent from patients is usually sufficient when giving information to relatives, but written consent should be obtained when communicating with employers and in any legal matters. Patients must be aware of the purpose of disclosure, the obligation a doctor has to the third party and that this may include disclosure of personal information.

CASE STUDY 7.14 BREACHING CONFIDENTIALITY WHEN A THIRD PARTY MAY BE AT RISK (1)

Instruction: *This 40-year-old man is due to undergo a renal biopsy. He tells you that he is hepatitis C positive but instructs you not to share this information with anyone else. Please discuss this with him (Case box 7.14).*

Case Box 7.14   **Breaching Confidentiality when a Third Party may be at Risk (1)**

The examiners are assessing your awareness of the broad range of issues. Crucially, they would want to see you explore the ethical dilemma of respecting confidentiality whilst considering your duty to others who may be at risk.

1. There are similarities to Case study 7.13. Again, a patient has asked you to respect confidentiality, and here this duty is weighed against potential risk to colleagues, especially the doctor performing the biopsy and those performing phlebotomy. Again, start by reassuring him that you will try to help.

2. It is always preferable to gather information before reaching conclusions and deciding on a course of action. The next step is to ask more about his hepatitis C. How does he know that he has hepatitis C? How did he contract it? What investigations and treatments has he had so far? Who has been looking after him? He may feel that these are irrelevant questions and that you do not need this information. You should explain that it may be important in building a better understanding of his kidney problem and that a renal biopsy can be dangerous if liver function is impaired.

3. It would be important to discuss the risks that hepatitis C could pose to the health care team. As part of this discussion, you might explore why he has told you of his diagnosis but instructed that others not be informed. Exploring any fears may give you the answer.

4. You should emphasise that whilst knowledge of his hepatitis status is important to those looking after him for the reasons mentioned above, it would remain strictly confidential and not be disclosed to anyone not involved in his immediate care.

5. If he remains firm in his decision and refuses to allow disclosure, you may conclude that failure to inform some of your colleagues will place them at serious risk. It is then possible to breach confidentiality on the grounds of risk to others and on a strictly 'need to know' basis. You should inform the patient of what you propose to do.

The examiners are aware that such a discussion is difficult. They would not be looking for a 'model answer' but be checking that you are aware of the range of issues provoked and are able to handle the problem sensitively and professionally. They would be more concerned if you found such a case clear-cut and chose one of two extremes—agreeing to the patient's instructions or informing him that you intended to breach confidentiality without having had careful discussion around it.

What are the broad steps you might take when handling information that concerns risk to others which a patient prefers not to disclose?

- Gather information—always get all the facts you need first of all!
- Attempt to discover the patient's reasons for not wanting to disclose
- Discuss your concerns about the potential risk to others
- If the patient still refuses disclosure, explain that you may need to talk to colleagues on a 'strictly need to know' basis. Discussion with your medical defence organisation may be appropriate.

CASE STUDY	7.15 BREACHING CONFIDENTIALITY WHEN A THIRD PARTY MAY BE AT RISK (2)

Instruction: *This 32-year-old man has presented to your general medical clinic with weight loss and admits to a history of intravenous drug misuse and having multiple sexual partners. He is now living with his girlfriend, who is pregnant. You mention the possibility of HIV infection and he admits to having suspected this but adds 'If I had AIDS I would want to kill myself, doctor'. He also says that he feels angry. Please talk to him (Case box 7.15).*

Case Box 7.15	Breaching Confidentiality when a Third Party may be at Risk (2)

1. It takes time to come to terms with the possibility of a serious diagnosis like cancer or HIV infection, and very often anger is a secondary emotion, the primary one being fear.
2. Remember that at this stage you are not talking to him about having HIV infection, but about the importance of testing for it.
3. Again, you should attempt to explore his fears, and find out why he would want to kill himself. It may be that to him HIV is a 'death penalty' and that he does not fully understand its natural history and current treatments.
4. It may be appropriate to offer him a referral to trained HIV counsellors for further discussion of the implications of the test and its possible result.

Does his partner have a right to know?

A patient who has decided not to tell contacts at risk must recognise that this decision may have serious outcomes for these contacts and that breach of confidentiality would be a potential step you might have to take. Here, the partner and the fetus would be at risk and would warrant screening for HIV and the hepatitis B and C viruses were this patient positive. There are also implications for the obstetric team. The difficulty is that this patient has not yet been tested. Although he has not refused to be tested, he has threatened self-harm should the test be positive. Hopefully, exploring his views and reaching a shared understanding of the problem may persuade him of the value of being tested and sharing the problem with his partner.

CASE STUDY | **7.16 BREACHING CONFIDENTIALITY IN THE PUBLIC INTEREST**

Instruction: *This previously well 51-year-old man was brought into hospital after a road traffic accident from which he has no recollection. He was said to be 'twitching on arrival' in the emergency department. Subsequent neurological and cardiac investigations have been normal but the consultant neurologist told him that he would not be able to drive for a year. He is very anxious about this because his work involves driving and asks for your advice. Please talk with him (Case box 7.16).*

Case Box 7.16 | **Breaching Confidentiality in the Public Interest**

1. Express concern for his situation.
2. Get the facts and aim for shared understanding. Find out more about his job, what it entails and what losses he might incur through not being able to drive.
3. Beware of providing conflicting advice but offer to speak to the neurologist yourself about the decision.
4. Explain that such a decision would have been made for his safety and the safety of others.
5. Remember that patients have a right to a second opinion, although it may be appropriate to advise patients that some decisions are likely to be uniform amongst doctors, particularly where bound by a professional or legal framework.
6. Be aware that this may develop into an angry patient scenario (Case study 7.12).

A patient you are seeing in clinic with epilepsy last had a seizure 9 months ago and continues to drive. What are the implications?

An epileptic patient who continues to drive has his or her own autonomy and right to confidentiality. Yet breach of this confidentiality may be more important in the greater interests of benefit to society. Such a dilemma would start with obtaining the facts. Ask yourself what is the problem for the patient, for you as the doctor and for society? Your decision should embrace the implications to each party involved and the guiding ethical principles as applied to each. The DVLA publishes a booklet on driving rules in medical conditions. Current rules for drivers (of non-heavy goods or public vehicles) are that they must have been seizure free for more than 12 months or free of daytime seizures for more than 3 years if seizures are purely nocturnal. These rules apply on or off antiepileptic drugs. Patients should not drive for 6 months following any dose adjustment.

CASE STUDY   **7.17 CONFIDENTIALITY WHEN TALKING WITH RELATIVES AND OTHER THIRD PARTIES**

Instruction: *A 34-year-old patient with muscular dystrophy is admitted to your general medical unit with lobar pneumonia. He is stable but has a number of signs that are associated with a poor prognosis (diminished conscious level, hypotension and leucopenia). His carer, who is not a relative, asks how he is. Please speak to the carer (Case box 7.17).*

Case Box 7.17   **Confidentiality when Talking with Relatives and other Third Parties**

1. Your primary responsibility is to the patient, whose medical details remain confidential. It is very easy to forget this when a patient is unable to speak. It is equally important, however, to respect the concerns of a third party and the valued information they can often provide.

2. Introduce yourself and establish the carer's identity. You might say 'I'm sure you will understand that out of respect for (patient's name), I need to be sure to whom I'm speaking'.

3. Use listening skills (pages 106–107) with the third party to obtain information the patient cannot give you. You will frequently find that the third party knows, or has suspected, a lot more than you think about the condition of the patient.

4. The case records may be a valuable source of information. They may even demonstrate the patient's willingness for information to be shared with the third party.

5. Show respect for the carer's expertise (and experience with this particular patient), and acknowledge the interdependence between your patient and his carer.

6. Involve the carer as far as you can in making decisions, without compromising the autonomy of the patient. Asking 'What do you feel he would want us to do?' is not asking the carer to make a decision but inviting their valued insights to help guide your own decision making.

A woman says that her elderly mother, under your care with pneumonia, has been increasingly forgetful at home over the last 8 months, has neglected her personal hygiene and has twice put herself at risk by leaving the gas cooker on. She asks you to 'make sure that she is not allowed to return to her own home once she has recovered from her pneumonia'. How would you respond?

> The principles are similar to those above, listening to the daughter and obtaining as much useful information as possible to add to your assessment. What the daughter is telling you is very likely true, and may prompt formal psychogeriatric assessment. However, you should avoid reaching a diagnosis on the basis of a third party description alone. Others useful sources of information might be the patient's GP, district nurse or health visitor.

CASE STUDY 7.18 CONFIDENTIALITY AND TELEPHONE INFORMATION

Instruction: *This 80-year-old man has just recovered from a stroke. He lives independently and is to be discharged from your ward later this week. One of the nurses on your ward asks if you'll speak to his daughter. You are asked by a woman over the phone, 'What has happened to my father?'. Please answer her (Case box 7.18).*

Case Box 7.18 Confidentiality and Telephone Information

1. The first task is to establish the caller's identity. If in doubt, suggest taking their telephone number and calling back. You might then check in the phone book or from ward records that the identity of the caller and the number given match (assuming they are phoning from home). The degree to which you are happy to accept the identity of the caller will depend upon a number of things. Clearly, if you have met the daughter on the ward before, recognise her voice, and know that her father has always been happy to share his medical problems with her, you will be less guarded. Poor candidates make no attempt to ascertain with whom they are speaking.

2. Your willingness to give information is the next step your examiners will assess. Good candidates, assuming they have no prior knowledge that the patient consents to the divulging of information to his daughter, would explain why they could not without his permission. A less satisfactory response would be to explain that information cannot be disclosed but without any explanation that it is in respect of his right to confidentiality. Poor candidates might offer the caller information without hesitation.

The daughter now requests that you not tell him anything more about his condition without her prior permission—'he is a worrier'. Would you agree to this?

> You should not be willing to withhold information from him based solely on his daughter's wishes. You should explain to her that he has

a right to know what has happened to himself (respecting his autonomy) and to make his own decisions based on that information. You could reassure her that you would not force information on him, explaining only as much as he appeared to want to know.

You might also suggest that discussion by phone is not ideal and offer to speak to her if she comes in to hospital to visit her father. Avoid stating your legal rights in these sorts of situations. Relatives never warm to being told 'I'm in my rights not to tell you'. Phrases like 'I share your concerns', 'I understand how concerned you must be', or 'I appreciate how you must feel' offer empathy and show that you are listening.

CASE STUDY | **7.19 CONSENT FOR INVESTIGATION**

Instruction: *You wish to perform a diagnostic lumbar puncture on this 25-year-old woman with fever of unknown origin. Please obtain her consent (Case box 7.19)*

A task such as this requires communication skills (including those for explaining an investigation), a sound ethical framework, knowledge of the suspected diagnosis and knowledge of the diagnostic procedure.

Case Box 7.19 | **Consent for Investigation**

1. Introduce yourself.
2. Refer to Case box 7.2 for explaining an investigation.
3. Explain why you feel the lumbar puncture is necessary (knowledge of disease).
4. Explain the nature of the procedure including any associated discomforts and risks (knowledge of diagnostic procedure).
5. Explain any alternatives. You would need to explain the disadvantages of not reaching a diagnosis, but also that performing the investigation may not lead to a diagnosis. There is, of course, value in a negative test.
6. Show respect for autonomy. Never say 'This is what we must do'. Rather, explain that in your opinion a particular course of action seems to be in the patient's best interests.
7. Invite questions.
8. Seek permission to proceed with an open question. 'How does that sound?' rather than 'So, do you consent to this test?'

What are the necessary requirements for valid consent?

Consent is firmly seated upon the principle of respect for patient autonomy. For consent to be valid:

1. A patient should be properly *informed*
2. The patient should understand that information and be *competent* to give consent?
3. Consent must be given *voluntarily*, without coercion.

What is meant by implied consent and express consent?

> Because touching a patient without consent can constitute *battery*, consent is needed even when taking a patient's pulse or examining the chest. Yet doctors seldom obtain consent specifically expressed (see also page 395) for such routine tasks and in law patients could not successfully sue doctors most of the time. This is because the Courts accept the concept of implied consent. If a patient offers their wrist whilst the doctor takes the pulse, consent is implied by their behaviour. However, the fact that a patient is in hospital does not constitute implied consent to examination, investigation or treatment.

What is battery?

> A procedure performed without consent may be grounds for battery. Generally, if a person touches another without consent, this constitutes battery, for which damages may be awarded. Unlike negligence (page 415), proof of harm is not necessary for damages to be awarded.

What exceptions are there to informed consent?

> Where a patient is judged not to be mentally competent informed consent may not be possible.

CASE STUDY	**7.20 CONSENT FOR TREATMENT**

Instruction: *This 65-year-old diabetic gentleman has diabetic nephropathy as evidenced by microalbuminuria. You wish to start an ACE inhibitor. Please seek his consent (Case box 7.20).*

> Rights are so basic yet so easily ignored. This is especially true of the right to consent to treatment or refuse it. In theory, consent should always be obtained for any treatment. In practice, there is often

Case Box 7.20	**Consent for Treatment**

1. Introduce yourself.
2. Refer to Case box 7.3 for explaining a treatment.
3. Explain why you feel the ACE inhibitor would be beneficial (knowledge of disease and its treatment).
4. Explain the important side effects (knowledge of drug).
5. Explain any alternatives, and the risks or benefits and likely outcomes of these.
6. Show respect for autonomy. Rather than saying 'This is what we must do', explain that in your opinion the course of action seems to be in the patient's best interests.
7. Invite questions.
8. Seek permission to proceed with an open question.

implicit understanding that consent for examination, investigation or treatment is *implied* by a patient (page 402). Although such assumptions seldom result in problems, legal justification for them is not inevitable.

What is meant by competence or capacity to consent?

For a patient to give valid consent (page 401) to a procedure or treatment, she or he must be *competent* (or, in legal terms, *have the capacity*) to do so. The key aspects of competence are given in Case study 7.21.

Competent patients should be given information from which to make an informed choice. If an apparently competent patient is refusing treatment that is strongly in their best interest, then it is very important to understand and explore the reasons and to make sure that the patient is fully informed. At the end of the day if a patient is competent he or she has the right to refuse.

An example would be that of a Jehovah's Witness patient declining blood products for whom a blood transfusion might be life saving. Respect for such a patient's autonomy (self-determination) means that you must accept that they can refuse treatment. Your acceptance of this autonomy may mean that the patient will die. Naturally, in a case as extreme as this, it would be sensible to seek corroboratory agreement from colleagues and even your medical defence organisation.

CASE STUDY | **7.21 CONSENT AND CAPACITY**

Instruction: *This 75-year-old woman was admitted to hospital with pneumonia. A hard mass was discovered arising from her rectum whilst under your care, most probably a carcinoma. She is asymptomatic. She refuses to consider any further investigations or treatments. Please speak with her (Case box 7.21)*

What are the key aspects, based on case law, of capacity to give or refuse consent?

- That the patient is able to *understand and retain information* about the treatment proposed, alternative options, the treatment's possible benefits and risks and the consequences of non-treatment
- That the patient *believes the information* to be truthful
- That the patient is able to *weigh up the information* in order to reach a decision.

Incompetence (in legal terms *incapacity*) must be proven. All adults are assumed by law to be competent (or have capacity) unless proven otherwise. Further, a person is not globally competent or incompetent. Competence or capacity is 'function specific'.

How may doctors be negligent in obtaining consent?

Patients need information to make decisions about whether or not to undergo procedures and treatments. In particular, they need information about the nature of treatment, its benefits and risks, and possible alternatives. Doctors may be *negligent* if they fail to provide sufficient information before consent is obtained.

Box 7.21	Consent and Capacity

1. Management may become acceptable to patients after underlying beliefs, concerns or expectations have been explored. It is possible that she already suspects this to be an incurable condition and has made a decision to 'let nature take its course' rather than submit to further time in hospital with tests. She may have experienced a similar situation with another family member or friend in the past. But has she been given enough information to make an informed decision? What does she know about the natural history, investigations and treatment options for colorectal cancer? It may be that she imagines too many painful tests. It may be that she imagines only chemotherapy, about which she has heard so many dreadful things, but would consider an operation. It may be that she feels she has had a good life, has no living relatives and has 'had her innings'.

2. There are many 'maybes'. The point is that before respecting her wishes (autonomy) for no further tests, you must try to understand precisely what her position is and help to inform her. Her decision may already have been made. But you should try to discover the reasons she made it and whether or not she has sufficient information at her disposal to make an informed decision. She may choose not to receive any more information, but ideally informed consent to no treatment should be obtained and based upon discussion of the acceptability and effectiveness of the various options.

3. Try to provide information about risks and benefits and possible outcomes of the various options open to her. This includes discussion that she likely has a growth which can only be confirmed by investigations, and that only with such investigations could it be determined how it be best treated. Discussion about the potential for early palliative surgery should she have an incurable condition may be appropriate.

4. It would be worth asking her what she thinks her relatives might think about her decision. Your duty is to respect her wishes, but when a decision has been made to refuse management of a potentially serious condition, a patient should be encouraged to share it with relatives.

5. She should be assured that she may seek more information or change her mind at any time.

How might doctors be guided when making decisions for a patient who has lost capacity to make decisions?

- Doctors may act in what they see as the best interests of the patient and may be afforded some protection in their decision by the Bolam test (page 415).
- Doctors may be guided by an advance directive (Case study 7.26) if made at a time when the patient was competent.
- Those close to the patient may be sources of information but cannot give or withhold consent—in other words, there is no proxy in English law for an adult patient who has lost the capacity to make decisions.

Who are 'those close to a patient'?

The phrase includes a partner, a family member, a professional or other carer or an informal advocate. In Scotland it also includes a 'proxy decision maker' appointed under the *Adults with Incapacity (Scotland) Act 2000*, a 'nearest relative' or a 'person claiming an interest' such as a public guardian or mental welfare commissioner (as referred to in the Act or under Scottish mental health legislation). In England and Wales under mental health legislation, a 'nearest relative' or 'guardian' may have been appointed. A proxy decision maker (not an accepted legal term in England or Wales) may be a welfare attorney, welfare guardian or a person authorised under an intervention order, and may be authorised to make medical decisions on behalf of an adult with incapacity.

CASE STUDY | 7.22 REFUSAL TO GIVE CONSENT

Instruction: *This 32-year-old woman has been diagnosed with Graves' disease. The endocrinologist has discussed the various treatment options and would like her to start oral treatment in the first instance. She tells you, the medical SHO, that she has decided to take homoeopathic treatment. Please discuss this option with her (Case box 7.22)*

Case Box 7.22   Refusal to Give Consent

1. You may not have the facts in front of you, but feel she 'needs' more than homoeopathic treatment. However, it is vital to start off in a non-confrontational manner, aiming to understand why she feels the way she does.
2. Try to explore her reasons for choosing homoeopathy. It may be that she has experience of homoeopathic remedies for other conditions. It may be something much more simple—perhaps she was ready to consider carbimazole before the endocrinologist mentioned the dangerous side effect of leucopenia. It may be that she would have considered other forms of treatment.

3. Explain the reasons why her consultant prefers the carbimazole option. Try to talk to her about Graves' disease, its complications, the benefits and risks of treatment and the likely natural history without treatment.
4. You might tell her that you are unaware of any effective homoeopathic treatments but that you are willing to look at any information she can provide. Is it possible, if she is adamant that homoeopathic treatment will help her, that she would consider conventional treatment as well? Failing this, might she accept switching to conventional treatment within a certain time frame if her approach does not work?
5. Tell the examiners that you would also inform your consultant of this conversation and document your advice in the case records.

You have been seeing a 50-year-old patient with tuberculosis in the respiratory clinic. He suggests that he wishes to pursue homoeopathic treatment rather than continue with antibiotics. How would you respond?

1. There comes a point where collusion with a patient is wrong, clinically, ethically and legally. Here, you have not just to consider this man's autonomy, but risks to other members of the public from his active tuberculosis.
2. As before, rather than approaching this dilemma in a dogmatic way, listening to the patient's reasons, beliefs and concerns may avoid confrontation. Perhaps the importance of antibiotic therapy has never been fully explained. Perhaps he has learned (mistakenly) from idle conversation or the internet that homoeopathy can help a wide range of respiratory conditions. Listening and simple explanation may be sufficient to persuade him of his misconception. Perhaps he feels the antibiotics should have worked by now and is concerned it could be something else because he's still coughing. Perhaps he is frustrated that he cannot return to work and needs to vent his feelings.

| CASE STUDY | 7.23 DO NOT RESUSCITATE (DNR) ORDERS AND WITHOLDING/WITHDRAWING LIFE-PROLONGING TREATMENTS |

Instruction: *Please discuss a DNR order with this 75-year-old gentleman, who despite domiciliary oxygen is admitted every few weeks with worsening exacerbations of severe COPD (Case box 7.23)*

Under what circumstances may a DNR order be considered?

The British Medical Association, Royal College of Nursing and UK

Case Box 7.23	DNR Orders

1. This requires sound communication skills, in particular listening and eliciting and explaining skills.
2. The setting must be private, and you should have plenty of time without the likelihood of interruptions.
3. An opening sentence followed by a warning shot can be useful:

   D: *Mr (patient's name), you and I got to know each other a little during your last admission. There is something important I would like to discuss with you.*

4. Pace your explanation slowly and carefully, allowing him to assimilate what you are saying:

   D: *You were with us 4 weeks on the ward last time and I know you were very uncomfortable with disturbed sleep, a lot of drugs with side effects, and a lot of blood tests. Your breathing was a bit better when you went home but now you're back in hospital again sooner than either of us hoped. Someone with a lung condition as bad as yours may suddenly take a turn for the worse. In fact, the heart may even stop beating. If that were to happen, there would not be time to ask you what you would like us to do. If we were to restart your heart, we might only be prolonging a situation which you find intolerable. This is not an easy thing to talk about, but we would hate to do the wrong thing.*

5. Dealing with emotions before facts is very important, acknowledging any distress caused.

   D: *I can see that you are distressed by this discussion. I find it very hard to confront you with painful facts like this.*

6. After discussion, if you feel that he is ready for your questions, you might ask:

   D: *If your heart were to stop beating, would you want us to try to restart it for you?*

7. You may need to seek confirmation if he indicates that he would not wish CPR:

   D: *I can see how distressing it is to face up to how ill you are. I can see that it's a hard decision for you, but you have said that life is so bad that you wouldn't want your heart to be restarted. Have I understood you correctly?*

8. There should follow a promise of continuing support of doctors and nursing staff in doing everything possible to help his condition.

Resuscitation Council guidelines broadly agree that it is appropriate to *consider* a DNR decision in the following circumstances:

1. Cardiopulmonary resuscitation (CPR) is unlikely to be successful (futile).
2. CPR is not in accord with a competent patient's recorded and sustained wishes.
3. CPR is not in accord with a valid advance directive (for a patient who is not competent).
4. Resuscitation is likely to be followed by a length and quality of life that would not be in the best interests of the patient.

Under what circumstances may a DNR order be made without consulting a patient?

Discussions about circumstances in which CPR should not be attempted can be difficult and distressing for all concerned. However, failing to give patients or, where appropriate, those close to the patient, opportunity to be involved in reaching a decision can cause more distress at a later stage than if handled sensitively at the outset. In most circumstances a patient should be involved in a DNR decision. Where a patient is already seriously ill with a foreseeable risk of cardiopulmonary arrest, or in a poor state of health nearing the end of their life, decisions about whether to attempt CPR in particular circumstances should ideally be made in advance as part of an overall care plan.

A DNR order may sometimes be made without consulting a patient if there is no likelihood that resuscitation would be successful (futility) or if the patient is not able to make such a decision (unconscious or not competent to do so) or if the patient's quality of life is extremely poor (a very grey area, because doctors cannot be judges of a patient's quality of life). None of these criteria is straightforward; for example, there is no easy definition of futility. Those close to a patient (page 405) may be involved in a DNR decision if the patient is unable to speak for her or himself or so wishes, but the first duty remains to the patient.

Do you know of any guidance documents about withholding and withdrawing life-prolonging treatments?

A GMC document specifically addresses this subject. A growing range of treatments (e.g. CPR, dialysis, artificial ventilation, artificial nutrition and hydration) countered with the fact that life has a natural end presents dilemmas to doctors, patients and their families.

What are the guiding principles on the subject of withholding and withdrawing life-prolonging treatments?

1. *Presumption for prolonging life in a patient's best interests.* Prolonging life will usually be in a patient's best interests if treatment is not excessively burdensome or disproportionate to expected

benefits. Not continuing or not starting a potentially life-prolonging treatment is in a patient's best interests when there is no net benefit. Life has a natural end and doctors should not strive to prolong the dying process with no regard to a patient's wishes.

2. *Adult patients who can decide for themselves*: Competent patients have the right to decide how much weight to attach to the benefits, burdens and risks, and overall acceptability of any treatment. They have the right to refuse treatment.

3. *Adult patients who cannot decide for themselves*: Any valid advance refusal of treatment made when a patient was competent (had capacity, page 403) and on the basis of adequate information must be respected. Where a patient lacks capacity, assessment of the benefits, burdens and risks, and overall acceptability of any treatment must be made on their behalf by the doctor, taking into account what is known to the doctor and any information from those closest to the patient.

4. *Choosing between options: difference of view about best interests*: Applying these principles may result in different decisions in each case, since patients' assessments of likely benefits, burdens and risks, and the weights and priorities given to these, will differ according to their values and beliefs. Where a patient lacks capacity, the doctor, health care team or those close to the patient may have different views, prompting independent or legal advice.

5. *Concerns about starting then stopping treatment*: Where decided that treatment is not in the best interests of a patient, there is no ethical or legal obligation to provide it and therefore no need to distinguish between not starting treatment and withdrawing treatment. Where a patient lacks capacity to make decisions and there is uncertainty about appropriateness of treatment, treatment that may be of some benefit should be started until clearer assessment can be made. This is particularly important in emergencies, when more time is needed for detailed assessment, or where there is doubt about the severity of a condition or the benefit of particular treatment.

6. *Artificial hydration and nutrition*: This is an especially difficult area since treatment benefits and burdens may not be well known. The term refers to techniques such as the use of nasogastric tubes, percutaneous endoscopic gastrostomy tubes and subcutaneous and intravenous hydration. It does not refer to oral hydration and nutrition, which are generally regarded as part of nursing care.

7. *Non-discrimination*: Priority must be based on clinical need whilst seeking to make best use of resources. Discrimination must not be allowed on the basis of, for example, age, disability,

race, colour, culture, belief, sexuality, gender, lifestyle or social or economic status.

8. *Care for the dying*: Patients who are dying should receive the same respect and standard of care as other patients.

9. *Conscientious objections*: Doctors with a conscientious objection to a decision may withdraw from care of a patient but must ensure that another suitably qualified colleague takes over their role without delay.

10. *Accountability*: Doctors are responsible to their patients, society, the GMC and the courts.

What framework is there for putting the above into practice?

1. *Clinical responsibility for any decision* rests with the consultant or general practitioner.

2. Thorough *assessment* of the *diagnosis* and *likely prognosis* must precede any decision.

3. *Options for treatment* must be based on clinical evidence about efficacy, side effects and other risks. A considered judgement should be reached on the likely clinical and personal benefits, burdens and risks of each treatment (or non-treatment) option. A clinician with relevant experience should be consulted if the responsible doctor has limited experience of the condition, if there are doubts about the range of options, if there are serious differences of opinion within the health care team, or if withholding or withdrawal of artificial nutrition or hydration is being considered for a patient with a very serious condition but who is not imminently dying and whose views cannot be determined.

4. Seeking the wishes of patients who *can decide for themselves* is essential.

5. For patients who *cannot decide for themselves*, the correct course of action may have been decided previously through a valid advance directive. Without this, an assessment of capacity to decide must be made through professional guidelines and tests of capacity and, if in doubt, legal advice.

6. *Communicating* and *recording* of decisions and *review of decisions at appropriate intervals* are essential.

One of your patients, a dying man with end stage renal failure, diabetes and peripheral gangrene has a hypoglycaemic attack. Would you treat him?

This would depend upon any prior wishes he may have made. He may have told his doctors to 'let him go' if he takes any turn for the worse. He may, alternatively, have declined treatment for his renal failure and requested a comfortable death. But a scenario such as hypoglycaemia may not have been anticipated or explicitly discussed. A common response to a potentially fatal change in condition that has not been previously discussed is to treat the current episode and later discuss with the patient what they would wish were it to recur. This said, since hypoglycaemia, unlike other potentially fatal changes in his condition, is caused by the medication and easily reversed, there may be legal risks in not treating, whatever the patient says.

CASE STUDY	7.24 PALLIATIVE CARE

Instruction: *This lady has breast cancer with cerebral metastases. She asks you how many of her anticonvulsant pills she would need to take to end her life. Please talk with her (Case box 7.24).*

Case Box 7.24	Palliative Care

1. Palliative care is a speciality in which patients frequently become despondent. It is essential to try to elicit their specific fears.
2. In terms of decision making, you are bound by ethical principles and a legal framework. Invariably, but not exclusively, your own moral beliefs will be in concert with these principles and the law.
3. We sometimes hasten death in clinical practice. The crucial distinction is *intention*, which may be to hasten death or relieve suffering. Frequently, doctors set out to relieve pain and suffering but see that life may be shortened. Foreseeing is not necessarily the same as intending. This has been tested in law and held to be permissible and in keeping with the duties of a doctor. It is one aspect of the doctrine of double effect, which makes a distinction between harms that are intended and harms that are foreseen but not intended. A scenario commonly encountered is where high doses of morphine are used to relieve pain yet may shorten life by reducing respiratory drive. A foreseeable consequence is that of hastening death, but the intention is to relieve pain.
4. In the scenario given, telling the patient how many anticonvulsant pills would be required in order to kill herself could be tantamount to assisting suicide and a criminal act. Your communication skills should endeavour to elicit key aspects of her suffering as she sees them and explore alternative ways of relieving them.

Consider a patient dying of lung cancer who develops pneumonia. A ventilator may prolong life but may also delay an inevitable death. What courses of action are there?

Broadly, there are five options at the end of life:

1. The sanctity of life view—to ventilate and therefore prolong life whatever else may apply
2. To withhold life prolonging treatment—to withhold ventilation

3. To withdraw life prolonging treatment—to ventilate then withdraw from ventilation
4. Assisted suicide
5. Active euthanasia.

Option 1 is uncommon. Options 2 and 3 are commonly accepted medical practice. Options 4 and 5 are illegal and widely accepted as unethical and immoral.

CASE STUDY	7.25 FUTURE CARE

Instruction: *A 52-year-old lady with multiple sclerosis is wheelchair bound and unable to feed herself. She has a percutaneous gastrostomy. She is recovering in hospital from her third episode of pneumonia this year, and on this occasion required ventilation in an ITU for 2 days. A nurse at a multidisciplinary meeting asks whether she will be considered for this 'next time she has pneumonia'. Please respond to the nurse's question (Case box 7.25)*

Case Box 7.25	Future Care

It is the competent patient's right to be involved in any decision about investigation or treatment or place of care. You cannot decide what you will do for this patient without talking with her. In such a discussion you would have to explore her fears and her quality of life as she sees it. This is best achieved with open questions such as:

● What are your thoughts about the future?
● What do you feel about your illness?
● What aspects of life still give you pleasure?
● What frightens you most about the future?

How might decision making be aided when a patient is not competent (page 403) to decide?

In the case of a patient who is not competent, doctors can sometimes respect requests about terminal illness management made by that patient at a time when he or she was competent. Such requests may be clarified by *advance directives*. Clearly, requests that could not be respected for a competent patient could also not be respected for a patient who is not competent, such as a request for assisted suicide. It is also very important to establish that the patient was not only competent but also fully informed at the time of making a request.

Because of the difficulties encountered when a patient is not competent, it is good practice to discuss with a terminally ill patient when competent what their wishes about future management are and what you can and cannot do for them.

CASE STUDY	7.26 ADVANCE DIRECTIVES

Instruction: *This 79-year-old retired GP asks you what you know about advance directives (advance statements, living wills). Please tell her what you know (Case box 7.26).*

What do you know about the persistent vegetative state (PVS)?

- A patient shows no behavioural evidence of awareness of self or the environment. There is a spectrum from unawareness to awareness.
- There is brain damage, usually of known cause, consistent with the diagnosis.
- There are no reversible causes present and at least 6 months and usually 12 months have passed since the onset.

Important issues in managing a patient with PVS include diagnosis and deciding on its permanence, decision to withdraw treatment (even with a valid advance directive this may need to be decided in the courts and legal advice is essential) and the process of withdrawing treatment.

Case Box 7.26   Advance Directives

1. Advance directives (or 'advance statements' or 'living wills') are statements made by adults at a time they are competent (or have legal capacity) to decide for themselves about treatments they wish to accept or refuse, in circumstances in the future where they are no longer able to make decisions or communicate their preferences. To make an advance directive, a patient should have sufficient information to understand the consequences of any decision as well as being legally competent (having capacity).
2. The premise of an advance directive is that patients have the right to consent to or refuse treatment.
3. There are different types of advance directive. *Instruction directives* set down a patient's wishes in highly specific circumstances. Defining circumstances is clearly difficult. It may be difficult to draw conclusions, for example, from an advance directive made in the event of a stroke, where the particular type of disability has not been stated. *Value directives* provide more general guidelines.
4. Advance directives may not always be legally binding or unambiguous, although an informed advance directive can potentially be regarded in the same way as contemporaneous consent or refusal and ignoring it could constitute negligence or battery. Advance refusal of treatment made when a patient was competent, on the basis of adequate information about the

implications of his/her choice, is legally binding and must be respected where clearly applicable to the patient's present circumstances and where there is no reason to believe that the patient has changed his/her mind.

5. Advance directives are most useful with reference to specific treatments. Broad statements about life saving treatments may be open to interpretation. What, for example, constitutes treatment? Does treatment include feeding a patient in a persistent vegetative state? Where a specific treatment is requested, doctors are not bound to provide it, if in their professional view it is clinically inappropriate.

6. Advance directives must be free from coercion and not the result of illness, fatigue or drugs.

7. Advance directives cannot authorise a doctor to do anything illegal.

8. Patients are free to amend their advance directive at any time.

9. The British Medical Association and the Royal College of Physicians have produced guides and statements on advance directives.

| CASE STUDY | 7.27 MEDICAL ERROR |

Instructions: *You have given a 62-year-old man an incorrect result following his recent endobronchial lung biopsy. You told him that the lesion was benign yesterday evening, and on this morning's ward round are surprised to see that the filed report suggests a carcinoma. Please tell the examiners how you might respond to this (Case box 7.27).*

| Case Box 7.27 | Medical Error |

Areas to include in your response include:

1. Establishing the facts: Double checking today's report, including the name and patient details. Is the report really correct or a clerical typing error? Which consultant or doctor performed the biopsy and who reported the result?

2. An open discussion of the mistake with your consultant. Is it your mistake alone or is there joint accountability? Is there failure of the system?

3. Possible discussion with your medial defence organisation.

4. An open discussion of the mistake with the patient and an apology. An apology in this scenario would seem weak solace in respect of the gravity of the error, but is essential.

What are the conditions for negligence?

- That the doctor owes a *duty of care* to the patient
- That the doctor was in breach of the appropriate *standard of care* imposed by the law
- That the breach in the duty of care *caused* any harm in question, meriting compensation.

Causation—that the failure of care caused the harm—is the most difficult criterion to prove. Any damages awarded aim to meet losses incurred by a patient, but not exceed it. In other words, punitive damages are not awarded. The law further requires that a patient must sue a doctor within 3 years of an act of alleged negligence.

What is an appropriate standard of care?

An appropriate standard of care is ordinary care, which is sometimes determined by the Bolam test.

What is the Bolam test?

The Bolam test considers whether or not a doctor's actions are consistent with a responsible body of medical opinion. The name refers to a real case in which a judge declared that a doctor is not guilty of negligence if he or she has acted in accordance with the practice accepted as proper by a responsible body of colleagues skilled in the same practice.

CASE STUDY   7.28 'UNFIT' COLLEAGUE

Instruction: A medical SHO colleague on your ward appears to have an alcohol problem. He has turned up to work numerous times in the last month smelling of alcohol, often leaving for a few hours in the morning, feeling sick. You are aware of two mistakes he has made which you feel are due to his alcohol habit. What would you do (Case box 7.28)?

Case Box 7.28   'Unfit' Colleague

1. Explain to the house officer that you realise something is wrong and invite him to talk about it.
2. Explain to the house officer about duties to patients.
3. Explain that he has a duty to seek help and that if he will not do so, then you have a duty to consider discussing the problem with a third party if you feel that patients could be at risk.
4. Offer to go and seek help with your colleague.

There is a question of when, whatever the house officer says, you should inform other people and who these should be. The whole area of patients at risk and of 'whistle blowing' is a moving target. The GMC and medical defence organisations provide updates.

Would you take the same approach if it were your consultant, rather than a fellow SHO, whom you suspected?

Consultants are subject to the same guidelines for safe practice!

CASE STUDY | **7.29 POTENTIALLY CRIMINAL INCIDENT**

Instruction: *This 19-year-old man asks you, the SHO, to delete the fact that he takes occasional recreational drugs from his records. He says that he has not told his GP and regrets having said 'yes' when the receiving JHO asked him about this. Please respond to him (Case box 7.29).*

Case Box 7.29   **Potentially Criminal Incident**

Areas to include in your discussion include:

1. Why he is in hospital.
2. The patient's reasons for the request. He may have concerns about insurance forms asking about HIV risks, or about employment implications, or about his partner finding out.
3. The potential clinical importance of this information, e.g. risks of transmissible infectious diseases.
4. Assurance of the confidentiality of his case records.
5. The ethical framework. Autonomy, beneficence, non-maleficence and justice apply not only to the patient but to you, your colleagues and society. For clinical, medicolegal and often moral reasons you cannot modify a patient's record and in this situation must consider the far-reaching implications to you and society. Is it fair to society that insurance companies could at a later date pay out a large sum to this patient, whose non-declaration of his risk factors was aided by your amendment of the record?

What do you know about the Access to Health Records Act?

- This gives patients the general right to see their medical records, obtain copies thereof and have the records explained to them.
- It only applies to records after 1 November 1991.
- A doctor may deny access (it is not that the whole record should be withheld but only specific information within it) on the grounds that it is 'likely to cause serious harm to the physical or mental health of the patient or any other person, or could lead to the identification of another individual (other than the health professional) who has been involved in the care of the subject'.
- An application must be in writing and made by a patient, person authorised by the patient, person appointed by the Court or an executor.
- When application for access is made by an individual on behalf of a patient who is incompetent or deceased, no information can be given that the patient had considered to be confidential and the

holder is not required to explain why any part of the record has been withheld.

- Viewing of the records should be provided within 21 days (40 days for records at least 40 days old).
- A reasonable fee may be charged.

REFERENCES AND FURTHER READING

The legal framework and interpretation of legal cases relevant to many of the issues in this chapter are often highly complex. Further, it is important to recognise that there are differences between Scottish and English Law. The various medical defence organisations have taken particular interest in providing legally orientated information to medical practitioners and in particular have produced texts and materials in the areas of confidentiality and consent. Ethical principles, rather than the complexities of the law, should be tested at this Station of PACES.

Many hospital and NHS Trusts have clinical ethics committees or other arrangements for access to clinical ethics support and advice. Other useful starting points are the BMA Ethics Department and the National Network of Clinical Ethics Committees, contactable through ETHOX (The Oxford Centre for Ethics and Communication in Health Care Practice). Online. Available: www.ethox.org.uk

British Medical Association guides (various guides are updated on medical ethics). Online. Available: www.bma.org.uk.

British Medical Association. Decisions about cardiopulmonary resuscitation. Information leaflet for patients published 2002 by BMA. Online. Available: www.bma.org.uk

DVLA, Swansea SA99 1DG. At a glance guide to the current medical standards of fitness to drive. Online. Available: www.dvla.gov.uk/ at_a_glance/aag_contents.htm

General Medical Council (GMC) booklets on *Duties of a Doctor*, covering issues such as Good Medical Practice, Consent and Confidentiality, Research. Online. Available: www.gmc.org

General Medical Council. Withholding and Withdrawing Life-prolonging Treatments: Good Practice in Decision-making. GMC August 2002. Online. Available: www.gmc.org

Hope T. Consent. Medicine 2000; 28: issue 10:5–9.

The Law Society/British Medical Association. Assessment of Mental Capacity: Guidance for Doctors and Lawyers. The Law Society/BMA 1995.

Lockwood G. Confidentiality. Medicine 2000; 28: issue 10:10–13.

Maguire P. Breaking bad news: talking about death and dying. Medicine 2000; 28: issue 10:34–35.

Neighbour R. The inner consultation. Lancaster: MTP Press; 1987.

Parker M, Hope T. Ways of thinking about ethics. Medicine 2000; 28: issue 10:2–5.

Savulescu J. End of life decisions. Medicine 2000; 28: issue 10:13–17.

Schofield T. Patient centred consultations. Medicine 2000; 28: issue 10:22–24.

Tate P. The doctor's communication handbook. Oxford: Radcliffe Press; 1984.

Skin, Locomotor System, Eyes, Endocrine System

8. SKIN

EXAMINATION: SKIN

Pattern recognition

The skin case is an opportunity to easily pick up points. Sadly, many candidates struggle with it, but recognising and interpreting is as relevant here as in any other system. Examiners do not examine in their specialist area and a general physician's knowledge of dermatology is all that you need. In other words, you do not need to know very much!

Pattern recognition is important—'I have seen this pattern before', e.g. photosensitivity; 'I recognise this morphology', e.g. psoriasis, lichen planus, dermatomyositis—and can be improved by studying a basic dermatology atlas. In PACES there are a limited number of diseases you should need to recognise, and they are detailed in this book.

Skin comprises an inner dermis of collagen and elastic tissue lying on subcutaneous fat, and an outer continuously replenishing epidermis extending from a basal layer of cells with scattered melanocytes to a top layer of protective keratinocytes. These continuously degenerate and slough off to be replaced by cells from beneath. The epidermo-dermal junction is demarcated by a basement membrane. Skin disease can originate in any of these structures and skin, the only visible organ, can be a 'window to the world' of systemic disease.

Skin cases tend to be rapid cases in which you are expected to:

1. Look at the distribution of a rash
2. Describe the lesions
3. Comment on differential diagnoses.

Distribution of skin lesions

You will likely be asked to examine a particular region—'the scalp, face, mouth, hands, nails or shins'. If not, work from scalp to sole. Always attempt to describe the distribution of skin lesions as well as their morphology, noting particularly if they are bilateral or symmetrical. As a general rule, *endogenous* causes are more likely to produce bilateral lesions and *exogenous* causes are more likely to produce a more random distribution.

Description of skin lesions

Central to dermatology is your ability to *describe* skin lesions (Box 8.1).

Box 8.1   Skin Terminology

- A **macule** is a flat area of discoloration which may range from pale (loss of melanin) to brown or black (increased melanin). Many macules are red, indicating vascular dilatation or an inflammatory process. Large macules are sometimes called **patches.**
- A **papule** is a raised lesion < 1 cm in diameter. A **nodule** is a raised lesion > 1 cm in diameter.

- A **plaque** is a raised lesion with a flattened top, or plateau.
- A **vesicle** is a fluid filled lesion or 'blister' < 0.5 cm in diameter. Larger blisters are called **bullae**. A **pustule** is a vesicle filled with neutrophils, but this may not necessarily indicate infection.
- **Telangiectasia** are dilated, superficial blood vessels (capillaries, postcapillary venules). Their occurrence may be idiopathic or associated with cold weather/outdoor exposure or conditions such as pulmonary hypertension, scleroderma, SLE, rosacea, lupus pernio or necrobiosis lipoidica diabeticorum.
- **Discoid** lesions are flat and disc like, the term sometimes overlapping with **nummular**, referring to coin like lesions.
- **Annular** lesions are ring shaped.
- **Reticular** lesions have a 'net like' appearance. Examples include erythema ab igne (Granny's tartan) and livedo reticularis. The latter may be associated with connective tissue disease and malignancy but may be physiological.
- **Atrophy** means loss of tissue. Loss of dermis or subcutaneous fat usually leaves a depression in the skin. Loss of epidermis causes wrinkling and a translucent, hypopigmented appearance.
- **Lichenification** refers to a characteristic thickening of the skin (resembling lichen on rocks or trees) often produced by chronic inflammation or rubbing.
- An **erosion** is an area of lost epidermis that generally heals without scarring. **Excoriations** are linear erosions often produced by scratching. **Ulcers** are areas of skin loss involving the dermis and **fissures** are slits through the whole thickness of skin.

| CASE STUDY | **8.1 PSORIASIS/PSORIATIC ARTHROPATHY** |

Instruction: *Examine this patient's knees and any other areas of skin you think appropriate. Discuss your findings and propose some management options.*

RECOGNITION

There are numerous *well demarcated pink/red plaques* of varying sizes with *silvery white scaling surfaces* (sometimes said to resemble limpets) (Fig. 8.1). The predominance of erythema or scaling can vary from patient to patient. Scratching of the scales may result in a *waxy* appearance, although the lesions are not usually itchy. The *Auspitz sign* (page 424, do not perform) would be present.

The plaques are most prominent on *extensor surfaces (elbows, knees)*/on the *scalp* and *hairline*/behind the *ears*/at the *umbilicus*. Ensure that you check all of these sites, and look at the nails for *pitting* and *onycholysis* and the joints of the hands for *arthropathy*.

INTERPRETATION

Confirm the diagnosis

The appearance of the plaques is usually diagnostic.

Fig. 8.1 *Psoriasis. Reproduced with permission from M.A. Mir (1995) Atlas of Clinical Diagnosis. W.B. Saunders, London*

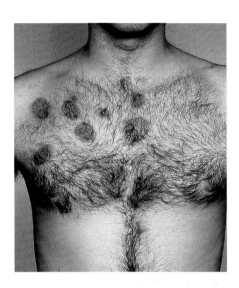

Assess other systems

Psoriatic arthropathy affects up to 10% of patients with psoriasis and may precede or follow skin disease by months or even years. There are, in theory, five types, although overlapping pictures are common:

1. **Asymmetrical distal interphalangeal joint arthropathy.** This is relatively uncommon but is the form most strongly associated with psoriasis. Affected digits often show nail changes such as *pitting*.
2. **Rheumatoid like hands.** This is the commonest arthropathy and is seronegative. *Exclude rheumatoid nodules at the elbows* and *look for psoriatic plaques*.
3. **Asymmetrical large joint mono- or oligoarthropathy.** Tell the examiners you would ask about large joint pain or swelling.
4. **Spondyloarthropahy** and **sacroiliitis.** Tell the examiners you would ask about low back pain (Case study 9.2).
5. **Arthritis mutilans.** A very uncommon, severely destructive form.

Assess severity

● Extent of plaque psoriasis ● Presence of variant psoriasis (Box 8.2) ● Presence of arthropathy.

Evidence of decompensation

● Extensive psoriasis (e.g. erythrodermic) can compromise the skin's barrier and metabolic function.
● Arthropathy may cause functional decompensation.

Assess function

As well as the physical effects of arthropathy, consider the psychological implications of severe skin disease.

Look for/consider associated diseases

If there is arthropathy, consider the tendency for HLA B27 spondyloarythropathies to overlap, common features being sacroiliac discomfort and enthesopathies such as plantar fasciitis.

DISCUSSION

What causes psoriasis?

The cause is unknown. Psoriasis often appears in early adult life, frequently precipitated by physical (e.g. trauma, pregnancy, infection, drugs, steroid withdrawal) or psychological stress and attenuated by sunlight. There may be a family history. There is an association with HLA Cw6 and, in psoriatic arthropathy, HLA B27.

What is the pathophysiology?

There is increased epidermal turnover. Histologically, increased nuclei are seen above the basal layer. This results in thickening of the epidermis with thick keratin deposition. However, the rapid turnover prevents adequate differentiation into normal keratin and the keratin that is produced is scaly and readily removed to reveal a red vascular layer beneath (*Auspitz sign*). The redness of lesions is caused by dilated blood vessels. The aetiology is unknown, but probably represents an immune response to the triggering agent.

An equivalent process in the nail leads to thickening, pitting and onycholysis.

In pustular psoriasis there is abundant migration of neutrophils into the epidermis causing multiple small, sterile pus deposits, mostly in the palms and soles.

What is Koebner's phenomenon?

Koebner's phenomenon is a feature of psoriasis in which lesions often appear at sites of minor trauma. Sometimes this is the first sign of psoriasis. Other causes of Koebner's phenomenon include:

● Lichen planus ● Bullous pemphigoid ● Vitiligo ● Certain viruses (e.g. wart viruses, molluscum contagiosum).

What psoriatic variants do you know of?

Mostly psoriasis is a condition producing chronic, stable plaques. Some variants do occur (Box 8.2).

What treatments are commonly used in psoriasis?

1. Topical treatments include:
   (i) Emollients.
   (ii) Coal tar ointments and pastes, which may be easier to apply in hospital. These are safe and effective for stable plaques but

Box 8.2	Psoriasis Variants

1. *Pustular psoriasis* is often chronic, with erythematous palms and soles turning an 'autumn brown' colour and scattered with 'raindrops' of pustules. Occasionally, it becomes generalised.
2. *Guttate psoriasis* produces lesions which look like drops of rain or paint, and is common in adolescence. It may be associated with infection, e.g. streptococcal pharyngitis.
3. *Flexural psoriasis* is less common and tends to produce more erythema than scaling.
4. *Erythrodermic psoriasis* is a severe, sometimes life threatening form with generalised erythema.

---

salicylic acid may also be needed to dissolve the keratin of thick lesions.

(iii) Short contact dithranol. Dithranol is used in incremental concentrations as first line treatment for stable plaques. It stains plaques and hair and must not be applied for longer than directed, usually 30 minutes.

(iv) Calipotriol, a vitamin D analogue used for mild to moderate stable plaques. High doses (in extensive psoriasis) may cause hypercalcaemia.

2. Steroids are used topically but tachyphylaxis is a major drawback.
3. Narrow band (311–313 nm) UVB phototherapy is often effective for widespread or guttate psoriasis.
4. Methotrexate and other immune modulatory drugs are used in severe, refractory disease. Indications include failure of topical treatment for extensive plaque posriasis and treatment of generalised pustular and erythrodermic psoriasis.
5. Scalp psoriasis can be difficult to treat. Salicylic acid, dithranol and steroids are sometimes used.

CASE STUDY	8.2 DERMATITIS

Instruction: *Look at this patient's skin. Discuss your findings.*

RECOGNITION	

The skin is *red, swollen and blistering* or *dry, thickened and leathery, with erythema, scaling and evidence of scratching.* Both extremes are *itchy.*

Dermatitis and eczema are interchangeable terms. The term 'eczema' means skin 'boiling over'. There are many types of dermatitis and the clinical appearance can fall anywhere between the two extremes. Pathologically, there is breakdown in the skin's horny barrier and there may be oedema high in the dermis. Any blisters tend to have a honeycomb, multiloculated core, not typical of other blistering diseases such as pemphigus.

INTERPRETATION

Confirm the diagnosis

Although you are unlikely to meet infectious conditions in PACES, in practice:

1. Acute 'dermatitis' may be due to scabies, often intensely itchy and worse after hot showers or baths and at night. Burrows of the scabies mite *Sarcoptes scabei* may be seen.
2. *Tinea pedis* should be considered before diagnosing foot dermatitis. *Tinea* is often unilateral, dry, scaly and interdigitate.

Look for/consider causes

Dermatitis may have endogenous or exogenous causes (Table 8.1)

Bilateral dermatitis is more likely to have an endogenous cause and unilateral dermatitis an exogenous cause (but contact dermatitis commonly affects both hands if dipped in chemical irritants).

Tell the examiners the features of the history that you would explore, especially atopy (hay fever, asthma) and occupation.

1. Allergic contact dermatitis

This is a type IV hypersensitivity reaction (page 203) to a previously tolerated substance. In contrast to irritant contact dermatitis, it may be a sudden reaction to a trace quantity of allergen and may become widespread, disseminating to areas of the body that have not been recently exposed. Nickel is a common culprit in many everyday items such as clothing (including underwear), keys and money. Patch testing can be used to screen for common triggers.

Contact dermatitis of the eyelids is commonly provoked by cosmetics (including the 'hypoallergenic' cosmetics), occupational chemicals such as epoxy resins, nail varnish and aminoglycoside eye drops (Figure 8.2).

2. Irritant contact dermatitis

This usually results from daily, regular exposure to a trigger factor (therefore more readily identifiable). Soaps and solvents are common

TABLE 8.1   Causes of dermatitis

Endogenous	Exogenous	Unclassified
Atopic	Contact (irritant or allergic)	Juvenile plantar
Discoid (nummular)	Photosensitivity	Lichen simplex
Venous	Napkin	Asteatotic
Seborrhoeic		
Pompholyx		

triggers, as is chronic wear and tear to the skin. There is frequently subclinical skin damage before it begins to *dry, crack* and develop a *smooth, shiny atrophic appearance*. It may become oedematous and blister. Early intervention is the key to successful treatment—the more chronic the process, the less likely it is to remit and if it does it can rapidly reappear with re-exposure.

3. Photosensitive dermatitis

True sun induced dermatitis is rare. Much more common are other forms of dermatitis aggravated by sunlight and other photodermatoses such as polymorphic light eruption.

4. Atopic dermatitis

This comprises at least 50% of all dermatitis and there is evidence that its prevalence, like asthma, is increasing. It often starts at a few months of age, when a trial of milk and egg exclusion may be warranted, but it may continue to wax and wane through adult life. The house dust mite (HDM) is the main trigger, its faeces contributing significantly to the weight of old pillows! It likes moist, sweaty atmospheres, preferring beds to curtains and carpets, but cannot survive in high, dry atmospheres above 3000 m. Atopic dermatitis, like asthma, may improve at this altitude. Patients changing their bedding should be warned that improvement may take 6–9 months. Radioallergosorbent tests (RAST) identify allergen specific IgF in serum. Skin prick testing involves introducing allergen into the skin, where it interacts with IgE bound to mast cells and causes histamine release and a consequent 'wheal and flare' (oedema and erythema) response.

Atopic dermatitis tends to affect the *flexors*, which may become *lichenified*. There is frequently superimposed staphylococcal infection, impeding complete or sustained response to steroids. *Herpes simplex type 1* may cause rapid worsening of dermatitis, especially atopic (*eczema herpeticum/'Kaposi's varicelliform eruption'*).

5. Discoid dermatitis

Infection (staphylococcal superantigen theory) is thought to be the basis for these intensely itchy coin shaped lesions on the limbs, often distributed symmetrically, of middle aged to elderly patients, and antibiotics may be of benefit.

6. Venous dermatitis

There is evidence of venous stasis with *swelling, sclerosis* or *atrophy* on the lower leg (often starting at the medial malleolus), with *haemosiderin* deposition from extravasated blood causing a *brownish discoloration*. There may be *ulceration*.

7. Seborrhoeic dermatitis

Erythematous plaques or patches tend to affect the *scalp, preauricular areas, nasolabial folds, glabella* or *eyelids*. Despite the

Fig. 8.2   *Contact dermatitis. Reproduced with permission from M.A. Mir (1995) Atlas of Clinical Diagnosis, W.B. Saunders, London*

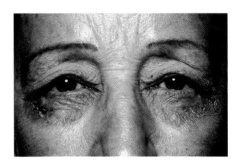

name, the lesions are dry, often with a *scaling* surface and are not associated with excess sebum production. Seborrhoeic dermatitis may be part of a spectrum which includes dandruff.

Blepharitis (Fig. 8.2), which causes itchy lids, crusting of the lid margins with a dandruffy appearance and broken lashes, is strongly associated with seborrhoeic dermatitis or staphylococcal infection (another differential diagnosis being contact dermatitis). The conjunctivae are often glistening and swollen. There may be excess lipid secretion with foaming of the lid margins. There may also be otitis externa.

There is likely a genetic predisposition to seborrhoeic dermatitis, mediated by several factors including hormonal and dietary factors. It may be an inflammatory response to *Pitysporum ovale*, a yeast present in the human scalp.

8. Pompholyx

These *intensely itchy blisters on the palms* may be seasonal or occur without an obvious trigger. Contact dermatitis affecting the palms is also sometimes referred to as pompholyx.

9. Juvenile planter dermatosis

This produces a *shiny, glazed appearance* to those aspects of the *soles* of the feet in contact with footwear. It seems to be increasing in prevalence. *Tinea pedis* should be excluded by microscopy of skin scrapings before reaching this diagnosis.

10. Neurodermatitis

There is *chronic lichenified skin* (lichen simplex chronicus). The trigger is usually historical, the signs due to habitual rubbing and scratching.

11. Asteatotic dermatitis (eczema craquelé)

This causes a *dry, crazy paving* pattern of fissuring, especially on the limbs.

Assess function

Always consider occupational causes of contact dermatitis and whether or not dermatitis could have an impact on occupation.

Which treatments are used in dermatitis?

Treatment options for the range of types of dermatitis (after removing any identifiable cause) include emollients/emollient bathing, topical steroids, topical/systemic antibiotics (secondary infection is a common cause of failure of response to steroids) and antihistamines. Ultraviolet light has been used in refractory cases. Antifungal creams and shampoos may help seborrhoeic dermatitis.

Tacrolimus ointment may be used for moderate to severe eczema unresponsive to conservative measures.

Ointments and creams vary in their grease : water ratio. The epidermis can absorb both greasy and aqueous preparations. Generally, greasy ointments are best for dry, scaling skin and watery creams for crusted weeping lesions. Pastes may be used for sustained action or occlusion.

Name some skin conditions which are itchy

Primary skin diseases causing itch include all types of dermatitis, lichen planus, blistering disorders especially dermatitis herpetiformis (pemphigoid doesn't itch), fungal infection or mite infestation, flea/tick bites and ichthyosis (dry skin with fish like scales, with a genetic basis or associated with malignancy).

Systemic causes include cholestasis, uraemia, diabetes, hyper/hypothyroidism, polycythaemia rubra vera, lymphoma, parasitophobia and certain drugs.

CASE STUDY   8.3 LICHEN PLANUS

Instruction: *Look at this patient's wrists/ankles and discuss what you see.*

There are *well demarcated, polygonal, raised plaques on the flexor surfaces*, especially the *wrists* and *ankles* (Fig. 8.3). Their *flat tops* are *shiny* with a *violaceous colour*, interrupted by milky *white streaks—Wickhams's striae*. They are very likely *intensely itchy*. There may be Koebner's phenomenon. These lesions usually resolve over a period of months to leave brownish macules.

Confirm the diagnosis

Lichenification is a feature of many skin diseases such as eczema and itchy drug eruptions. The shiny, purplish flat tops of lichen planus, and their distribution, usually aid diagnosis.

Fig. 8.3   *Lichen planus*

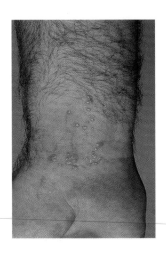

Assess other systems

Look for:

1. *White, 'net like' lesions* on the *oral mucosa*, often with *ulceration* (Fig. 8.4). Other causes of white oral lesions include leukoplakia (hyperkeratotic lesions associated with *Epstein–Barr virus*) and candidiasis, both more common in HIV infection.

2. *Atrophy* and *longitudinal grooves* of the *nail plates*. Sometimes nails disappear altogether.

DISCUSSION	

What causes lichen planus?

The cause is uncertain. There is no family history and no definite association with stress.

Fig. 8.4   *Lichen planus (intraoral). Reproduced with permission from M.A. Mir (1995) Atlas of Clinical Diagnosis. W.B. Saunders, London*

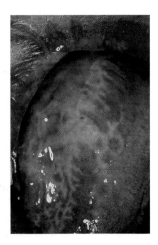

What is the pathophysiology?

The epidermis is thickened, with increased keratin. The white streaks imply a thickened granular layer and underlying cellular infiltrate. The basal layer is infiltrated with T lymphocytes in a band pattern.

How may it be treated?

Moderately potent topical (occasionally systemic) steroids are effective. Lichen planus is self-limiting but tends to relapse and remit over months or even years.

Which other skin diseases may arise in the epidermis?

● Psoriasis.
● Dermatitis.
● Pityriasis rosea. Pityriasis is Greek for 'bran' and refers to a fine scaly appearance. In pityriasis rosea the scales are on top of pale pink oval patches. There is often a 'herald patch'. Pityriasis rosea affects young adults, is of unknown cause, and is self-limiting.
● Pityriasis versicolor. White macules on tanned skin or pale brown patches on non-tanned skin, in the absence of inflammation or vesicles, suggest yeast infection.
● Fungal infections.

What is meant by the term erythema?

Erythema is the result of reactions in blood vessels in the skin, resulting in red macules, papules or vesicles. The vast array of causes includes:

● Psoriasis ● Dermatitis ● Toxic erythema (drugs, infection)
● Erythema associated with connective tissue disease
● Erythema multiforme ● Erythema nodosum.

What is erythema multiforme?

The pathophysioloy is unknown but there is vasodilatation, inflammation and degeneration within the epidermis. Causes include *Herpes simplex* and *Mycoplasma* infections, infectious mononucleosis, HIV, sulphonamides, penicillin, SLE, polyarteritis, Wegener's granulomatosis and sarcodiosis.

Crops of *maculopapular erythema* occur on the *limbs and trunk*. Lesions may expand, leaving a pale centre, the classic *target lesion*. *Bullae/vesicles* and/or *necrosis* may develop within the targets of the lesions and in the mucous membranes. The severe bullous form is *Stevens–Johnson syndrome*.

| CASE STUDY | 8.4 PEMPHIGUS AND PEMPHIGOID |

Instruction: *Inspect this patient's skin and discuss the possible causes.*

RECOGNITION

Pemphigoid

There are *tense blisters* of *variable size* (much more variable than pemphigus, from a few millimetres to a few centimetres) on the *trunk and flexor surfaces*. Some of these are *surrounded* by *patches* of *red skin*. Oral lesions are less frequent than in pemphigus.

Pemphigus

There is a *bullous eruption* (in a middle-aged/elderly patient) comprising *flaccid, thin walled blisters* on the *trunk* 1–2 cm in diameter (Fig. 8.5). Many have *burst*, leaving *red, exuding, tender patches*. *Oral erosions* are common and may precede the rash.

INTERPRETATION

Confirm the diagnosis

- Pemphigoid blisters are tense and pemphigus blisters flaccid
- Inspect the mouth for erosions (Fig. 8.6).

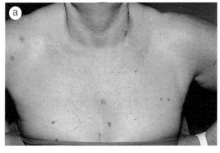
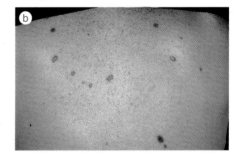

Fig. 8.5   *(a,b) Pemphigus (trunk)*

Fig. 8.6   *Pemphigus (intraoral)*

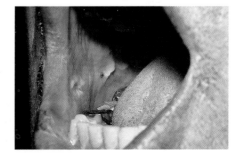

Assess severity

- Note if the lesions are widespread or confluent
- Note any cushingoid features (prolonged steroid treatment).

Evidence of decompensation

- Pemphigus is more serious than pemphigoid
- Pemphigus and pemphigoid may be complicated by secondary bacterial infection.

DISCUSSION

What else do you know about pemphigoid?

It tends to affect the elderly. Deeply seated tense bullae appear on both normal skin and on pre-existing areas of erythema, and mostly affect the flexor surfaces and trunk. There are autoantibodies at the dermo-epidermal junction.

Treatment is with steroids ± immunomodulatory steroid sparing agents. Pemphigoid tends to relapse and remit. Chronic scarring may affect the mucous membranes with small bullae that break down to leave erosions, followed by adhesions, affecting the conjunctivae, mouth, pharynx and genitalia.

What else do you know about pemphigus?

Pemphigus refers to a group of disorders affecting adults, with widespread superficial epidermal blisters. Pemphigus often affects mucous membranes, but with erosions rather than blistering. Pemphigus vulgaris, the commonest type, often begins in the mouth, becoming a chronic progressive disease with widespread superficial bullae arising from normal skin. The bullae are easily broken, and even rubbing of normal skin can cause sloughing of the epidermis (Nikolsky sign). There are autoantibodies against the desmosomes which bridge adjacent epidermal cells.

Pemphigus is a serious disease with high morbidity despite treatment with steroids and immunomodulatory drugs.

List some other blistering skin conditions

- Dermatitis herpetiformis
- Chickenpox
- Erythema multiforme/Stevens–Johnson syndrome
- Drug eruptions
- Epidermolysis bullosa (refers to a group of hereditary disorders causing blistering of the skin, palms and soles and especially the oro-pharyngo-oesophageal mucosae)
- Porphyria cutanea tarda
- Dermatitis (e.g. pompholyx)
- Allergy (e.g. insect bite)

- Pustular psoriasis
- Impetigo
- *Herpes simplex/zoster.*

What is dermatitis herpetiformis?

This refers to symmetrical, highly itchy vesicles or urticarial plaques on the trunk and extensor surfaces, buttocks and occasionally the face and scalp, and is associated with gluten sensitive enteropathy (coeliac disease). Dapsone is the treatment of choice.

What types of drug induced rash do you know of?

- Exanthematous
- Urticarial
- Blistering (e.g. Stevens–Johnson syndrome)
- Fixed drug eruptions (macules, papules or blisters tending to occur at the same site with each exposure)
- Drug induced vasculitis
- Photosensitivity (e.g. amiodarone).

What is urticaria?

This term refers to wheals (oedema) surrounded by flares of erythema. It may be caused by drugs, heat, cold, pressure, water, food substances, infections, insect bites or dermatographism. More severe reactions may lead to angio-oedema.

Urticaria pigmentosa refers to itchy red-brown macules/papules which are the dermal manifestation of systemic mastocytosis.

CASE STUDY | **8.5 ALOPECIA AREATA**

Instruction: *Look at this patient's scalp. Discuss your findings.*

RECOGNITION

Alopecia areata causes *diffuse, patchy hair loss* and *does not scar* (the hair follicles are not destroyed) and *'exclamation mark' hairs* may be seen 'sprouting in the desert'.

INTERPRETATION

Assess other systems

Alopecia areata is associated with nail pitting, vitiligo and autoimmune disease.

DISCUSSION

Which treatments may be tried?

Steroids or phototherapy.

List some other causes of non-scarring alopecia

● Male pattern (androgenic) baldness ● Stress ● Hypopituitarism
● Thyroid disease ● Hypoparathyroidism ● Diabetes mellitus
● Pregnancy ● Drugs (e.g. cytotoxics, antithyroid drugs,
anticoagulants, ciclosporin).

List some causes of scarring alopecia

● Psoriasis ● Dermatitis ● Lichen planus ● Fungal and other
infections ● Trauma and burns ● Lupus erythematosus
● Morphea ● Sarcoidosis.

CASE STUDY | **8.6 FACIAL RASH**

*Instruction: Look at this patient's facial rash. Describe what you see and comment on
your differential diagnosis and the likely cause.*

RECOGNITION

There is a *'butterfly distribution' malar rash* (Fig. 8.7).

INTERPRETATION

Look for/consider causes

1. Systemic lupus erythematosus (SLE)

There are *raised or flat patches of malar erythema, sparing the
nasolabail folds.* Other areas such as the forehead and neck are often
affected. The may be marked *photosensitivity.* There may be *mouth
ulcers.*

Fig. 8.7   *Malar rash*

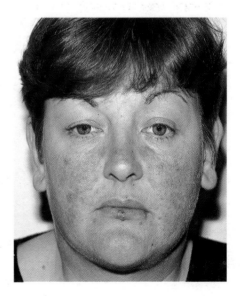

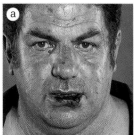
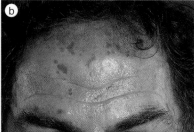

Fig. 8.8   *(a,b) Lupus pernio*

2. Discoid lupus erythematosus (DLE)

DLE is skin limited disease, with *well defined erythematous papules or plaques on light exposed areas* including the *head, neck, hands* and *arms*. The lesions are *scaling* and hyperkeratosis of hair follicles gives these scales a dotted, 'nutmeg' appearance. If you were to remove the scales and inspect their undersurface, you would see spicules projecting from them. This is known as follicular keratosis or plugging (also known as the 'carpet track' sign) and no other scaling condition does this—it is specific to lupus.

There may be *patches of depigmentation.* Once affected areas heal and the scab falls off, the skin beneath is often scarred, hypopigmented and atrophic.

Mostly affected are the *cheeks, nose and forehead*. Like SLE, the rash is *photosensitive*, and more common in females.

3. Rosacea (and acne vulgaris)

This is discussed in Case study 8.7.

4. Lupus pernio

There are *purple/red/violaceous plaques on the nose, cheeks and earlobes* with *telangiectasia over and around the plaques* (Fig. 8.8). The plaques may have a yellowish translucency. They tend to flatten with time.

Lupus pernio is a manifestation of sarcoidosis, tending to represent the chronic inflammatory, granulomatous end of the spectrum compared with erythema nodosum (Case study 8.11).

5. Lupus vulgaris

This is the skin manifestation of tuberculosis and is rare in the UK. The lesion has an 'apple jelly' consistency when a translucent slide is rested upon it.

6. Dermatomyositis

This may cause a malar rash (not usually in isolation) and is discussed in Case study 8.8.

7. *Seborrhoeic dermatitis*

Seborrhoeic dermatitis may cause a nasolabial/malar rash (pages 427–428).

8. *Pulmonary hypertension/mitral stenosis*

DISCUSSION	

List some skin signs of common connective tissue diseases

Skin signs are common in connective tissue disease (Box 8.3). In PACES, connective tissue disease may appear at the Skin or Locomotor Station.

Box 8.3	Common Skin Signs in Connective Tissue Disease

Rheumatoid disease

Rheumatoid disease may cause *cutaneous/nail fold vasculitis and infarction, nodules* (both associated with rheumatoid factor positivity) and *pyoderma gangrenosum*. Rheumatoid disease is discussed in Case study 9.1.

SLE

SLE commonly causes *malar erythema, sparing the nasolabail folds*. SLE is discussed above and in Case study 9.3.

Scleroderma

Scleroderma (*face*) causes *dilated capillaries (telangiectasia), smooth, shiny, tight skin* and *perioral skin puckering*.

Scleroderma (*hands*) causes *sclerodactyly, nail fold erythema due to dilated nail fold capillaries (telangiectasia), nail fold infarction, ragged cuticles, digital ischaemia, pulp atrophy, calcinosis* and *Raynaud's phenomenon*.

Scleroderma is discussed in Case study 9.5.

Dermatomyositis

Dermatomyositis causes a *heliotrope rash* (especially of the eyelids), *Gottron's papules* and *nail fold erythema*. Dermatomyositis is discussed in Case study 8.8.

Raynaud's phenomenon

Cold white hands (ischaemia), which turn *blue (stasis)* then *red (reactive hyperaemia)* with pain may be due to scleroderma, SLE, dermatomyositis, mixed connective tissue disease, cold exposure, beta-blockers, and other vasospastic (especially smoking) or vaso-occlusive conditions. It may be idiopathic, especially in young females.

What treatments may be used for the rash of SLE/DLE?

Treatments include moderately potent topical steroids and hydroxychloroquine. Sunscreens are essential.

CASE STUDY   **8.7 ROSACEA**

Instruction: *Look at this lady's face and discuss your findings.*

RECOGNITION

There is an *erythematous, 'acneiform' papular eruption* on the *flush areas* of the face—*cheeks* (and sometimes *nose/chin/forehead*) (Fig. 8.9). The erythema is marked, with prominent dilated blood vessels (*telangiectasia*). There are *pustules* within the eruption.

A variant, often seen in elderly men, is rhinophyma, with thickened erythematous skin of the nose and enlarged follicles.

INTERPRETATION

Confirm the diagnosis

Rosacea may not spare the nasolabial folds and its pustules are characteristic, usually distinguishing it from other facial rashes:

- The rash of SLE (and DLE) spares the nasolabial folds and pustules are not a feature. Scaling, follicular plugging and scarring are features of DLE but not rosacea.
- Acne vulgaris causes comedones (blackheads) without telangiectasia, and its distribution is generally wide. Acne vulgaris and (acne) rosacea may, however, coexist.

Fig. 8.9   *Rosacea*

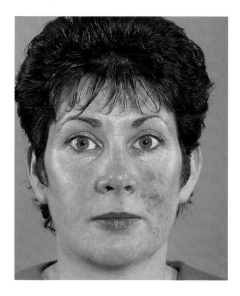

- Lupus pernio and lupus vulgaris are not pustular. The surface of the thickened nose in lupus pernio, although telangiectactic, is smooth and lacks the rugose peau d'orange surface of rhinophyma.
- The rash of dermatomyositis is characteristic and not pustular.
- Seborrhoeic dermatitis (pages 427–428) involves the scalp, nasolabial folds or eyelids. Scaling is characteristic but does not normally occur in rosacea. However, seborrhoeic dermatitis and rosacea may coexist.

Assess function

The rash can be psychologically damaging.

DISCUSSION

What causes rosacea?

Rosacea tends to affect females (especially the 30–50 year age group) more than males, although rhinophyma is more common in males. Precipitating factors include heat, sun, alcohol, spicy foods, emotion/embarrassment and steroids. There is a *Demodex folliculorum* theory, implicating pilosebaceous follicular mites as an underlying cause, but the cause is not clear.

There is episodic flushing with erythema, telangiectasia and papules/pustules in the earlier stages. Later, there is sebaceous hyperplasia, but seborrhoea and comedones are not a feature. Rosacea is generally symmetrical.

How is rosacea treated?

Steroids should not be used. They are not effective in the long term and tend to cause skin addiction and 'flares' of severe rebound erythema which do not easily settle. Avoidance of precipitating factors is seldom helpful except for the use of sunscreens. Topical treatments include metronidazole or erythromycin gel, with an emollient. Systemic treatments include tetracycline (often prolonged as low-dose maintenance treatment), minocycline and doxycycline. Isotretinoin is usually beneficial.

Rosacea tends to run a protracted course, often recurring after treatment.

What is acne vulgaris?

The aetiology and pathology of acne and rosacea are not related.

Acne vulgaris is a chronic inflammatory disorder of the pilosebaceous structure, characterised by comedones (non-inflamed lesions), erythematous papules, pustules and nodules (inflamed lesions) and scarring. Scarring tends to be hypertrophic and keloid (trunk) or 'ice pick' (cheeks). Acne vulgaris affects the face, back and chest.

Sebaceous glands are also distributed in areas not associated with hair follicles, including the eyelids (whose follicles are separate structures). Sebaceous glands contain holocrine cells, which secrete triglycerides, fatty acids, wax and sterols as sebum.

Acneiform lesions develop from sebaceous glands associated with hair follicles, mostly distributed on the face, back, chest and anogenital region. In acne vulgaris there is primarily an increase in androgen dependent sebum production, although testosterone levels are not increased. Pilosebaceous duct proliferation is central to increased sebum production. There is thickening (cornification) of the keratin lining of the duct, associated with an increase in sebum lipid content and keratinocyte comedogenesis. The colour of 'blackheads' is mainly due to melanin, not dirt. There is also an increase in *Proprionibacterium acnes* ± other bacteria in the duct and inflammation around the sebaceous gland.

CASE STUDY	8.8 DERMATOMYOSITIS

Instruction: *Please examine this patient's face and hands, describe what you see and interpret the findings.*

RECOGNITION	

This is a *heliotrope* (referring to the distinctive lilac colour of the flower so named) *rash* around the *eyelids* (Fig. 8.10a). It may also affect the malar region, limb extensors, knuckles and trunk (Fig. 8.10b).

Gottron's papules may be present on the dorsum of the hands (notably metacarpophalangeal joints and and interphalangeal joints) and occasionally elsewhere.

Nail fold erythema due to *dilated capillaries (telangiectasia)* is often present, and the cuticles may be ragged.

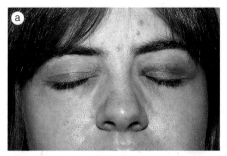
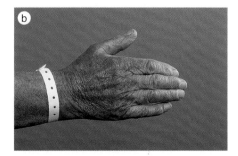

Fig. 8.10   *(a,b) Dermatomyositis*

Assess other systems

> Look for symmetrical weakness in a proximal muscle distribution. The patient may be unable to rise from a squatting position or raise their arms above their head. These findings suggest associated *polymyositis* (page 357).

Which conditions may be associated with dermatomyositis?

> Dermatomyositis is occasionally associated with neoplasms, notably colorectal, ovarian, breast or lung.

CASE STUDY **8.9 ORAL LESIONS**

Instruction: *Look at this patient's mouth and comment on your findings.*

Hereditary haemorrhagic telangiectasia (HHT)

> There are *dilated capillaries/venules of the lips and tongue* and *around the mouth* (Fig. 8.11), *nail beds, hands* and frequently elsewhere. There may be evidence of recent epistaxis.

Fig. 8.11   *Hereditary haemorrhagic telangiectasia. Reproduced with permission from M.A. Mir (1995) Atlas of Clinical Diagnosis. W.B. Saunders, London*

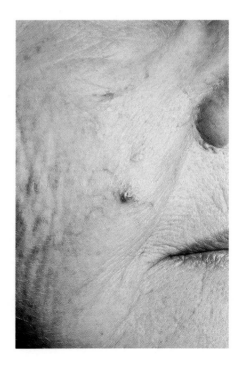

Peutz–Jehgers syndrome (PJS)

> The *lips* are *pigmented*.

Other

> Other mouth lesions you could encounter in PACES include:
>
> - Perioral dermatitis ● Lichen planus (Case study 8.3)
> - Leukoplakia ● Candida ● Pemphigus (Case study 8.4)
> - Addison's disease pigmentation (Case study 11.7).

INTERPRETATION

Confirm the diagnosis

> The circumoral and mucosal pigmentation of PJS is usually less diffuse than that of Addison's disease.

Evidence of decompensation

> In HHT there may be *arteriovenous malformations (AVMs)*—direct connections between arteries and veins—throughout the gastrointestinal tract, liver, lungs and nervous system. Note any:
>
> - Pallor (iron deficiency anaemia due to gastrointestinal haemorrhage) ● Hepatic bruits ● Dyspnoea/tachypnoea/ cyanosis (polycythaemia) ● Chest bruits ● History of subarachnoid haemorrhage.
>
> Tell the examiners that you would ask about neurological problems. These may result from an intracranial AVM or from an embolic stroke arising from a pulmonary AVM.

DISCUSSION

What causes HHT?

> HHT refers to a group of autosomal dominant diseases genetically linked to chromosomes 9 and 12. In some families the implicated gene encodes endoglin, a protein on endothelial cells which binds the cytokine transforming growth factor beta (TGF-β).

In which other conditions are telangiectasia found?

> - Common on the face with prolonged cold outdoor exposure
> - Pulmonary hypertension (mitral stenosis) ● Post radiotherapy
> - Rosacea ● Scleroderma ● Dermatomyositis ● Necrobiosis lipoidica diabeticorum.

What is PJS?

> An autosomal dominant disorder characterised by mucocutaneous melanosis (lentigo) and gastrointestinal hamartomas. Gastrointestinal bleeding and malignancy may complicate PJS.

Give a differential diagnosis for mouth ulcers

● Aphthous ulcers ● Traumatic ulcers ● Lichen planus ● Oral candidiasis ● *Herpes simplex* ● Stevens–Johnson syndrome ● Pemphigus ● Carcinoma ● Behçet's disease ● Crohn's disease.

CASE STUDY | **8.10 HAND AND NAIL LESIONS**

Instruction: *Look at this patient's nails and comment on the possible cause*

Hand cases tend to appear at the Neurology Station (e.g. wasting of small muscles) or the Locomotor Station (e.g. rheumatoid arthritis, scleroderma). More common nail abnormalities are described here.

RECOGNITION

Psoriasis

There is *pitting* and *onycholysis*.

Lichen planus

Occasionally lichen planus may cause *atrophy of the nail plate* (which may disappear altogether or exhibit longitudinal furrows) and the cuticle may advance forwards.

Nail lines

Beau's lines are *transverse* depressions representing altered growth rate and are a non-specific sign of previous illness or physiological change. *Onychomedesis* refers to shedding of the nail, which may occur in severe illness.

    Longitudinal depressions or ridges may occur in lichen planus, alopecia areata and Darier's disease (dystrophy with a series of longitudinal streaks which end in triangular shaped nicks at the free margin).

Clubbing

Clubbing progresses through the following phases:
1. *Swelling of the soft tissues of the terminal phalanx* (*fluctuant nail beds* – page 9)
2. A permanently *increased angle between the nail plate and the posterior nail fold* (this defines clubbing)
3. *Increased curvature of the nails* due to soft tissue hypertrophy (*Shamroth's sign* may be used to confirm 2 and 3: by asking the patient to approximate the dorsal aspects of the terminal phalanges there is a wide, deep angle or window.)
4. *HPOA* (page 17), representing the most extreme form.

Leuconychia

The nails appear *white*.

Koilynychia

The nails (especially the fingernails) are *brittle* and *concave* or 'spoon-shaped'.

INTERPRETATION

Confirm the diagnosis

Psoriasis

Psoriasis is discussed in Case study 8.1.

Lichen planus

Lichen planus is discussed in Case study 8.3.

Look for/consider causes

Beau's lines

Tell the examiners that you would ask about systemic illness.

Clubbing

Tell the examiners that clubbing may be caused by:
- Chronic suppurative lung disease — bronchiectasis, cystic fibrosis
- Lung cancer ● Cryptogenic fibrosing alveolitis ● Infective endocarditis ● Congenital cyanotic heart disease ● Chronic liver disease ● Inflammatory bowel disease.
    Clubbing may also be congenital or idiopathic.

Hypoalbuminaemia

Tell the examiners that you would consider chronic liver disease (Case study 3.3).

Koilonychia

Tell the examiners that you would consider iron deficiency anaemia (page 455).

DISCUSSION

What causes the nail changes in psoriasis?

Nails comprise a nail bed, on top of which grows the highly keratinised nail plate (between the posterior and lateral nail folds and anterior free margin) from the nail matrix beneath the lunula and cuticle. Psoriasis causes keratin thickening (page 424) of the nail. Loss of minute plugs of normal keratin results in characteristic *pitting* and sometimes the thickened, dystrophic nail separates from its nail bed (*onycholysis*).

List some other causes of pitting

    ● Alopecia areata ● Dermatitis.

List some other causes of onycholysis

    Other causes of *onycholysis* (often with discoloured, thickened, hyperkeratotic but brittle, dystrophic nails) include:

    ● Fungal infection (onychomycosis)
    ● Trauma
    ● Dermatitis
    ● Peripheral vascular disease
    ● Thyrotoxicosis (in this case referred to as Plummer's nails)
    ● Idiopathic, sometimes associated with excessive wetting of nails and chronic bacterial paronychia.

What is onychogryphosis?

    Hypertrophy of the nail plate, often resulting from chronic trauma.

What other causes of nail discoloration do you know of?

    ● Dystrophic nails of any cause often have a yellow/brownish tinge.
    ● A yellow/brownish discoloration may also occur in chronic renal failure, which may also produce 'half and half nails' in which the proximal halves are pale and the distal halves pink.
    ● Tetracyclines may stain nails yellow and some antimalarials imbue them with a blue tinge.
    ● Wilson's disease may give the lunula a blue tinge.
    ● Subungual melanoma (melanin may also cause brown longitudinal streaks) should be excluded in patients with isolated pigment discoloration beneath a nail.
    ● Yellow nail syndrome (associated with pleural effusion, bronchiectasis, nephrotic syndrome, malignancy, lymphoedema, thyroid disease and rheumatoid disease) gives rise to yellow, curved nails.

CASE STUDY	8.11 SHIN LESIONS

Instruction: *Examine this patient's legs and discuss your findings.*

RECOGNITION	

Erythema nodosum

    There are *erythematous* (progress through the colour changes of a bruise), *warm, nodular* (flatten with healing) *lesions over the anterior aspect of both shins* (Fig. 8.12). They may be single or multiple, of various sizes, and may occur elsewhere. Ask if they are *tender* (before you examine them!).

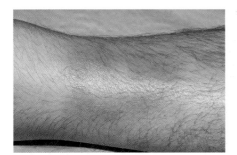

Fig. 8.12   *Erythema nodosum*

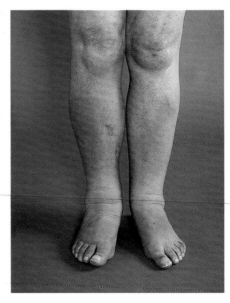

Fig. 8.13   *Pretibial myxoedema*

The lesions evolve slowly, changing from acute red nodules to residual bruises over a period of weeks.

Pretibial myxoedema (PTM)

There are *elevated symmetrical shin lesions* (Fig. 8.13). Such lesions may occur at other sites. They are *coarse, purplish red or brown*, with *well defined edges*. The *skin is shiny*, with an *orange peel appearance*. The lesions may be asymptomatic or painful. Coarse hairs tend to occur in the vicinity of the lesions.

Necrobiosis lipoidica diabeticorum (NLD)

There are *well demarcated (often oval) non-scaling plaques* on the shins (Fig. 8.14a). Characteristically they occur on the legs but they may occur anywhere else. They have a *shiny, atrophic surface, red/brown margins* and *yellow waxy centres. Surface telangiectasia* is characteristic. Trauma often results in persistent ulceration (Fig. 8.14b).

Pyoderma gangrenosum

Pyoderma gangrenosum may begin as nodular erythema or a sterile pustule, but develops into often large areas of *painful necrotic ulceration* with *purplish hypertrophic/overhanging edges* (Fig. 8.15). There may be plaques and pustules within the lesion. Healing often leaves a papery scar. Pyoderma gangrenosum can occur at any site, but the face and legs are common sites.

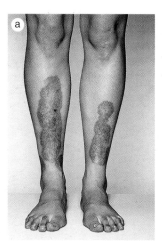 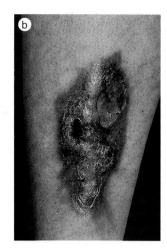

Fig. 8.14   *Necrobiosis lipoidica diabeticorum: (a) plaques on the shins (reproduced with permission from M.A. Mir (1995) Atlas of Clinical Diagnosis. W.B. Saunders, London); (b) ulceration*

Fig. 8.15   *Pyoderma gangrenosum. Reproduced with permission from M.A. Mir (1995) Atlas of Clinical Diagnosis. W.B. Saunders, London*

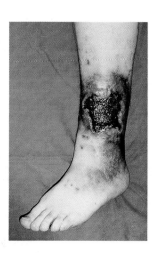

INTERPRETATION

Look for/consider causes

- The causes of erythema nodosum and pyoderma gangrenosum are given below.
- Pyoderma gangrenosusm should always be in the differential diagnosis of any non-healing ulcer.

Assess other systems

- PTM is specific to Graves' disease (Case study 11.1).
- NLD may prompt discussion of diabetes (Case study 4.18).

DISCUSSION

What are the causes of erythema nodosum?

- *Streptococcus* (sore throat), *Salmonella* or *Campylobacter* (enteritis), primary tuberculosis, fungi, leprosy
- Sarcoidosis, commonly with arthralgia and bilateral hilar lymphadenopathy
- Oral contraceptive pill, sulphonamides, tetracyclines, penicillin
- Ulcerative colitis, Crohn's disease
- Lymphoma/malignancy
- Pregnancy.

What is the histology of PTM?

The superficial layer of the skin is infiltrated with mucopolysaccharides and hyaluronic acid. Keloid scarring occurs post biopsy.

How does NLD arise?

NLD affects < 0.5% of diabetes patients and there is, in essence, degeneration and thickening of collagen bundles within the dermis with a palisading granuloma (similar to another condition, granuloma annulare, which may also occur in diabetes). Lesions progress slowly and seldom resolve. There is no effective treatment but topical or intralesional steroids occasionally help. Lesions often recur at the sites of skin grafts.

What are the causes of pyoderma gangrenosum?

- Ulcerative colitis, Crohn's disease
- Rheumatoid disease, ankylosing spondylitis
- Chronic active hepatitis, primary biliary cirrhois, sclerosing cholangitis
- Lymphoproliferative and myeloproliferative disorders
- Diabetes mellitus, thyroid disease, sarcoidosis.

List some skin manifestations of diabetes

- Infection ● Arterial foot ulcers ● Vitiligo ● Lipoatrophy.

List some causes of leg ulceration

- Chronic venous insufficiency ● Peripheral vascular disease
- Vasculitis ● Neuropathy (often with Charcot's joints)
- Pyoderma gangrenosum ● Sickle cell disease ● Malignancy.

| CASE STUDY | 8.12 NEUROFIBROMATOSIS (NF) |

Instruction: *Look at this patient's skin and examine for any other salient features before discussing your findings.*

RECOGNITION

There are multiple (more than six) *café au lait spots*, each > 5 mm (15 mm in postpubertal patients) in diameter (Fig. 8.16).

There are multiple *neurofibromas*. These may be soft or firm mobile subcutaneous lumps or nodules along peripheral nerves.

Neurofibromas comprise all elements of a peripheral nerve. From sensory twigs they arise as subcutaneous nodules, and from peripheral nerve trunks as fusiform enlargement (plexiform neurofibromas).

INTERPRETATION

Assess other systems

Look for:

● Lisch nodules in the iris. These are melanocytic hamartomas, appearing as well defined dome shaped elevations on the surface of the iris, clear to yellow/brown in colour. They may only be visible on slit lamp examination.
● Axillary or inguinal freckling.

The diagnosis is NF type 1.

Evidence of decompensation

Tell the examiners that complications can arise from:

Fig. 8.16   *Neurofibromatosis. Reproduced with permission from M.A. Mir (1995) Atlas of Clinical Diagnosis. W.B. Saunders, London*

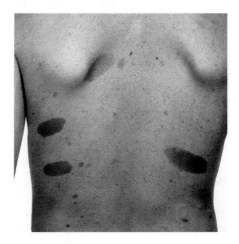

- Spinal cord or peripheral nerve compression (from neurofibromas or skeletal abnormalities) ● Kyphoscoliosis ● Optic gliomas
- Astrocytomas and meningiomas ● Renal artery stenosis
- Phaeochromocytomas.

DISCUSSION

What is the genetic basis of NF?

NF type 1 is associated with chromosome 17.
NF type 2, associated with chromosome 22, is associated with bilateral acoustic neuromas. Café au lait spots are less frequent.

List some other causes of hyperpigmentation

- Peutz–Jeghers syndrome ● Addison's disease ● Haemosiderin deposition ● Haemochromatosis/chronic liver disease
- Uraemia ● Amiodarone.

CASE STUDY   8.13 TUBEROSE SCLEROSIS (TS)

Instruction: *Look at this patient's skin and discuss your findings.*

RECOGNITION

There are multiple small skin lesions on this young man's face. There are several flesh coloured or pink papules on the nose and cheeks. These are *angiofibromas* (once incorrectly called adenoma sebaceum). *Shagreen patches* may be present, often on the trunk. There may also be *hypopigmented 'ash leaf' macules. Periungual fibromas* arise from the proximal nail folds of the fingers or toes.

INTERPRETATION

Assess other systems

Tell the examiners that you would ask about seizures (intracranial tumours and calcification may cause seizures and learning difficulties).
Tell the examiners that you would also consider:

- Eye involvement (retinal hamartomas) ● Renal involvement (cysts) ● Cardiac involvement.

DISCUSSION

What is the genetic basis of TS?

An autosomal dominant condition in which hamartoma formation occurs in multiple organs including the skin, central nervous system, eyes, kidneys and heart.

CASE STUDY	8.14 ANAEMIA

Instruction: *Please ask this 50-year-old anaemic man some questions and then examine him. Discuss your findings.*

RECOGNITION

Ask about

- Sources of blood loss, especially rectal bleeding, dyspepsia and alarm symptoms (page 126); menorrhagia in females
- Drugs (e.g. NSAIDs, warfarin)
- Alcohol
- History of malabsorption (Crohn's disease, coeliac disease)
- History of autoimmune disease (e.g. thyroid disease)
- History of gastrectomy
- Diet (e.g. veganism).

General signs of anaemia

There is *pallor* of *conjunctival membranes, buccal membranes, palmar creases* and *nail beds.*

INTERPRETATION

Look for/consider causes

Acquired anaemias:

- Iron deficiency anaemia (*ridged brittle nails, koilonychia* or spoon shaped nails, *angular stomatitis, dysphagia*)
- Megaloblastic anaemia (*atrophic glossitis*) (pages 455–456)
- Haemolytic anaemia (*?jaundice*) (pages 456–458)
- Anaemia of chronic disease (page 458)
- Aplasia (page 458)
- Myeloproliferative (page 71) and myelodysplastic (page 70) disease
- Secondary marrow infiltration (*splenomegaly, hepatosplenomegaly, lymphadenopathy, petechial* or *purpuric rash*).

Inherited anaemias:

- Sickle cell disease (*deformed digits, dactylitis, skin ulceration*) (Case study 8.15)
- Thalassaemia (skeletal enlargement due to marrow hyperplasia, e.g. jaw, limbs) (Case study 8.15).

Evidence of decompensation

1. Severe anaemia of any cause may cause high output *cardiac failure.*

2. Megaloblastosis may occur outwith the bloodstream. Overt subacute combined degeneration of the cord (SACDC) is rare, but there may be paraesthesia and impaired vibration sense. Hypothyroidism can also cause paraesthesia by compression of the median nerves.

3. Marrow infiltration of any cause can cause leucopenia (*sepsis*) and thrombocytopenia (*petechiae*).

Look for/consider associated diseases

Pernicious anaemia may be associated with the spectrum of autoimmune conditions. Look for obvious ones (*Graves' ophthalmopathy, hypothyroid face, rheumatoid hands, lupus rash*).

DISCUSSION

What is anaemia?

Low haemoglobin concentration, which may occur if haemoglobin synthesis fails or if red blood cells (RBCs) are prematurely destroyed.

What are the components of a RBC and how might alteration in any of these components give rise to anaemia?

RBCs are approximately 8 μm in diameter and biconcave with an area of central pallor. Their shape enables them to squeeze through tight capillaries. There is normally only minimal *anisocytosis* (variation in size) and *poikilocytosis* (variation in shape). Some other clinically important RBC variants are listed in Box 8.4.

The three integral components of a RBC are its:

1. Membrane

This bears blood group antigens and comprises a lipid bilayer and underlying protein skeleton. Alterations in lipid can cause macrocytosis without anaemia. Alterations in cytoskeletal molecules (e.g. spectrin, ankryn) can cause haemolysis and anaemia.

2. Metabolic components

The main energy creating pathways are the Embden–Meyerhof pathway and the hexose monophosphate shunt. Energy is used by the RBC to maintain osmotic stability by membrane pumps. Enzymopathies (page 461) within these metabolic pathways can give rise to haemolytic anaemia.

3. Haemoglobin

The haemoglobin molecule comprises four *haem* groups (as a tetramer) and *globin*.

Each haem group is a binding site for oxygen. Other haem containing molecules include myoglobin and the abnormal

| Box 8.4 | Clinically Important Red Blood Cell (RBC) Variants |

Acanthocytes
These are spiky RBCs occurring in certain disorders of lipid metabolism which affect the membrane (abetalipoproteinaemia)

Basophilic stippling
This occurs when RNA remains in the RBC due to defective Hb synthesis; seen in thalassaemias and lead poisoning

Burr cells
These are irregularly shaped RBCs with spikes (hence Burr cells are sometimes called echinocytes) seen in chronic renal failure

Dimorphic blood film
This refers to two populations of red cells, seen after treatment/transfusion in iron deficiency or megaloblastic anaemia, or when these two conditions coexist

Elliptocytes
These are ellipse shaped RBCs, seen in hereditary elliptocytosis

Heinz bodies
These are inclusions of oxidised haemoglobin seen in G6PD deficiency

Howell–Jolly bodies
These are nuclear remnants which are normally removed by the spleen, hence they are present post splenectomy and in hyposplenic states such as coeliac disease and sickle cell disease

Hypochromic RBCs
Pale staining (hypochromasia) is due to defective haemo-globinisation, notable in iron deficiency and thalassaemia

Macrocytic RBCs
These are large RBCs present because of dyserythropoiesis (abnormal synthesis of RBC) or because RBCs are released early into the circulation (*left shift*, a term also used when cells of the white cell line are released early into peripheral blood as in sepsis); seen in megaloblastic anaemia, liver disease, hypothyroidism and pregnancy

Megaloblastosis
This refers to macrocytosis resulting from deficient synthesis of nuclear material in B_{12} or folate deficiency

Microctic RBCs
These are small RBCs, because of defective haemoglobination, seen in iron deficiency anaemia, thalassaemia and sideroblastosis

Pencil cells
These are elongated cells, seen in iron deficiency

Polychromasia

This refers to variable haemoglobinisation of RBCs, seen particularly when reticulocytes are present in the peripheral blood, giving the blood film a blue tinge because the ratio of nuclear remnant material to haemoglobin is higher than usual

Reticulocytes

These are young RBCs, normally comprising < 1% of peripheral RBCs, but 'churned out' when erythropoiesis is increased in compensation for peripheral destruction (as in haemolysis)

Schistocytes

These are fragmented RBCs, seen in intravascular haemolysis, often as part of microangiopathic haemolytic anaemia (MAHA). Strands of fibrin are laid down in small vessels and RBCs get chopped in half (*helmet cells*) or into multiple irregular fragments as they gush through. All of the features of haemolysis (page 457) are present. Causes include disseminated intravascular coagulation (DIC), thrombotic thrombocytopenic purpura (TTP), haemolytic uraemic syndrome (HUS) and severe hypertension

Sickle cells

These are the characteristic sickle (curved blade) shaped RBCs in sickle cell disease

Spherocytes

These are small, dense cells without central pallor, seen when the RBC membrane has been damaged and subsequently resealed, as in hereditary spherocytosis

Target cells

These RBCs have a ring of pallor between central and peripheral staining, seen when haemoglobinisation is inadequate as in iron deficiency, thalassaemia, liver disease and hyposplenism

Tear drop cells

These are seen in myelofibrosis

methaemoglobin (ferric Fe^{3+}) and carboxyhaemoglobin. Iron usually exists in its ferrous (Fe^{2+}) form.

Haemoglobin is normally glycosylated as a result of binding to glucose during the 120 day life span of the RBC.

Normal adult haemoglobin (HbA) comprises two α and two β *globin polypeptide chains*. There is normally a trace of HbA2 ($\alpha2, \delta2$) and sometimes a trace amount of fetal (HbF) haemoglobin ($\alpha2, \gamma2$). In the *haemoglobinopathies, abnormal polypeptide chains are produced (sickle cell disease) or normal polypeptide chains are produced in decreased amounts (thalassaemias).*

What do you know about iron uptake, transport and storage?

- The average diet contains 15 mg of iron daily, of which about 1 mg is absorbed into the circulation from the duodenum and jejunum, increasing to a maximum of 3–4 mg in deficiency states. The HFE gene product (page 60) is one of the proteins responsible for its uptake.
- Iron is transported in plasma bound to transferrin, and cells which require iron express receptors to which transferrin delivers its iron. In iron deficiency, the number of transferrin receptors, and hence the total iron binding capacity (TIBC), increases.
- Iron is stored in the liver and reticuloendothelial system (RES), and incorporated into haemoglobin in the bone marrow.

How might you confirm reduced iron status?

Peripheral blood film

- Hypochromia ● Microcytosis ● Pencil cells ● Occasional target cells.

Serum markers

- Low serum iron ● Raised transferrin and TIBC ● Low transferrin saturation ● Low ferritin (may be raised if coexistent chronic inflammatory disease).

Bone marrow (BM) aspiration

- Normal cellularity
- Perls stain showing absence of erythroblast iron stores and of siderotic granules.

  BM examination is the traditional gold standard but has been largely superseded by *soluble transferrin receptor assays*. These are particularly useful in patients with chronic disease and suspected iron deficiency, in whom the classical markers of iron deficiency may be altered.

What other conditions can cause microcytosis?

- Thalassaemias (Case study 8.15).
- Sideroblastic anaemia, characterised by the presence of ring sideroblasts in BM, which arise as a result of failure to incorporate iron into haemoglobin. It may be congenital or acquired (primary as in the myelodysplastic syndromes or secondary to drugs or toxins, notably lead poisoning).

What is megaloblastic anaemia?

Megaloblastic anaemia is characterised by *macrocytosis* and *megaloblastic erythropoiesis*. The underlying common denominator is faulty DNA synthesis resulting from deficiency of vitamin B_{12} or folate.

What other conditions can cause macrocytosis?

● Haemolysis (because abundant reticulocytes of larger diameter than mature RBCs enter the peripheral blood) ● Liver disease ● Hypothyroisism ● Pregnancy.

List some causes of vitamin B$_{12}$ deficiency

● Pernicious anaemia or gastrectomy causing lack of intrinsic factor (IF, page 133)
● Malabsorption (e.g. Crohn's disease, ileal resection, stagnant loops, bacterial overgrowth)
● Nutritional deficiency (e.g. veganism).

List some causes of folate deficiency

● Dietary deficiency (e.g. elderly, alcoholics)
● Malabsorption (e.g. coeliac disease, Crohn's disease)
● Drugs (e.g. anticonvulsants)
● Increased utilisation in pregnancy or haemolysis
● Abnormal metabolism (e.g. methotrexate, which inhibits dihydrofolate reductase).

What abnormalities may appear on the blood film in megaloblastic anaemia?

● Oval macrocytes ● Poikilocytes ● Hypersegmented neutrophils (> 5 lobes to nucleus).

BM examination, seldom necessary with vitamin B$_{12}$ and folate assays (serum/red cell, the latter an estimate of body stores), shows increased cellularity, loss of fat spaces and accumulation of early cells—erythroid precursors, 'giant' metamyelocytes and megaloblasts. At all stages nuclei are primitive with an open 'lacy' chromatin pattern.

What is pernicious anaemia?

Pernicious anaemia is the most common cause of vitamin B$_{12}$ deficiency and is due to *chronic atrophic gastritis (CAG)*. There are two types of CAG (Box 8.5). The stomach has three regions, the *fundus* and *body*, both containing *parietal cells* which *secrete acid and intrinsic factor (IF, page 133)* and *peptic cells* which *secrete pepsinogen*, and the *antrum*, which contains *gastrin (page 127)* producing *G cells*.

What is haemolytic anaemia?

Haemolysis refers to destruction of peripheral RBCs earlier than their normal life span of 120 days. Anaemia results if the marrow response fails to compensate for this destruction.

> **Box 8.5** **Chronic Atrophic Gastritis**
>
> **Type A CAG** (autoimmune) spares the antrum and is associated with pernicious anaemia, autoantibodies against parietal cells causing IF deficiency and hypergastrinaemia due to G cell hyperplasia. The natural history of Type A CAG from its origin to anaemia is likely years. Type B CAG is much more common.
>
> **Type B CAG** (not autoimmune) is usually associated with *Helicobacter pylori* and low serum gastrin because of antral destruction. Acute gastritis may occur as a result of *H. pylori* infection or irritants such as NSAIDs or alcohol.

Most causes of haemolysis are *extravascular* (RBCs are destroyed in the RES), an accentuation of the normal destruction process. Some causes are *intravascular*, giving rise to red cell fragmentation.

What are the laboratory findings in haemolytic anaemia?

- Unconjugated hyperbilirubinaemia (jaundice is common)
- Increased urinary urobilinogen (page 47)
- Reduced or absent serum haptoglobins
- Increased serum lactate dehydrogenase (LDH)
- Reticulocytosis (bone marrow compensation)
- Bone marrow erythroid hyperplasia
- Polychromasia (reticulocytosis) of the peripheral blood film.

What are the causes of haemolytic anaemia?

Immune haemolysis (usually extravascular triggers)

This includes:

- Autoimmune haemolytic anaemia (AIHA)
- Drug induced haemolysis
- Alloimmune transfusion incompatibility reactions or haemolysis of the newborn.

In AIHA the Coomb's direct antiglobulin test is positive. In this test, the autoantibody coating the surface of RBCs is detected directly by application of an antiglobulin:

- *Warm AIHA,* in which the autoantibody reacts best at 37°C, may occur in SLE and lymphoproliferative disorders. There is often marked spherocytosis.
- *Cold AIHA,* in which the autoantibody reacts best at < 37°C, may occur in *Mycoplasma* infection and infectious mononucleosis.

Intravascular haemolysis

Causes include:

- Prosthetic heart valves
- 'March' haemoglobinuria

- DIC/TTP/HUS (page 466)
- Paroxysmal nocturnal haemoglobinuria, a condition in which the RBC membrane is abnormally sensitive to complement lysis because of aberrant membrane anchored proteins which normally inhibit lysis.

What do you know about anaemia of chronic disease?

Anaemia of chronic disease occurs in a wide variety of inflammatory, infectious and neoplastic disorders. Anaemia of chronic renal failure is probably in part attributable to anaemia of chronic disease as well as reduced levels of erythropoietin (EPO).

Anaemia of chronic disease typically occurs with adequate iron stores but is characterised by:

- Reduced serum iron and transferrin ● Normal or raised ferritin.

Other types of anaemia frequently coexist and the blood film may show normochromic, normocytic RBCs or hypochromic, microcytic RBCs. The transferrin receptor assay (page 455) is useful in identifying iron deficiency anaemia in such patients.

What are the causes of normochromic normocytic anaemia?

- Chronic disease ● Pregnancy ● CRF ● Bone marrow failure.

What is aplastic anaemia?

This is pancytopenia due to marrow hypoplasia, which may be idiopathic or a consequence of drugs (chloramphenicol, gold), chemicals or infection.

What are the porphyrias?

Porphyrias are enzyme disorders of haem synthesis leading to accumulation of various pre-haem molecules (porphyrin precursors or porphyrins).

Hepatic porphyrias, including *acute intermittent porphyria (AIP)*, may cause intermittent abdominal pain, neuropsychiatric sequelae, tachycardia and hypertension. These may be precipitated by drugs or infection. In addition, *variegate porphyria* causes fragile skin. Most people with the AIP defect never develop symptoms.

Porphyrins, which cannot be metabolised by the liver, accumulate in the urine in AIP (even between attacks) turning it red on light exposure, and in the faeces in other forms.

Porphyria cutanea tarda (PCT) usually occurs secondary to chronic liver disease, especially from alcohol. It causes skin photosensitivity and pigmentation with blistering, especially of the face.

All porphyrias cause photosensitivity except AIP.

Lead poisoning causes accumulation of porphyrins by inhibiting several steps in haem synthesis. Features of lead poisoning include abdominal pain/constipation, motor neuropathy, a blue gum line and sideroblastic anaemia with basophilic stippling.

8.15 SICKLE CELL DISEASE (SCD)

Instruction: *Please examine this patient's hands and legs. He suffers from numerous episodes of abdominal pain. You may briefly examine any other systems you feel relevant before discussing your findings.*

RECOGNITION

The *digits are of various lengths, deformed*, and there may be active finger swelling (*dactylitis*). The patient appears anaemic. There are also numerous areas of *skin ulceration*.

INTERPRETATION

Confirm the diagnosis

Tell the examiners that you would like to ask about a history of bone pain, strokes, priaprism, and precipitating factors such as infection and dehydration.

Assess other systems

This could include:

- Abdominal palpation for hepatomegaly or splenomegaly
- Ophthalmoscopy for retinal infarcts or neovascularisation
- Telling the examiners that you would like to check the urinalysis for haematuria.

DISCUSSION

What is the underlying abnormality in SCD?

Valine is substituted for glutamine at position 6 on the β globin chain, giving rise to the haemoglobin S gene. Sickle cell haemoglobin (HbS) molecules derived from this gene tend to polymerise.

The rate of polymerisation is accelerated by:

- Hypoxia
- An increased concentration of intracellular haemoglobin
- A decreased concentration of fetal haemoglobin (HbF).

Polymerisation renders the RBC less pliable and it deforms into its characteristic sickle shape.

The HbS gene occurs widely throughout Africa and in countries with African immigrant populations and also in parts of the Mediterranean, Middle East and India.

What types of SCD are there?

The spectrum of SCD is shown in Box 8.6.

Box 8.6	The Spectrum of Sickle Cell Disease (SCD)

1. Heterozygote (AS) sickle cell trait
Inheritance of the HbS gene from one parent and a normal β globin gene from the other results in this harmless carrier state.

2. Homozygous (SS) sickle cell anaemia
This occurs when HbS is inherited from both parents, and it tends to be severe.

3. Sickle cell/haemoglobin C (SC) disease
This occurs if HbS is inherited from one parent and HbC from the other. The HbC gene is the second commonest haemoglobin gene abnormality in West Africa. HbSC disease tends to be mild but important microvascular complications can occur.

4. Sickle cell/β thalasssaemia
This is designated $β^+$ if 20–30% of HbA (normal adult haemoblobin) is present and $β°$ if no HbA is present. $β^+$ tends to be mild clinically but $β°$ severe.

What are the clinical consequences of severe SCD?

1. Haemolysis, because RBCs fail to negotiate tight capillaries resulting in anaemia, jaundice and a predisposition to pigment gallstones.
2. Vaso-occlusive or sequestration crises due to sickle cells impeding blood flow. Complications of occlusion can include:
   (i) Painful bone crises and dactylitis
   (ii) Skin ulcers
   (iii) Splenic infarcts and tendency to sepsis from encapsulated organisms
   (iv) Retinal infarcts
   (v) Impaired renal tubule concentrating ability
   (vi) Renal papillary necrosis and chronic renal failure
   (vii) *Salmonella* osteomyelitis
   (viii) Aseptic necrosis of the humeral and femoral heads
   (ix) Priapism
   (x) Strokes
   (xi) Hepatic infarcts
   (xii) Growth impairment
   (xiii) Pregnancy complications
   (xiv) Pulmonary emboli.
3. Aplastic crises may also occur, often due to *parvovirus B19*.

Severe SCD causes autosplenectomy but milder forms may cause splenic sequestration without infarction and the spleen may be palpable because of 'congestion'. Where there is hyposplensim, there may also be an elevated white cell and platelet count.

Against which organisms should asplenic individuals be vaccinated?
> *Pneumococcus, Meningococcus* and *Haemophilus.*

What might the peripheral blood film reveal in sickle cell anaemia?
> ● Anaemia (Hb 6–10 g/dl) ● Reticulocytosis ● Target cells
> ● Howell–Jolly bodies due to autosplenectomy.

> Definitive diagnosis requires haemoglobin electrophoresis.

What are the principles of treatment?
> Treatment of crises includes oxygen, hydration, analgesia and
> antibiotics. Numerous therapies are being evaluated which may
> reduce polymerisation.

What are the important inherited anaemias?
> 1. **Anaemias due to membrane abnormalities.** *Hereditary
>   spherocytosis* is caused by abnormalities of membrane proteins
>   rendering the RBC excessively permeable to sodium influx. Some
>   of the RBC membrane is spliced by the spleen/RES to leave small
>   spherical cells without central pallor (spherocytes). Ultimately,
>   spherocytes are haemolysed by the RES. Osmotic fragility tests
>   reveal increased susceptibilty to lysis compared to normal RBCs.
> 2. **Enzymopathies.** *Glucose-6-phosphate dehydrogenase (G6PD)
>   deficency* is by far the most important enzymopathy worldwide.
> 3. **Haemoglobinopathies.** *SCD* and *thalassaemias*, both autosomal
>   recessive disorders.

How do thalassaemias arise?
> Thalassaemias are due to *inefficient rate of production of normal
> globin chains (compare with SCD in which normal globin chains fail to
> be produced—page 454).* Depending upon which pair of globin
> chains, α or β, has inefficient production, α *thalassaemias or* β
> *thalassaemias* result. α thalassaemias are more common than β
> thalassaemias. Thalassaemias are most common in patients of Far
> and Middle Eastern origin.

What types of a thalassaemia are there?
> There are two α genes on each chromosome such that normal
> individuals have four copies of the α gene (unlike just two copies of
> the β gene). There are four possible genetic abnormalities
> (Box 8.7).

What types of β thalassaemia are there?
> β *thalassaemias* are common in patients of Mediterranean, Middle
> and Far Eastern origin, and over 180 different mutations of the gene
> have been described which decrease the output of β globin chains,
> either completely or partially.

Box 8.7   ## Types of α Thalassaemia

1. Deletion of one gene, resulting in an **asymptomatic carrier state** with a normal blood film
2. Deletion of two genes, resulting in the **α thalassaemia trait** with mild hypochromic, microcytic anaemia
3. Deletion of three genes **(HbH disease)** in which there is anaemia (Hb 7–10 g/dl), splenomegaly and the presence of 'golf ball cells' on the blood film due to precipitation of β globin chains in the red cell. The reduced rate of α chain synthesis generally leads to an excess of β and γ chains
4. Deletion of all four genes **(Hb Bart's disease)** causing *hydrops fetalis* and stillbirth.

There is just one β gene on each chromosome such that normal individuals have only two copies of the β gene (unlike four copies of the α gene). There are two common genetic abnormalities (Box 8.8).

Box 8.8   ## Types of β Thalassaemia

Thalassaemia major

Homozygotes (inheriting the same or different β thalassaemia genes from each parent) develop thalassaemia major. This is characterised by:

- Severe anaemia (Hb 2–8 g/dl; much being HbF) resulting from deficiency of β chains
- Compensatory excess of α chains, which damage RBCs
- Hypertrophy of ineffective marrow leading to bone expansion and skeletal abnormalities
- Extramedullary haemopoiesis and hepatosplenomegaly
- Failure to thrive, which is almost inevitable
- A blood film showing severe hypochromia and microcytosis, target cells and reticulocytosis
- A need for repeated blood transfusions which downregulate marrow dyserythropoiesis but lead to secondary haemochromatosis.

Thalassaemia minor

Heterozygotes have the thalassaemia trait (thalassaemia minor). Individuals may be mildly anaemic during times of stress but otherwise have merely a hypochromic, microcytic blood film

CASE STUDY	8.16 PURPURA/BLEEDING

Instruction: *Look at this patient's skin. What diagnoses would you consider?*

RECOGNITION

1. There is *purpura*. Purpura refers to spontaneous extravasation of blood from the capillaries into the skin.
2. There are *petechiae* (tiny purpuric spots).

INTERPRETATION

Look for/consider causes

1. *Blood vessel/connective tissue problem (purpura)*
   - Age (purpura especially on forearms)
   - Cushing's syndrome (Cushing's face)
   - Rheumatoid arthritis (rheumatoid hands)
   - Vasculitis
   - Rarely, scurvy (bleeding gums with perifollicular haemorrhages and 'corkscrew' hairs)
   - Inherited causes include hereditary haemorrhagic telangiectasia (HHT), Ehlers–Danlos syndrome (EDS), osteogenesis imperfecta and Marfan's syndrome.

2. *Platelet problem (petechiae)*

   Platelet problems result in prolonged *mucosal bleeding (epistaxis, genitourinary, gastrointestinal)* spontaneously or after minimal trauma and *petechiae* are characteristic (Box 8.9).
   Thrombocytopenia may be due to:

   1. Decreased marrow production:
      (i) Myelodysplasia
      (ii) Aplasia
      (iii) Leukaemia and bone marrow infiltration
      (iv) Drugs, alcohol
      (v) Viruses (e.g. parvovirus B19)
      (vi) Hereditary.
   2. Increased peripheral destruction:
      (i) Hypersplenism
      (ii) Autoimmune thrombocytopenic purpura (ITP) in which autoantibody–platelet complexes are sequestered in the spleen
      (iii) Autoantibodies in SLE, chronic lymphocytic leukaemia (CLL), HIV
      (iv) Drugs
      (v) Disseminated intravascular coagulation (DIC).

Platelet dysfunction may be acquired, as in renal failure, or inherited, as in the rare Glanzmann's disease, in which GPIIbIIIa (Fig. 8.12) receptors are undetectable.

3. Coagulation problem (purpura)

Coagulation problems tend to cause *muscle and joint bleeding* (Box 8.9). Important causes of coagulopathy are:

- Impaired liver synthetic function ● Anticoagulants
- Haemophilia A or B.

DISCUSSION

How does blood normally clot?

Evolution taught blood to clot, but to prevent unhindered clotting of the entire vasculature, coagulation must adopt a balanced ride on the see saw whose copartner is anticoagulation. Central to these processes is the endothelium, no longer thought of as inert but as a dynamic 'gamespitch' whose molecular 'players' are in continuous engagement to achieve a draw.

Normal haemostasis (Fig. 8.17) is a function of:

1. **Blood vessel integrity**. Healthy blood vessels *vasoconstrict* and synthesize/activate molecules when the endothelium is breached and subendothelium exposed (as in trauma or acute coronary syndromes).
2. **Platelet activation, adhesion and aggregation**. Platelets are *activated* by subendothelial molecules which are exposed when the endothelium is damaged. Platelets also secrete molecules (such as ADP) from granules in their own cytoplasm which sustain this process of activation. Platelet glycoprotein receptors (GPRs) mediate *adhesion* to subendothelial tissue—GPIbR to subendothelial von Willebrand's factor (vWF) and GPIaIIbR to collagen—and subsequent *aggregation* (GPIIbIIIaR to fibrinogen) to form the early haemostatic plug. Fibrinogen is derived from the coagulation pathway.
3. **Coagulation**. The coagulation mechanism consolidates the platelet 'plug' into an insoluble fibrin clot. A series of inactive coagulation factors are activated (intrinsic and extrinsic pathways), resulting in a final common molecule, fibrin.

How does the bleeding tendency in a platelet problem differ to that of a coagulation problem?

This is explained in Box 8.9.

What is Henoch–Schönlein purpura (HSP)?

An IgA mediated vasculitis which may give rise to skin purpura, gastrointestinal vasculitis, arthropathy and IgA nephropathy.

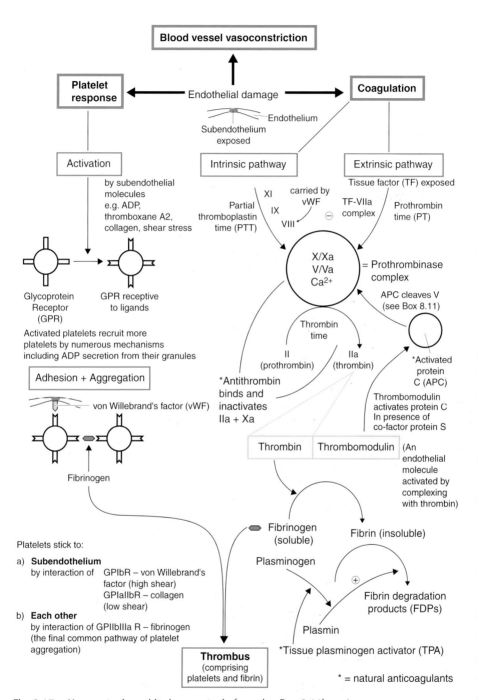

Fig. 8.17   *Haemostasis and its homeostasis (see also Box 8.11)*

Platelet Problem Versus Coagulation Problem

- Platelet problems result in prolonged *mucosal bleeding (epistaxis, genitourinary, gastrointestinal)* spontaneously or after minimal trauma. *Petechiae* are characteristic. This is because small endothelial lesions fail to seal
- Coagulopathies tend to cause *muscle and joint bleeding*. Recurrent haemarthroses lead to *joint deformity*. Patients are also at risk of *visceral and intracranial bleeds*. Excessive bleeding from small cuts is not typical, however. This is because platelet activation, adhesion and aggregation are sufficient to seal small endothelial lesions. Haemostasis of a larger wound requires fibrin reinforcement and hence a fully functional coagulation pathway

What are the Ehlers–Danlos syndromes (EDS)?

An inherited and heterogeneous group of disorders of collagen synthesis. The three broad clinical features are:

1. Purpura and skin fragility with poor 'tissue papery' wound healing
2. Skin 'stretchiness' which later becomes lax with excessive folds and wrinkles
3. Joint hypermobility/kyphoscoliosis.

Mitral valve prolapse and aortic dissection may occur.

What is osteogenesis imperfecta?

A group of collagen disorders with similar features to EDS but characterised by bone fractures, defective dentition and blue sclera (underlying choroid visible beneath thin collagen sclera). Aortic regurgitation may occur.

What do you know about Marfan's syndrome?

This results from autosomal dominant mutations of the fibrillin gene on chromosome 15. Fibrillin is the supporting framework for elastin deposition and is especially important for ligaments, blood vessel (notably aorta) integrity and lens support. Clinical features are shown in Box 8.10.

What do you know about disseminated intravascular coagulation (DIC) and the haemolytic uraemic syndrome (HUS)–thrombotic thrombocytopenic purpura (TTP) spectrum?

DIC causes exuberant haemostatic/antihaemostatic activity precipitated by cytokines in the systemic inflammatory response to sepsis. A similar mechanism is seen in the HUS–TTP spectrum and in severe hypertension. Platelets and coagulation factors are consumed by the haemostatic process and intraluminal fibrin strands damage

Box 8.10	Clinical Features of Marfan's Syndrome

- Tallness (arm span > height, pubis–sole > pubis– vertex)
- Spidery fingers, 'arachnodactyly', which are hypermobile (a clenched thumb overlaps the ulnar border of the hand)
- High arched palate
- Upward subluxation of lens in 50–75% (seen with a slit lamp)
- Blue sclera
- Underdeveloped muscles
- Pectus excavatum
- Multiple spontaneous pneumothoraces
- Kyphoscoliosis
- Mitral valve prolapse, aortic regurgitation and aneurysm tendency.

RBCs, causing microangiopathic haemolytic anaemia (MAHA). The cardinal features are thrombocytopenia, MAHA, haemolysis and a tendency to renal or neurological sequelae. TTP may be acute or chronic and autoantibodies against the cleaving protease for von Willebrand's factor (vWF) may be important in the pathogenesis of acute TTP.

DIC causes prolongation of the prothrombin time (PT) and partial thromboplastin time (PTT) – see Fig. 8.17.

CASE STUDY	8.17 HAEMOPHILIA (A OR B)

Instruction: *This young man has multiple joint deformities. Please examine his skin rash.*

RECOGNITION	

Haemophilia causes *muscle and joint bleeding*. The presence of purpura in the setting of joint deformity strongly suggests the diagnosis.

INTERPRETATION	

Confirm the diagnosis

Coagulopathy may be due to liver disease (*signs of chronic liver disease*, Case study 3.3) or over-anticoagulation but the haemophilias cause *recurrent* haemarthroses, which lead to *functional joint deformity*.

Tell the examiners that you would like to know about a family history of bleeding.

Evidence of decompensation

Tell examiners that patients are also at risk of *visceral and intracranial bleeds*. Intracranial bleeds and transfusion acquired viruses (acquired mostly prior to the advent of screening programmes) are the commonest causes of death.

DISCUSSION

What causes haemophilia A?

It is an X linked recessive (males affected, females carriers) disorder causing deficiency of factor VIII. It may occasionally result from an acquired autoimmune antibody (inhibitor) to factor VIII.

How would you assess the severity of haemophilia?

Haemophilia may be *severe* (factor VIII level < 2%) causing spontaneous bleeds, *moderate* (2–10%) causing traumatic bleeds or *mild* (> 10%) usually with bleeding only after major trauma. Factor VIII assays are available.

What is haemophilia B?

Haemophilia B is almost identical to haemophilia A but due to factor IX deficiency.

How are blood coagulation studies affected in haemophilia?

- The partial thromboplastin time (PTT) is prolonged – see Fig. 8.17. The PTT corrects with the addition of normal plasma in a 50 : 50 mix in hereditary haemophilia. Where there is an inhibitor (acquired disease), factor VIII in normal plasma is attacked by an autoantibody and thus the PTT will remain prolonged despite such a mix.
- The bleeding time (BT) is normal (< 10 minutes).

What do you know about von Willebrand's disease (vWD)?

It is caused by a quantitative or qualitative defect in von Willebrand's factor (vWF), with various modes of inheritance. Therefore males or females may be affected.

vWF has two roles (Fig. 8.17). It acts as a subendothelial binding molecule for platelets and is a carrier molecule for factor VIII in the bloodstream. vWF deficiency therefore causes platelet type bleeding and a secondary factor VIII deficiency, although the latter is seldom of clinical significance unless vWF disease is severe.

The BT is prolonged and the PTT is prolonged or normal.

What do you know about acquired coagulopathy?

Liver disease (decreased synthesis of vitamin K dependent coagulation factors II, VII, IX and X) and warfarin are the commonest causes.

Mention some transfusion and antihaemolytic products you use on the wards

1. Fresh frozen plasma (FFP) is a source of coagulation factors that is stored frozen and thawed prior to use. It is indicated in coagulopathy in an emergency or when no specific therapy is

available (bleeding in haemophilia or acquired coagulopathy).
2–4 units are usually given.

2. Platelet transfusion may be considered for platelet counts
   < 10–20×10^9/L (< 50 if bleeding or invasive procedure planned).

3. Packed RBCs are used for active bleeding. 1 unit of packed RBCs
   should raise the Hb by 10 g/L in an average adult.

4. Cryoprecipitate contains some clotting factors, vWF and
   fibrinogen. It may be indicated in hypo/dysfibrinogenaemia, e.g.
   liver disease or haemophilia or vWD where other treatments are
   unavailable (seldom the case these days).

5. Desmopressin (synthetic ADH) is used for disorders with a
   prolonged bleeding time and mild bleeding (haemophilias, vWD,
   chronic renal failure).

CASE STUDY	8.18 DEEP VEIN THROMBOSIS

Instruction: *Please examine this patient's leg and report your findings.*

RECOGNITION	

There is unilateral *calf redness* and *swelling* with *pitting oedema*. The
main differential diagnosis is soft tissue infection.

INTERPRETATION	

Look for/consider causes

Tell the examiners that you would ask about risk factors for venous
thromboembolism (VTE). Here is a golden opportunity to invite
discussion of prothrombotic disorders (below). Other risk factors include
immobility, surgery/trauma, malignancy, chronic inflammatory diseases,
pregnancy, the combined oral contraceptive pill, hormone replacement
therapy and obesity.

Evidence of decompensation

Tell the examiners that you would be concerned about propagation of
thrombus and pulmonary emboli. Compression ultrasound is the non-
invasive investigation of choice for confirming deep vein thrombosis
and determining its extent. Diagnosing pulmonary embolus is
discussed in Case study 2.7.

DISCUSSION	

What do you know about prothrombotic disorders?

These disorders, sometimes called *thrombophilias*, may be inherited
or acquired.

Inherited thrombophilias (Box 8.11)

| Box 8.11 | **Inherited Thrombophilias** |

Some of the enzymes in the coagulation cascade are inhibited by antithrombin.

The protein C anticoagulant system (Fig. 8.17) is activated by thrombomodulin (an endothelial molecule activated by complexing with thrombin as part of the homeostatic response to coagulation). Protein C (in the presence of its cofactor, protein S), a vitamin K dependent molecule, is activated by thrombomodulin to form activated protein C (APC). APC cleaves factor V.

Inherited thrombophilias include:

1. The presence of *factor V Leiden*, a mutant factor V molecule which has normal procoagulant properties but is resistant to cleavage by APC. The condition is also called APC resistance (APCR).
2. Deficiency of *protein C*.
3. Deficiency of *protein S*.
4. Deficiency of *antithrombin*.
5. *Prothrombin G20210A variant*, in which a single base change in the prothrombin gene is associated with an elevated plasma level of prothrombin.
6. Dysfibrinogenaemia, which is rare, and associated with a reduced plasma fibrinogen level.

It has been difficult to quantify risk attributable to inherited thrombophilias because thrombosis is a multifactorial disease. Many people with mutations will never have venous thromboembolic manifestations. Thrombotic risk in factor V Leiden heterozygotes, for example, is increased dramatically by smoking. Estimated increases in relative risk are given in Table 8.2.

Inherited thrombophilias tend to be associated predominantly or exclusively with venous thrombosis, unlike acquired thrombophilias and *hyperhomocysteinaemia* which can induce both venous and arterial thrombosis.

There are strong links between hyperhomocysteinaemia and vascular disease. The conversion of methylenetetrahydrofolate (MTHF) to methyltetrahydrofolate by the enzyme MTHF reductase (MTHFR) is central to normal homocysteine metabolism. The methyltetrahydrofolate generated by MTHFR is converted to tetrahydrofolate by the enzyme methyltetrahydrofolate:homocysteine methyltransferase, generating a methyl group which is transferred to homocysteine, converting homocysteine to methionine. This series of reactions is critical to normal DNA and RNA synthesis. A common mutation in the gene for MTHFR, in its heterozygous form, is associated with a moderate (20%) increase in serum homocysteine and a significantly higher risk of vascular thrombosis. Homocysteine is not metabolised exclusively to methionine. It is also metabolised to cysteine by the action of cystathione β synthase (CBS). Mutations in CBS give rise to the homocystinuria, in which homocysteine concentrations and thrombotic risk are very high.

TABLE 8.2 Risk of VTE attributable to inherited thrombophilia

	Increased risk of VTE	Prevalence in patients with VTE (%)	Prevalence in normal population (%)
Heterogeneous factor V Leiden mutation	3–8×	25–50	5
Protein C deficiency	10–15×	3	0.3
Protein S deficiency	10×	3	2
Antithrombin deficiency	25–50×	1	0.02
Prothrombin G20210A	3×	6	2
Dysfibrinogenaemia	Variable	Low	Rare

Acquired thrombophilias

Acquired thrombophilias include the antiphospholipid syndrome (APLS). Antiphospholipid antibodies associated with thrombosis and sometimes recurrent spontaneous first trimester miscarriage have long been recognised. They may also occur in conjunction with SLE. They include the lupus anticoagulant (LAC) and anticardiolipin (ACL) antibodies. APLS is a syndrome of thrombosis (venous or arterial), recurrent miscarriage, or both, in association with laboratory evidence of antiphospholipid antibodies. Why antibodies which react with phospholipid cause a prothrombotic tendency is not known.

Who should be considered for thrombophilia screening?

- Patients with spontaneous thrombosis, particularly if young or if pregnant
- Patients with thrombosis at an unusual site, e.g. sagittal sinus thrombosis
- Patients with recurrent thrombosis
- Patients with VTE and a history of VTE in a first degree relative.

Identifying a laboratory thrombophilic abnormality will not usually influence a patient's immediate treatment but may be of value in preventing further thrombosis and in counselling other family members, notably any family members contemplating pregnancy. A normal thrombophilia screen does not exclude prothrombotic defects which may be yet to be discovered and cannot be assumed to imply 'normal' or 'no increased risk' in the future or in other family members.

Which antithrombotic agents do you know of (refer also to Fig. 8.17)?

Antiplatelet agents

1. *Aspirin* blocks platelet activation by inhibiting thromboxane A2 via the cyclooxygenase pathway. Since there are many other platelet activators, aspirin's antiplatelet activity is limited.

2. Alternatives or adjuncts to aspirin include *clopidogrel*, which inhibits ADP induced platelet aggregation, and *dipyridamole*, which inhibits phosphodiesterase mediated platelet adhesion.

3. *Inhibitors of GPIIbIIIa receptors* are now used extensively in cardiovascular disease. They are powerful antithrombotics because they inhibit platelet crosslinking, the final common pathway of platelet aggregation.

Anticoagulants

1. *Warfarin* inhibits the procoagulant factors II, VII, IX and X but also the anticoagulant protein C. Since the half-life of protein C is short, a procoagulant state may precede wafarin's anticoagulant effect. This is seldom clinically significant but may cause problems in patients with underlying protein C underactivity and is responsible for the phenomenon of warfarin induced skin necrosis. Warfarin can interfere with diagnostic testing for protein C and S deficiency.

2. *Heparin* forms a high affinity complex with antithrombin and accelerates its action. Antithrombin inhibits both thrombin (factor IIa) and factor Xa when it binds to these. *Unfractionated heparin* is a long molecule which complexes with antithrombin, causing it to bind with and accelerate the action of both coagulation factors. Unfractionated heparin's anti-Xa : anti-IIa antithrombin binding ratio is 1 : 1. *Low molecular weight heparin (LMWH)* complexes with and accelarates mostly that region of antithrombin binding to Xa. In other words, LMWH exerts more effect on the proximal part of the pathway. This results in higher bioavailability, a longer half-life and lower propensity to thrombocytopenia. Monitoring of the PTT is not required. LMWHs are administered subcutaneously in the treatment and prophylaxis of deep venous thromboses, pulmonary emboli and acute coronary syndromes. Heparin can interfere with diagnostic testing for antithrombin deficiency.

3. Oral thrombin inhibitors are under evaluation for therapeutic use.

Thrombolytic agents

These agents lyse pre-existing thrombus, either by potentiating natural fibrinolytic pathways or mimicking natural thrombolytics (such as reteplase, a recombinant tissue plasminogen activator).

Is there a role for folic acid in cardiovascular disease prevention

High homocysteine levels contribute to arterial and venous thrombosis (meta-analysis—page 473—analysed 120 studies). Folate is integral to homocysteine metabolism (Box 8.11). Evidence suggests that lowering homocysteine levels by 3 μmol/L from current levels (achievable with folic acid—0.8 mg daily) reduces the risk of ischaemic heart disease by 16%, stroke by 24% and venous thromboembolism by 25%, and that folate should be considered for primary or secondary prophylaxis in people at risk. Testing homocysteine levels may not be necessary to institute therapy because of the high occurrence rate of hyperhomocysteinaemia in people with vascular disease.

REFERENCES AND FURTHER READING

British Society of Gastroenterologists. Guidelines for management of iron deficiency anaemia. Online. Available: www.bsg.org.uk

Electronic Dermatology Atlas. Online. Available: www.dermis.net

George JN. Platelets. Lancet 2000; 355: 1531–1539.

Prevention of Venous Thromboembolism. Scottish Intercollegiate Guidelines Network (SIGN) Edinburgh. March 2002. Online. Available: http://www.sign.ac.uk.

Provan AB, Weatherall DJ. Red cells II: acquired anaemias and polycythaemia. Lancet 2000; 355: 1260–1268.

Spivak JL. The blood in systemic disorders. Lancet 2000; 355: 1707–1712.

Thrombophilia. British Heart Foundation Factfile February 2002. Online. Available: www.bhf.org.uk.

Wald DS, Law M, Morris JK. Homocysteine and cardiovascular disease: evidence of causality from a meta-analysis. Br Med J 2002; 325: 1202–1206.

Walker ID, Greaves M, Preston FE et al. Investigation and Management of Heritable Thrombophilia. British Journal of Haematology 2001; 114: 512–528. Online. Available: http://bcshguidelines.com.

Weatherall DJ, Provan AB. Red cells I: inherited anaemias. Lancet 2000; 355: 1169–1175.

9. LOCOMOTOR SYSTEM

EXAMINATION: HANDS, ELBOWS, SHOULDERS, FEET, KNEES, HIPS, SPINE

Diagnosis in rheumatology

Common rheumatological symptoms are pain, stiffness and joint swelling.

1. *Diffuse pain not localised to joints* and *without stiffness* is often due to one of the chronic pain syndromes such as fibromyalgia. Polymyalgia rheumatica causes diffuse symptoms but is characterised by *stiffness*.
2. *Pain and stiffness localised to joints* may occur *without joint swelling*. Polyarthralgia without polyarthritis is typical of osteoarthritis, systemic lupus erythematosus (SLE) and viral infections. Osteoarthritis can also be associated with both soft tissue joint swelling and the more commonly encountered bony joint swellings such as Heberden's and Bouchard's nodes. Tendonitis may also give rise to pain in the region of a joint, and bursitis to swelling in the region of a joint.
3. *Pain and stiffness with joint swelling* (in PACES you are most likely to encounter joint swelling) *may be monoarticular or polyarticular.*

Monoarticular swelling is seen in:

● Palindromic rheumatism, usually short lived (days) and occasionally the first manifestation of rheumatoid arthritis

● Crystal arthropathy, which is usually brief

● Spondyloarthropathy

● Septic arthritis.

Polyarticular symptoms may be a transient feature of some viral infections, but where recurrent or persistent are likely to due one of the following:

● Rheumatoid arthritis
● Crystal arthropathy
● Spondyloarthropthy
● SLE.

Diagnosis in rheumatology may take time, the clinical picture often emerging over months or even years. When the history and examination meet a number of diagnostic criteria, serological tests (Box 9.1) can seek to confirm the diagnosis. Serological tests should not be used indiscriminately for patients with, for example, chronic pain, because they are only diagnostically useful in the context of defined clinical criteria.

General points for examining the locomotor system

Many rheumatologists use the *gait, arms, legs, spine (GALS)* system of general examination and then apply *inspection, palpation and movement (look, feel, move)* to each set of joints.

Look at

● The shape and position of the limbs and digits

● The skin for any scars, lumps or discoloration

● The joints for any swellings.

Box 9.1 Serological Tests

Antinuclear antibodies (ANAs)

ANAs can be detected by immunofluorescence which may show a predominantly *homogeneous*, *speckled* or *nucleolar* pattern. Further testing for extractable nuclear antigens (ENAs) may detect antibodies to specific nuclear components which provide supportive evidence of specific diseases:

- *Anti-ds* (double stranded) *DNA* antibodies: *SLE*
- *Anti-Sm* (Smith) antibodies: highly suggestive of SLE but present in < 20% of patients
- *Anti-RNP* (ribonucleoprotein) antibodies: *SLE*, 100% of patients with *mixed CTD*
- *Anti-Ro/SSA* (an RNA protein particle antigen) antibodies: *Sjögren's syndrome, SLE*
- *Anti-La/SSB* (an RNA protein particle antigen) antibodies: *Sjögren's syndrome*. In Sjögren's syndrome SSA becomes positive first since the SSA antigen is peripheral to the SSB antigen and exposed to autoantibodies first
- *Anti-Jo-1* (histidyl-transfer ribonucleic acid synthetase) antibodies: *polymyositis*
- *Antitopoisomerase* (formerly called anti Scl-70) antibodies: *diffuse scleroderma*
- *Antinucleolar* (various including anti-PM-Scl) antibodies: *diffuse scleroderma, polymyositis*
- *Anticentromere* antibodies: *limited scleroderma*/CREST.

Rheumatoid factor (RF)

Rheumatoid factors are antibodies against the Fc portion of IgG. They may be of any isotype but only IgM was traditionally detected by the now superseded latex agglutination test. An easy way to consider rheumatoid factor is to first consider that antibodies directed against other antibodies is a normal phenomenon. New antibodies are created continuously in response to an infinite variety of antigens in the environment; some antibodies, when newly formed, may also be seen by the immune system as foreign and 'anti-antibodies' are produced against them. Sometimes a cascade of antibody against antibody may be triggered.

Some of the anti-antibodies produced in this way are RFs and, hence, RFs are not specific to rheumatoid arthritis. They may be detected transiently after many acute infections, may be present in low titres in chronic infections, and are sometimes found in chronic inflammatory disorders like SLE and scleroderma. RFs are detectable in 5% of the normal population and in up to 25% of elderly people—simply because elderly people have been exposed for a longer time to the environmental stimuli which engender such antibodies. Up to 70% of patients with rheumatoid arthritis are RF +ve.

Feel

- The skin (warm, cold, dry, tender), and any skin swellings which may comprise fluid, soft tissue or bone

- The joints at rest. Examining joints *at rest* should precede examining *moving* joints.

Move

- The joints. Movements may be *active* (involving active muscle contraction) or *passive*. Joints may be flexed and extended, abducted and adducted, externally and internally rotated, supinated and pronated, inverted and everted, and circumducted. Only ball and socket joints (hip and shoulder) can do the latter.

In general:

● Pain and stiffness due to synovitis occurs with both active and passive movements.

● Pain due to tendonitis is worse with active movements.

● Pain due to movements of a tendon over an inflamed bursa (e.g. impingement in subacromial burisitis, pages 478, 480) occurs with passive and active movements.

Examining the hands

Examining the hands neurologically is detailed on pages 331–334.

1. Be careful about shaking your patient's hand. Ask if there is pain before examining, and preferably examine the hands rested on a pillow on your seated patient's lap.
2. Note functional aids such as walking sticks.
3. Examine the hands at rest, looking particularly at the joints. Note any *swelling of the distal interphalangeal (DIP) joints, proximal interphalangeal (PIP) joints, metacarpophalangeal (MCP) joints or wrists*. Note any deformities, in particular *swan neck and boutonnière deformities, Z shaped thumbs, ulnar deviation* and *wrist subluxation*. A mallet finger or thumb, in which the terminal phalanx cannot be extended, is caused by rupture of the extensor tendon, usually from trauma or rheumatoid arthritis.
4. Look at the nails for *pitting, nail fold erythema* or *telangiectasia, nail fold infarction* or *vasculitis*.
5. Look at the skin for *palmar erythema, vasculitis, digital ischaemia, purpura* (corticosteroids) or *scars* from arthrodeses or previous carpal tunnel release.

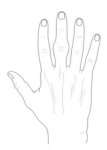

Fusiform swelling

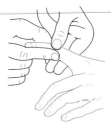

Palpation of interphalangeal joint for synovitis

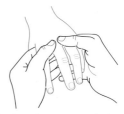

Palpation of metacarpophalangeal joint for synovitis

Fig. 9.1   *Examining for synovitis*

6. Look for *wasting* of the thenar or hypothenar muscle groups or both.
7. Feel the joints for evidence of *synovitis* (Fig. 9.1), or the bony *Heberden's* or *Bouchard's nodes* of osteoarthritis. *Active synovitis* of a joint results in *fusiform swelling*. Press both sides of the joint with the index finger and thumb of one hand and any swelling will 'bulge up'. Now press on the swelling (it has a spongy feel) with the fingers of your other hand. You should normally be

able to feel the bony margins of each MCP joint and the gaps between them, especially when the patient makes a fist, like mountain peaks and valleys. In inflammatory joint disease the valleys are filled with synovial fluid.

8. Now start to examine joint movements (Fig. 9.2). Some movements may not be possible—do not force your patient. Ask your patient to make the *'prayer sign'*, with wrists extended at 90°.

9. Ask them to do the *opposite*, with the dorsal surfaces of the *wrists* touching and *flexed* at 90°.

10. Ask them to *make a fist*, and then *tighten it*. If there is incomplete fist formation there may be a problem with the MCP, PIP or DIP joints or thickening of the flexor tendons.

11. Ask them to spread their *fingers apart*, a good test of the extensor tendons.

12. Ask them to *grip your fingers*. This allows you to detect flexor tendon thickening.

Stenosing tenosynovitis (trigger finger) may be a consequence of persistent inflammation. Both *de Quervain's tenosynovitis* (affecting abductor pollicis longus and extensor pollicis brevis) and *osteoarthritis of the carpometacarpal (CMC) joint* may cause pain around the base of thumb. *Finklestein's test* is positive in de Quervain's tenosynovitis—the wrist is deviated in an ulnar direction whilst the thumb is held flexed in the palm by the fingers (Fig. 9.3). This causes pain. Tenosynovitis is often associated with crepitation at the wrist. In osteoarthritis, grinding the extended thumb causes pain at the thumb base.

Examining the elbows

1. Ask about the location of any pain.
2. Look at the skin, in particular for *rheumatoid nodules* or *psoriatic plaques*. *Synovitis* or an *effusion* appears as a

Fig. 9.2
Hand movements

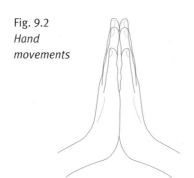

'Prayer sign', wrists extended

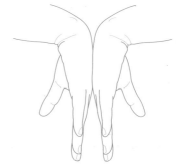

Wrists flexed

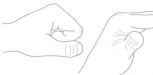

Making a fist, testing active flexion of the interphalangeal joints.

Note that active flexion of the metacarpophalangeal joints is best tested as shown here.

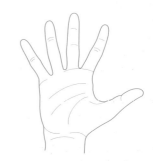

Spreading fingers apart to test extensor tendons

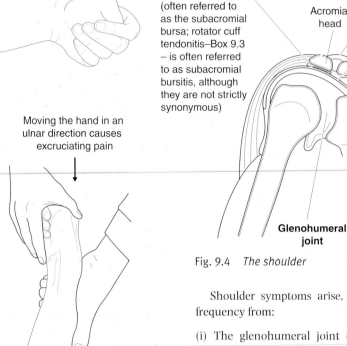

Moving the hand in an ulnar direction causes excruciating pain

Subacromial joint (often referred to as the subacromial bursa; rotator cuff tendonitis–Box 9.3 – is often referred to as subacromial bursitis, although they are not strictly synonymous)

Acromial head

Acromioclavicular joint

Rotator cuff tendon

Clavicle

Glenohumeral joint

Fig. 9.4   *The shoulder*

Fig. 9.3   *Finklestein's test*

bulge between the olecranon and the lateral epicondyle.

3. *Flex* and *extend* the joint, and *feel for crepitus.* Lack of complete extension is often overlooked. Remember to test *supination* and *pronation.*

Pain is often due to *epicondylitis*—a lateral (tennis elbow) epicondylitis causing pain over the lateral elbow and forearm or a medial (golfer's elbow) epicondylitis causing pain over the medial elbow and forearm. Both may be painful on gripping. *Olecranon bursitis* causes swelling at the point of the elbow.

Examining the shoulders

To know what you are examining for, you should be aware of basic shoulder anatomy (Fig. 9.4).

Shoulder symptoms arise, in order of frequency from:

(i) The glenohumeral joint (most commonly adhesive capsulitis; sometimes arthritis)

(ii) The subacromial joint (most commonly rotator cuff disease)

(iii) The acromioclavicular joint.

1. Ask your patient to point to any site of *pain,* although this is not a reliable guide for localising the structure from which it arises. The shoulder may hurt when moved, or at night, and pain may travel into the arm. Shoulder pain can be referred from thoracic viscera and from structures adjacent to the diaphragm. Neck pain is more likely to originate in the neck. More reliable is any clear pattern of loss of movement. Since removal of a garment requires external rotation at the glenohumeral joint, it is likely that difficulty with this movement (shrugging off a shirt) is due to a glenohumeral joint problem.

2. Look at the shoulder *contours,* especially at the supraspinatus and infraspinatus

Box 9.2   Adhesive Capsulitis (Frozen Shoulder)

Often occurring in middle aged patients, adhesive capsulitis is a disorder causing fibrosis (notably fibrosis and shortening of the coraco-humeral ligament) of the joint capsule with restricted movement, especially external rotation. It may start with pain over the insertion of the deltoid. Stiffness is often more severe after several months. 'Thawing' is typical within 12 to 18 months.

Plain X-rays are unhelpful. Magnetic resonance imaging (MRI) is the investigation of choice when trials of treatment are ineffective. Treatments include NSAIDs, corticosteroid injections into the joint capsule and physiotherapy.

Glenohumeral arthritis, more common over 50 years of age, is a less common glenohumeral problem and results in a stiff, often creaky joint.

---

muscles which overlie the upper and lower segments of the scapula. Flattening suggests rotator cuff muscle atrophy.

3. Look for any *swellings*. Although these are unusual, rotator cuff tears with bleeds, rheumatoid arthritis effusions, pseudogout and sepsis can all affect the shoulder. A chronic effusion occurs in a peculiar destructive apatite arthritis of the shoulder (Milwaukee shoulder).

4. Standing behind your patient, gently grasp both wrists and, flexing the elbows to 90°, attempt to *externally rotate* both arms ('hands behind head' action). Reduced movement and pain on the affected side almost certainly represents a glenohumeral joint problem, most likely adhesive capsulitis (Box 9.2).

5. *Attempt to abduct* the affected shoulder. Normally the scapula will swing out after about 70° of abduction. If scapular movement starts early, with pain, glenohumeral joint disease is confirmed and by definition a capsulitis. Another way of demonstrating the capsulitic restriction of movement is by fixing the scapula; otherwise, the shoulder may appear to abduct when in fact the scapula is creating the movement. In adhesive capsulitis all *passive* movements will be affected, and *internal rotation* ('hands behind back' action) can also be markedly restricted. The

glenohumeral joint can also be palpated. Feel for the humeral head and slide your finger into the anterior groove, which is tender in capsulitis but not in osteoarthritis. If examination to this point is normal, glenohumeral pathology is unlikely.

6. Returning to the original position with elbows flexed at 90° and held at the side, place your hands outside the patient's and ask them to push their hands outwards whilst keeping their elbows tucked in. This tests *active external rotation*, which is a function of the rotator cuff and is painful and restricted in *rotator cuff lesions* (Box 9.3) and subacromial joint pathology.

7. Check the *abduction arcs* (Fig. 9.5). Ask your patient to abduct their shoulder in the neutral (palm to leg) position. Restriction of movement as well as pain is usual in *rotator cuff lesions* (unlike chronic pain syndromes), and may be exacerbated by gentle resistance to abduction.

(i) *Pain in early abduction* suggests a *rotator cuff lesion. Pain usually begins at about 40° and continues to 120°. Rotator cuff tendonitis is more painful on active movement.*

(ii) *Late abduction* involves *scapula rotation on the thorax.* If there is *pain during a high arc of movement* (starting at

Box 9.3   Rotator Cuff Lesions ('Impingement Syndrome' or 'Rotator Cuff Tendonitis')

This is common under 50 years of age, and often occurs de novo or due to repetitive strain. In addition it may occur in rheumatoid arthritis in which chronic inflammation can lead to atrophy of the muscles of rotator cuff. Rotator cuff muscle tears also occur. *Supraspinatus tendonitis* is the most common problem.

The cuff initiates abduction. Its presence between the glenohumeral and subacromial joints (Fig. 9.4) holds the humeral head stable and means that abduction will reach a point of being stuck ('impingement') as the humeral head and acromion come together. Palpation (lateral) over the subacromial joint may also be painful.

Plain X-rays may show tendon calcification, and atrophy demonstrated by subacromial space narrowing (decreased vertical height between the humeral head and the acromion). Magnetic resonance imaging (MRI) is the investigation of choice. Treatments include intra-articular corticosteroid injections.

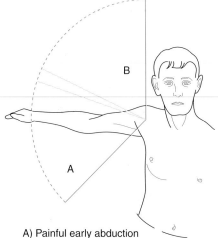

A) Painful early abduction suggests a rotator cuff lesion
B) Painful late abduction suggests acromioclavicular joint osteoarthritis

Fig. 9.5   *Painful abduction arcs*

90°, the patient unable to raise their arm straight up above their head to 180°, even passively), *acromioclavicular arthritis* should be considered.

Examining the feet

There are three main sets of joints:

1. The hindfoot, comprising the true ankle or *tibiotalar* joint (dorsiflexion by anterior tibialis and plantar flexion by gastrocnemius/soleus) and *talocalcaneal* joint. Hindfoot movements are examined by cupping the calcaneum in the hand and testing flexion/extension and inversion/eversion respectively (Fig. 9.6).
2. The midfoot joints, tested by stabilising the hindfoot (cupping the patient's ankle in dorsiflexion) and then inverting and everting the midfoot (Fig. 9.7).
3. The metatarsophalangeal and interphalangeal joints which flex and extend the toes. As well as noting movements, note any abnormal forefoot appearances such as hallux valgus, hallux rigidus or dactylitis.

Flexor and extensor tendonitis is common in inflammatory arthritis and overuse. Plantar fasciitis is common in the spondyloarthropathies.

Examining the knees

Proceed as outlined under the general examination points. The following points apply specifically to knee examination:

1. Look for any obvious *swellings* or *effusion* including *prepatellar and infrapatellar*

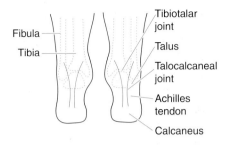

Fibula

Tibia

Tibiotalar
joint

Talus

Talocalcaneal
joint

Achilles
tendon

Calcaneus

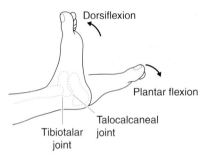

Dorsiflexion

Plantar flexion

Talocalcaneal
Tibiotalar   joint
joint

Dorsiflexion and plantar flexion involve
principally the tibiotalar joint

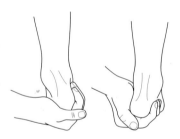

Inversion and eversion involve
principally the talocalcaneal joint

Fig. 9.6   *Movements of the hindfoot*

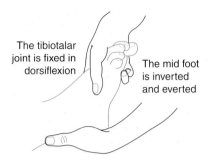

The tibiotalar
joint is fixed in
dorsiflexion

The mid foot
is inverted
and everted

The talocalcaneal joint is fixed by a
cupping hand

Fig. 9.7   *Movements at the midfoot*

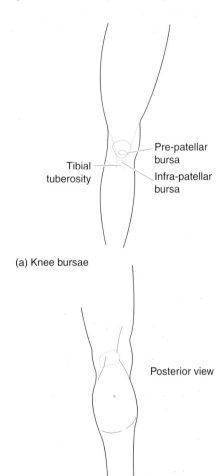

Tibial
tuberosity

Pre-patellar
bursa

Infra-patellar
bursa

(a) Knee bursae

Posterior view

(b) Popliteal cyst

Fig. 9.8   *Knee bursae: (a) sites of bursae;
(b) Popliteal cyst*

bursitis and *popliteal (Baker's) cysts* (Fig.
9.8). If the latter ruptures, swelling may
track into the calf.

2. With a *large effusion* the suprapatellar
pouch may be distended (Fig. 9.9).

3. The *patellar tap* tests for the presence of
fluid squeezed back into the joint space
from the suprapatellar bursa (Fig. 9.9).
Squeeze any excess fluid out of the

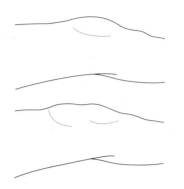

(1) With a large effusion the suprapatellar pouch may be distended

suprapatellar pouch with your thumb and index finger, sliding them distally from a point some 15 cm above the knee to the upper border of the patella. With your other hand feel for the presence of a click by jerking the patella quickly downwards. The click may not be present with either a small or a tense effusion.

4. The *bulge test* is performed by a sudden pincing movement of the upper hand, which displaces fluid inferiorly and is palpated by a bulging apart of the fingers of the lower hand (Fig. 9.9).

5. A small effusion may be detected by *fluid displacement* (Fig. 9.10). This is

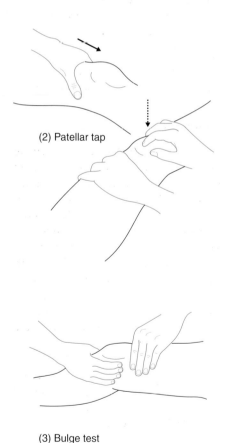

(2) Patellar tap

(3) Bulge test

Fig. 9.9   *Examining for a knee effusion (large effusion)*

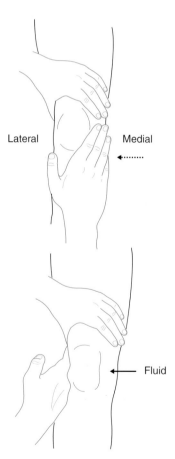

Lateral   Medial

Fluid

Fig. 9.10   *Examining for a knee effusion (small effusion)*

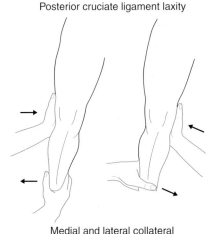

Tibial tuberosity

Pull to draw tibia forwards
(note excess movement)

Anterior cruciate ligament laxity

Normal tibial
tuberosity

Push (note any excess
movement and
depression from tibia
moving posteriorly)

Posterior cruciate ligament laxity

Medial and lateral collateral
ligament laxity

Fig. 9.11   *Examining the ligaments of the knee*

performed firstly by evacuating the suprapatellar pouch as for the patellar tap. The medial side is then stroked to displace any excess fluid in the main joint cavity to the lateral side of the joint. Then stroking the lateral side will move the excess fluid back across the joint resulting in visible distension medially.

6. The knees should be *flexed* and *extended*, and palpated for *crepitus* whilst so testing.
7. Finally, the stability of the cruciate and collateral ligaments should be tested (although these are more likely to be unstable in orthopaedic/sports injury disorders than disorders encountered in PACES) (Fig. 9.11).

Monoarthritis of the knee may occur in pseudogout and occasionally in rheumatoid arthritis of palindromic onset.

Examining the hips

Proceed as outlined under the general points for examining the locomotor system on page 474 and testing the movements outlined in Figure 9.12. The hips are less likely to be involved in inflammatory arthritis and are usually a source of pain rather than swelling. It is worth noting that *trochanteric bursitis*, associated with numerous inflammatory arthritides, produces pain over the lateral thigh and pelvis. Pure arthritis tends to produce anterior pain, sometimes referred to the knee.

A flexion deformity of the hip can be masked by the patient tilting their pelvis forwards and increasing the lumbar lordosis. *Thomas's test* can be used to obliterate the lumbar lordosis and unmask

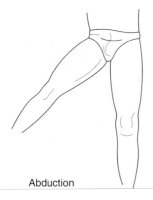

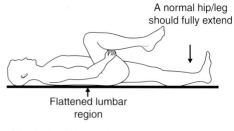

Fig. 9.13   *Thomas's test*

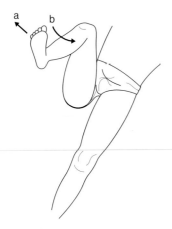

Abduction

(a) External rotation
(b) Internal rotation

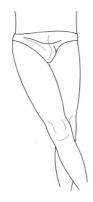

Adduction

Fig. 9.12   *Hip movements*

hip flexion (Fig. 9.13). The unaffected hip is flexed to its limit to straighten the lumbar spine. An affected hip rises from the couch to reveal the degree of abnormal flexion.

Examining the spine

Neurological examination of the limbs for signs referable to the spinal cord is described in detail in Chapter 6. General mobility of the back may be examined by observing (Fig. 9.14):

1. The overall shape and *posture*, looking for any deformities such as kyphosis, scoliosis or the typical 'question mark' posture of ankylosing spondylitis.
2. The degree of *forward flexion*.
3. The degree of *lateral flexion*.
4. The degree of *rotation*.

Nerve stretch tests for sciatic and femoral nerve impingement are an important part of spinal examination. In the *sciatic nerve stretch test* the supine patient's straight leg raising is limited by pain produced by tension of nerve roots supplying the sciatic nerve (L4–S2), commonly tensed over a prolapsed disc (commonly at vertebral level L4/5 or L5/S1—see pages 312–313 and 325–326). Pain may be in the back of the leg, sometimes radiating to the lumbar

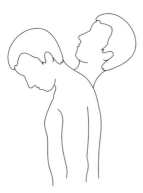

Neck flexion and extension

region. Tension is increased by dorsiflexion of the foot (which tugs the distal component of the sciatic nerve, the posterior tibial nerve) and relieved by flexion of the knee. In the *femoral nerve stretch* test the prone patient's femoral nerve roots (L2–4) are tightened by flexion of the knee, causing pain which radiates into the back. The femoral roots may be further tensed by extending the hip joint, which produces increasing pain.

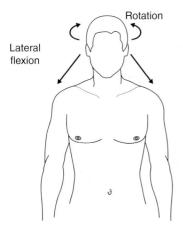

Neck lateral flexion and rotation

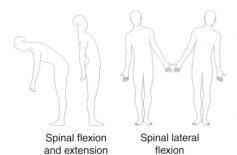

Spinal flexion   Spinal lateral
and extension   flexion

Fig. 9.14   *Spinal movements*

| CASE STUDY | 9.1 RHEUMATOID HANDS/RHEUMATOID ARTHRITIS (RA) |

Instruction: *Examine this patient's hands and discuss your findings.*

| RECOGNITION | |

There is *deforming polyarthritis* of both hands.

Swellings

1. There is often *marked soft tissue swelling* of the *MCP joints and wrists*.
2. The *PIP joints may be swollen* (it is useful to remember that the IP joint of the thumb behaves as a PIP joint). The DIP joints are spared.

There may be *active synovitis* with *fusiform spongy swelling* of joints.
   Soft tissue swelling around a joint is the hallmark of inflammatory joint disease and the associated stiffness is worse after inactivity and relieved by movement. *Pain, stiffness and warmth* are the other features of synovial inflammation, but erythema is rare. Pain originates predominantly from the joint capsule, abundantly supplied with pain fibres.

Deformities (Fig. 9.15)

- There may be *ulnar deviation* of the fingers due to subluxation/dislocation at the MCP joints (ulnar deviation may also be a consequence of displacement of the extensor tendons).
- There may be *swan neck* deformities of the fingers (flexion deformity of the DIP joint together with a hyperextended PIP joint).
- There may be *boutonnière deformities* of the fingers (extended DIP joint due to rupture of the central extensor tendon slip together with a flexed PIP joint).
- There may be *Z shaped thumbs* (flexed MCP joint with extended IP joint of thumb).

Other signs

- *Muscle wasting* is usually *generalised* and predominantly due to disuse. There is thenar and hypothenar wasting (compare with isolated median or ulnar neuropathies) and interosseous wasting is very common.
- *Palmar erythema* is common.
- *Cutaneous vasculitis* usually presents as crops of small brown spots at the nail folds, and as digital pulp infarcts. These findings occur in other connective tissue diseases, notably scleroderma (Case study 9.5).

Fig. 9.15   *Finger deformities in rheumatoid arthritis*

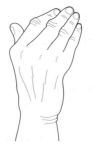

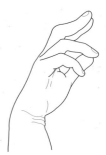

Ulnar deviation at the metacarpophalangeal joints

Boutonnière deformity

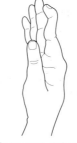

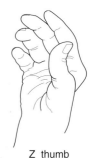

Z thumb

Swan neck deformity

| INTERPRETATION |

Confirm the diagnosis

- Do not confuse with *osteoarthritis*, which affects small and large joints and may be symmetrical. *Heberden's* (DIP joint) and *Bouchard's* (PIP joint) nodes are bony swellings, not soft synovial swellings. Osteoarthritis commonly affects the knees and hips.
- *Psoriatic arthritis* may mimic rheumatoid arthritis in the hand. Look at the *elbows* for *rheumatoid nodules*, which if present help confirm rheumatoid hands. Alternatively you may find *psoriatic plaques*, making psoriatic arthritis more likely. Psoriatic arthritis commonly involves the DIP joints and produces nail pitting. Rheumatoid nodules are soft tissue nodules, not to be confused with the tendon nodules of tendon xanthomata.

Assess other systems

Consider that your patient may have other *extra-articular features* of rheumatoid disease (Box 9.4). Generally these are associated with rheumatoid factor positivity. You would not have time to check for all but may need to discuss some of them.

Box 9.4	Extra-articular Features of Rheumatoid Disease

- **Neurological** manifestations include *carpal tunnel syndrome* (entrapment mononeuropathy due to synovial swelling at the wrist), *cervical myeloradiculopathy* and less frequently *hoarseness/stridor from cricoarytenoid arthritis* and *hearing difficulty* (synovial involvement of the ossicles). *Sensory polyneuropathies* may result from vasa nervorum involvement in vasculitis. *Mononeuritis multiplex* can cause *foot drops* and *wrist drops.*

- **Lung** manifestations include recurrent *pleuritic pain*, *pleural effusions*, *pulmonary fibrosis* and *pulmonary nodules*. Methotrexate can also cause fibrosis and nodules. In *Caplan's syndrome*, massive fibrotic nodules coexist with occupational coal dust exposure. These are more common autopsy than clinical findings. Lung disease tends to affect men more than women.

- **Cardiac** disease includes *pericarditis* and *pericardial effusion*. Up to 50% of patients at autopsy have a pericardial effusion. Effusions are commonly mild and asymptomatic.

- **Vasculitis** is *usually restricted to the skin*, e.g. *nail folds*. In its more aggressive form, it can cause peripheral neuropathy, mononeuritis multiplex, cutaneous ulceration, digital gangrene and even cerebral or mesenteric infarction. Coronary and renal vasculitis are extremely rare. High titres of rheumatoid factor are present with RA vasculitis.

- **Rheumatoid nodules** are also invariably associated with rheumatoid factor positivity. They tend to affect the extensor tendons of the hand (look also for a trigger finger due to thickening, usually without nodules, along the flexor aspect), and pressure points like the elbows, Achilles tendons and bridge of nose in wearers of spectacles. They may also occur in the lungs, and occasionally the pericardium and sclera.

- **Eye** signs occur in a minority of patients. They include *episcleritis* and *scleritis*. Recurrent scleritis (which should alert physicians to vasculitis) may progress to scleromalacia perforans. Anterior uveitis is associated with the spondyloarthropathies, *not* rheumatoid disease. *Keratoconjunctivitis sicca* affects 15–20% of patients.

- **Felty's syndrome** is the association of chronic rheumatoid arthritis, *splenomegaly* and *leucopenia*. Hypersplenism is not invariable and severe neutropenia (and even thrombocytopenia and anaemia) may occur in the absence of hypersplenism.

- **Systemic features due to the proinflammatory response** (page 199) but not specific to RA include *malaise, weight loss, anaemia, lymphadenopathy* and *amyloid* accumulation.

Assess severity

- Any of the above clinical features may be severe.
- Tell the examiners that depression is underappreciated in chronic disease.

Evidence of decompensation

Any of the above may lead to decompensation. Other important ones to remember are:

- Subluxation of the atlantoaxial joint. This is due to laxity of the transverse ligament of the atlas. Synovitis of the facet joints may also contribute to instability. Subluxation may be shown by flexion and extension X-rays, demonstrating an increased distance between the posterior aspect of the C1 vertebral body and the anterior aspect of the odontoid process of C2.
- Amyloid accumulation in the kidneys causing nephrotic syndrome.
- Osteoporosis, accelerated by immobility and steroids.

Numerous factors are associated with a less favourable prognosis in RA (Box 9.5).

Box 9.5	Factors Associated with a Less Favourable Prognosis in RA

- Rheumatoid factor positivity (70% of patients are positive)
- Many active joints at presentation
- Extra-articular disease, which affects about a third of all patients
- Severe disability at presentation
- Joint erosions early in course of disease
- High erythrocyte sedimentation rate (ESR) or C reactive protein (CRP) at presentation

A slowly progressive course used to be considered adverse but this was more relevant in the days when disease modifying antirheumatic drugs (DMARDs) were not introduced early in disease.

Assess function

Functional status can be assessed by a simple screen of pincer, grip and arm movements and by asking about routine movements such as:

- Fastening buttons ● Using keys ● Writing ● Taking coins out of pockets ● Holding cups ● Opening jars ● Cleaning teeth ● Combing hair ● Getting dressed ● Reaching into kitchen cupboards.

Tell the examiners that you would ask about symptoms of disease activity, including active joint pain and swelling, weight loss, overall activity during the day (what job does your patient do, and can they still work? 50% of patients are unable to work after 10 years) and afternoon tiredness. Rheumatologists tend to have specific ways of assessing disease activity which include:

- Health assessment questionnaires
- Physician global assessments/patient global assessments
- Patient pain assessments
- Tender joint scores
- Swollen joint scores
- Duration of morning stiffness
- ESR or CRP, and plasma viscosity.

Look for/consider associated diseases

Many organ specific autoimmune diseases are more common in patients with rheumatoid arthritis.

DISCUSSION

What causes RA?

It is a chronic inflammatory, autoimmune disease, mediated by proinflammatory cytokines like tumour necrosis factor alpha (TNF-α). There is a strong HLA DR4 association. It affects around 1% of people, its onset commonly in the fifth decade.

What patterns of onset are recognised?

The usual pattern of onset is insidious, over weeks to months, often starting with fatigue, anorexia and vague musculoskeletal symptoms. Less frequently it may appear over a week or two, and rarely over a few days. *Palindromic* refers to episodic features with complete resolution in between, such as acute, self-limiting swelling of a knee. *Extra-articular* onset is also recognised.

Which joints may be affected other than the hands?

These include:

- The *elbow* (flexion contractures)
- The *knee* (synovial hypertrophy, ligament laxity, chronic effusion, and sometimes popliteal cysts)
- The *cervical spine*
- The joints in the *foot* (typical features include eversion at the subtalar joint, plantar subluxation of the metatarsal heads, widening of the forefoot, hallux valgus and lateral deviation/dorsal subluxation of the toes).

Tenosynovitis and *bursitis* commonly accompany joint disease. Examples include rotator cuff tendonitis, subacromial bursitis, de Quervain's tenosynovitis, hand extensor and flexor tendonitis and trochantric bursitis.

Do you know of any diagnostic criteria for RA?

The American College of Rheumatology (ACR) criteria for diagnosing RA (you would not be expected to remember the criteria) are as follows:

1. Morning stiffness > 1 hour*
2. Swelling of at least three types of joint — PIP, MCP, wrist, elbow, knee, ankle, MTP*
3. Swelling of hand joints*
4. Symmetrical joint involvement*
5. Nodules
6. Rheumatoid factor positivity
7. Radiological features (e.g. joint erosions).

Four criteria are required (* must be > 6 weeks).

What radiological features of RA do you know of?

- Soft tissue swelling together with juxta-articular osteoporosis in early disease
- Joint space narrowing
- Joint erosions
- Cyst formation
- Joint destruction
- Subluxation/dislocation.

What other investigations may be useful in RA?

- CRP measurement
- Rheumatoid factor (always positive if vasculitis or nodules are present)
- Haemoglobin
- Synovial fluid analysis. This reveals an inflammatory arthritis but is not specific. Fluid is often turbid, with low viscosity, high protein concentration, low/normal glucose concentration, low C3 and C4 complement levels and an elevated white cell count (5–50 000 cells/ml). In practice, there is seldom a place for synovial fluid examination other than to exclude infection.

Which factors might contribute to anaemia in RA?

- Anaemia of chronic disease
- NSAID related gastritis/peptic ulceration
- Bone marrow suppression from DMARDs (Box 9.6)
- Splenomegaly in Felty's syndrome
- Megaloblastic anaemia (associated pernicious anaemia or methotrexate related folate deficiency).

What is Sjögren's syndrome?

Sjögren's syndrome refers to keratoconjunctivitis sicca (decreased lacrimal secretion) and xerostomia (decreased salivary gland secretion) in association with a connective tissue disease, usually RA.

| Box 9.6 | RA Treatments |

1. *NSAIDs* relieve pain, stiffness and swelling. Potential side effects are peptic ulceration, interstitial nephritis and worsening of asthma.
2. *Disease modifying antirheumatic drugs (DMARDs)*, especially sulfasalazine or methotrexate, are used to delay disease progression and reduce subsequent disability. DMARDs are tending to be introduced earlier in disease. In addition to symptomatic improvement (reduction in pain, morning stiffness and swelling), DMARDs can decrease inflammatory markers and, more importantly, improve outcome measures such as disability and radiological progression. Many DMARDs can cause bone marrow suppression and skin rashes. Gold and penicillamine may cause nephrotic syndrome. Penicillamine is associated with drug induced lupus and autoimmune disease. Leflunomide is a recently introduced DMARD.
3. Low dose oral *corticosteroids* attenuate the acute phase response but do not modify the disease course and unlike DMARDs are not routinely used.
4. *Novel ways of impeding cytokine activity*, such as monoclonal antibodies directed against TNF-α or its receptor, have had beneficial results. Treatment is very costly and resources limit it to selected patients with active disease unresponsive to DMARDs.

What do you know about RA treatments?

Treatment goals are pain relief, reduction of inflammation, limitation of joint damage, control of systemic disease and maintenance of function. No current therapy (Box 9.6) is curative.

| CASE STUDY | 9.2 ANKYLOSING SPONDYLITIS AND SPONDYLOARTHROPATHIES |

Instruction: *Examine this patient's spine and any other systems you feel relevant. Discuss your findings.*

| RECOGNITION | |

There is *kyphosis* with *restriction of spinal movement in all directions* (unable to look at the ceiling, rest head on wall, turn head from side to side) (Fig. 9.16) and a *positive modified Schober test:* mark the level of the posterior iliac spines and sacral dimples, and a point 10 cm above this in the midline (Fig. 9.17); when the patient flexes

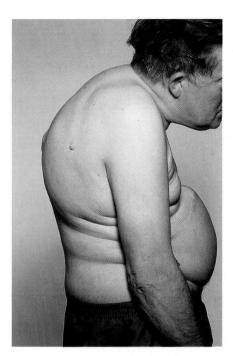

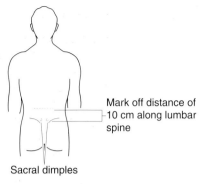

Mark off distance of 10 cm along lumbar spine

Sacral dimples

Modified Schober test to detect restricted lumbar flexion

Fig. 9.16   *Ankylosing spondylitis.
Reproduced with permission from M.A. Mir
(1995) Atlas of Clinical Diagnosis. W.B.
Saunders, London*

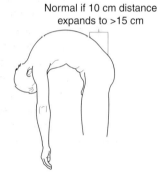

Normal if 10 cm distance expands to >15 cm

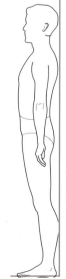

Fig. 9.17   *Modified Schober test and
wall–occiput test*

Wall–occiput test

forward, the distance between the two points normally increases to at least 15 cm but is less than this if the test is positive. Upper spine involvement is demonstrated by the *wall–occiput test* (Fig. 9.17).

INTERPRETATION

Confirm the diagnosis

1. Firstly, be sure this is a spondyloarthropathy. Some differentiating articular signs are shown in Table 9.1. Tell the examiners that you would ask about those features of back pain listed in Box 9.7. The back pain of spondyloarthropathies, unlike mechanical back pain, has typical features.
2. Secondly, remember that ankylosing spondylitis is the primary spondyloarthropathy, but there are several others.

TABLE 9.1   **Articular signs differentiating a spondyloarthopathy from rheumatoid arthritis and osteoarthritis**

Spondyloarthropathy	Rheumatoid arthritis	Osteoarthritis
Asymmetrical	Symmetrical	Asymmetrical/symmetrical
Peripheral arthritis affects large joints predominantly (knees, hips and ankles)	Peripheral arthritis affects small joints predominantly (MCPs and wrists)	Both small and large joints affected, especially hips, first carpometacarpal joint, knees and hips
Spondylitis and sacroiliitis (page 497)	Atlantoaxial subluxation	Lumbar and cervical 'wear and tear'

Box 9.7   **Typical Features of Spondyloarthropathy Back Pain**

● Worse when sitting, lying and resting
● Worse with prolonged immobility
● Improved by exercise
● Associated with prolonged (> 1 hour) morning stiffness.

These symptoms also tend to be true for joint symptoms in any inflammatory arthritis.

Assess other systems

Some 'A's are associated with ankylosing spondylitis. You should look for or mention these to the examiners, but apart from tendonitis/fasciitis and uveitis, they are rare.

● **A**chilles tendonitis and plantar fasciitis ● **A**nterior uveitis
● **A**ortic regurgitation and aortitis ● **A**pical lung fibrosis ● **A**-V heart block ● **A**myloidosis.

You could look briefly at the eyes and listen briefly to the aortic area in expiration and to the lung apices. Tell the examiners that you would ask about heel pain.

Evidence of decompensation

- Look for signs of severe aortic regurgitation (page 234) if you detect aortic regurgitation.
- Tell the examiners that you would arrange pulmonary function tests if you detect pulmonary fibrosis.

Assess function

Note the extent of postural deformity and stiffness. You could enquire about activities such as driving. Even being a passenger in a car can be difficult for patients with severe deformities.

DISCUSSION

What are the major spondyloarthropathies?

The spondyloarthropathies (Box 9.8) lack rheumatoid factor positivity and are associated with HLA B27. A family history is common. Environmental triggers likely interact with genetic susceptibility to provoke disease. HLA B27 is positive in 5–10% of the white population and in 90% of patients with ankylosing spondylitis, 70% of patients with Reiter's syndrome and up to 50% of patients with other spondyloarthropathies. Serology is not used widely in diagnosis, which should rely on clinical and radiological assessment.

Overlap of clinical features may occur between the spondyloarthropathies. For example, a patient with psoriatic arthritis may develop anterior uveitis. The European Study Group spondyloarthropathy criteria (embraced fully in the references by Khan MA, page 511) encompass the multisystem features for diagnosing a spondyloarthropathy – *inflammatory spinal pain* or synovitis (asymmetrical or predominantly lower limbs) *plus* one or more of *sacroiliitis, alternating buttock pain, positive family history, psoriasis, inflammatory bowel disease* or *enthesopathy.*

Box 9.8	The Major Spondyloarthropathies

1. Ankylosing spondylitis
2. Psoriatic arthritis/arthropathy
3. Reactive arthritis/arthropathy (including Reiter's syndrome)
4. Enteropathic arthritis/arthropathy.

Ankylosing spondylitis

Ankylosing spondylitis is the primary spondyloarthropathy (absence of features to suggest one of the other conditions, symmetrical pain). Age of onset is 15–40 years and the male : female ratio is 5 : 1.

The New York criteria for diagnosing ankylosing spondylitis are:

Clinical

- Limited movement of lumbar spine in three planes
- Pain in lumbar spine or at thoracolumbar junction
- Chest expansion < 2.5 cm.

Radiological

- Unilateral sacroiliitis (grades III–IV) or bilateral sacroiliitis (grade II) (Box 9.9)

Psoriatic arthritis

Psoriatic arthropathy affects up to 10% of patients with psoriasis and may precede or follow skin disease by months or even years. There are, in theory, five types of arthropathy (page 423). Radiologically, there may be erosions and severe joint destruction.

Reactive arthritis

Reactive arthritis refers to arthritis after any infection. It may be of small or large peripheral joint type with features of a spondyloarthropathy.

Reiter's syndrome

Reiter's syndrome, a form of reactive arthritis, often follows urethritis/cervicitis (e.g. *Chlamydia*) or dysenteric infections (e.g. *Shigella, Salmonella, Campylobacter, Yersinia* species). The classic triad is:

1. Arthritis
2. Urethritis
3. Conjunctivitis/anterior uveitis.

The classic triad is not always complete, however, and common findings include *mouth ulceration, circinate balanitis, persistent plantar fasciitis* and *keratoderma blennorrhagica* (hyperkeratotic vesicles, often on soles or palms).

Which articular/musculoskeletal features are shared by the spondyloarthropathies?
These are described in Box 9.9.

Which investigations may be useful in the investigation of a spondyloarthropathy?

- Diagnosis is based on clinical and radiological evidence.
- The X-ray features of established spondylitis and sacroiliitis are useful but X-rays in acute disease are normal. Symptomatic sacroiliitis can precede X-ray changes by years.
- ESR and CRP are often elevated in active disease.

Which treatments are beneficial for spondylarthropathy?

- A dramatic improvement with NSAIDs is typical in early disease.

Box 9.9 **Musculoskeletal Features of Ankylosing Spondylitis and the Spondyloarthropathies**

Spondylitis (inflammatory spine disease)

This is characterised clinically by an *insidious* onset, persistence for > 3 months, *morning stiffness* and *improvement with exercise*. Refer also to the *New York criteria* on page 496. *Enthesitis* (below) contributes to the process of spondylitis because destruction of the insertion sites of vertebral discs (outer fibres of annulus fibrosus) to vertebrae leads to squaring of the vertebrae. *Syndesmophytes* (reactive bone formations) may link vertebrae. Calcification within the anterior and posterior spinal ligaments gives rise to the characteristic but rare *bamboo spine*.

Sacroiliitis

This often causes *alternating buttock pain* (especially nocturnal). Sacroiliitis tends to be *symmetrical* in *ankylosing spondylitis* but *asymmetrical* or *unilateral* in the other spondyloarthropathies. Severity is graded radiographically by the extent of joint distortion (0 is normal, IV is fused, and the majority of patients with established disease have grades II or III).

Peripheral large joint monoarthritis or oligoarthritis

This tends to be *asymmetrical* and to affect the lower limbs (*hip, knee or ankle*). It may predate or follow spine disease by several years.

Enthesitis

Many symptoms in the spondyloarthropathies are due to enthesitis, which refers to inflammation (± fibrosis ± calcification ± ossification) at the insertion site (enthesis) of a tendon, ligament or joint capsule to bone. Heel pain, worse when starting to walk in the morning and associated with a 'burning sole' sensation is due to *plantar fasciitis* and is the commonest enthesopathy. Other sites include the insertion of the Achilles tendon to the calcaneus (*Achilles tendonitis*; calcaneal spurs may also develop), the capsular insertions of the costovertebral, sternoclavicular, manubriosternal and costochondral junctions, the capsules and ligaments around finger joints, and finger tendon sheaths.

Dactylitis

This refers to the *sausage swelling* of a digit which may result from a combination of joint swelling and tendon/tendon sheath swelling.

- Good posture, physiotherapy and home exercises including extension exercises are important.
- DMARDs (page 492) may help large joint arthritis, but seem to have less effect on spine (axial) disease. Anti-TNFα is of emerging benefit for axial disease.
- Ankylosing spondylitis does not 'burn out'. It persists through life and fatigue may be a major symptom that is difficult to treat.

CASE STUDY   9.3 SYSTEMIC LUPUS ERYTHEMATOSUS (SLE)

Instruction: *Examine this patient's face and any other systems you feel may be relevant. Discuss your findings and how you might further assess this patient.*

RECOGNITION

There are *raised or flat patches of malar erythema, sparing the nasolabail folds* (Fig. 9.18). There may be marked photosensitivity. There may be *mouth ulcers*.

INTERPRETATION

Confirm the diagnosis

The differential diagnosis of a facial rash is described in Case study 8.6.

Assess other systems

Be aware of the other possible manifestations of SLE for discussion. The ARC criteria (Box 9.10) can be a useful *aide-mémoire*.

Fig. 9.18   *Malar rash typical of SLE*

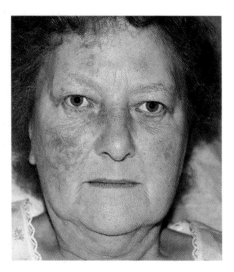

Box 9.10	American Rheumatism Council (ARC) Criteria for Diagnosing SLE

1. Malar rash (raised or flat red patches, nasolabial fold sparing)
2. Discoid rash (red papules on head and neck with scaling, follicular keratosis, atrophic scarring and depigmentation)
3. Photosensitive rash
4. Oral/nasopharyngeal ulcers (painless)
5. Arthritis (non-erosive, > 2 joints)
6. Serositis (pleural, pericardial or peritoneal)
7. Renal involvment (proteinuria)
8. CNS involvement (seizures or psychiatric)
9. Haematological involvement (autoimmune haemolytic anaemia, leucopenia $< 4 \times 10^9$/L, lymphopenia $< 1.5 \times 10^9$/L or thrombocytopenia $< 100 \times 10^9$/L)
10. Serological evidence—anti-dsDNA, anti-Sm (page 475)
11. ANA positivity.

Four criteria are required (only one skin manifestation may be used).

DISCUSSION

What causes SLE?

SLE is the archetypal autoimmune disease, with autoantibodies to many different types of tissue. The cause is not known. The female : male ratio is 9 : 1.

What are the common features of SLE?

The most common clinical features are arthralgia and rash. Arthritis in SLE is non-erosive.

Renal disease includes a range of types of glomerulonephritis. Low C3 and C4 suggests lupus nephritis. Peripheral and cranial neuropathies rarely occur. Raynaud's phenomenon, scarring alopecia, pulmonary fibrosis (including 'shrinking lung' syndrome), pulmonary hypertension, myocarditis and Libman–Sacks endocarditis may also occur, but are rare. There is an association with antiphospholipid syndrome (APLS).

What do you know about drug induced lupus?

Drug induced lupus (e.g. penicillamine) is more common in males, spares the CNS and kidneys, resolves on stopping the implicated drug and does not produce antibodies to dsDNA.

Which treatments may be used in SLE?

Treatment includes sunscreens, NSAIDs and antimalarials for arthritis and steroids/immunosuppression for lupus nephritis.

| CASE STUDY | 9.4 CRYSTAL ARTHROPATHY |

Instruction: *Examine this patient's feet/other joints/ears. Discuss your findings and any tests you would like to arrange.*

RECOGNITION

1. There is *swelling of the first MTP joint* (or knee, wrist, hand or other joints). The patient reports that the joint has been *exquisitely painful and tender* (ask before examining!). *Erythema with acute synovitis* is usually due either to crystal arthopathy or septic arthritis.

2. *Chronic tophaceous gout* is characterised by painless nodules of urate (tophi) in joints or soft tissues (helix, olecranon/patellar bursa, ulnar surface of forearm, Achilles tendon, etc.). Uric acid is less soluble at lower temperatures, which may explain the tendency for tophi to occur at sites exposed to cold.

INTERPRETATION

Confirm the diagnosis

Septic arthritis must always be considered as a cause of monoarthritis. There is usually fever and systemic upset.

Look for/consider causes

Most cases are idiopathic but gout may be due to *inborn errors* increasing purine levels or *increased purine/urate production* (myeloproliferative/lymphoproliferative disorders, chemotherapy, any cause of rapid cell lysis), *increased purine intake* (diet, alcohol), *decreased urate excretion* (renal failure, lactic acidosis, ketoacidosis) or *drugs* (diuretics, low dose aspirin).

Gout is most readily precipitated when serum urate levels are in a state of rapid flux, rather than by absolute levels. It can occur when the urate level is falling. Factors precipitating attacks include dehydration, alcohol, trauma, infection (lactic acid competes with urate excretion), diuretics and allopurinol.

Evidence of decompensation

Consider nephrolithiasis and renal failure due to urate crystals formed by prolonged hyperuricaemia and hyperuricuria.

DISCUSSION

What causes gout?

Gout is caused by sodium urate crystals in joints and soft tissues.

How is gout diagnosed?

- Synovial fluid suggests inflammation (often with a very high white cell count), and polarised microscopy reveals needle shaped, negatively birefringent intra- (especially acute attacks) and extra-cellular crystals.
- Serum urate levels can be misleading. They can be normal during an acute attack. Elevated levels with joint pain and swelling do not necessarily add up to a diagnosis of gout.
- X-rays may show punched out erosions distant from the joint margin and eventually joint destruction. Tophi are usually radiolucent but sometimes calcified.

What treatments are there for acute episodes?

Painful acute attacks last up to 3 weeks but are usually suppressed by NSAIDs. Oral colchicine may be used (0.5–1 mg 4–6 hourly for 24–48 hours) but causes diarrhoea. Occasionally a short course of systemic steroids is required to control the pain of acute attacks.

How are attacks prevented?

Having controlled the acute pain a decision should be made about the need for prophylaxis. Indications may include:

- Three or four acute attacks of gout/year (joints start to become irreversibly damaged by repeated attacks of inflammation) ● One attack of polyarticular gout ● Tophaceous gout ● Urate calculi.

The preferred agent for lowering uric acid levels is allopurinol. It should not be commenced during an acute attack. The dose should be adjusted in renal disease. It interacts with azathioprine (cytopenias). Concurrent prophylaxis in the form of NSAIDs or colchicine should be given until normouricaemia is achieved and for a month thereafter. Colchicine (0.5 mg twice daily) is an alternative long term prophylactic agent where allopurinol is contraindicated, but has no effect on hyperuricaemia and therefore joint/renal damage.

What do you know about pseudogout?

Calcium pyrophosphate deposition disease (CPDD) can mimic gout and often affects the knee but may be polyarticular. Pseudogout may be precipitated by intercurrent illness. The synovial fluid is similar to that of gout but the crystals are polymorphic, often rhomboid or rectangular, sometimes needle shaped, and positively birefringent. Treatment is as for the acute pain of gout, with NSAIDs. Intra-articular steroids can be very helpful in settling acute pain from a large joint in both gout and pseudogout. No prophylaxis is available for pseudogout.

What is chondrocalcinosis?

Chondrocalcinosis refers to calcium deposition in cartilage and may be a feature of gout, pseudogout, primary hyperparathyroidism, haemochromatosis and Wilson's disease.

| CASE STUDY | 9.5 SCLERODERMA |

Instruction: *Examine this patient's face and hands and discuss your findings.*

| RECOGNITION | |

Face (Fig. 9.19)

There are *dilated capillaries* (*telangiectasia*), and the *skin appears smooth, shiny and tight*. The nose may appear beaked. There may be *perioral skin puckering* with microstomia and restricted mouth opening.

Hands (Fig. 9.20)

The *skin over the fingers* is also *smooth, shiny and tight* (*sclerodactyly*). There may be *dilated nail fold capillaries* (*telangiectasia*), *nail fold infarcts, ragged cuticles, evidence of digital ischaemia with ulceration, infarcts and pulp atrophy* (± amputations), and *calcinosis* (with subcutaneous calcium deposits in the digits and fingertips).

| INTERPRETATION | |

Confirm the diagnosis

Scleroderma is a multisystem connective tissue disorder of unknown cause characterised by fibrosis of the skin and other organs. It is more common in females. There are various disease patterns, the two major ones being:

Fig. 9.19   *Scleroderma*

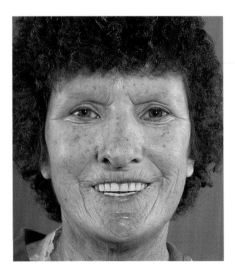

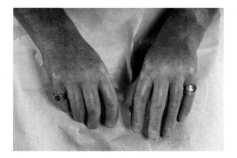 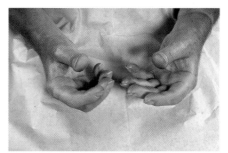

Fig. 9.20 *(a,b) Scleroderma*

1. *Limited scleroderma* (CREST syndrome), in which skin involvement is limited to the face, neck and distal limbs. CREST refers to **c**alcinosis, **R**aynaud's phenomenon, o**e**sophageal dysmotility, **s**clerodactyly and **t**elangiectasia. It usually begins with Raynaud's phenomenon, which is much more common than in SLE, affecting almost all patients with skin disease. Tell the examiners that you would ask about:
   (i) Cold white hands (ischaemia) which turn blue (stasis) then red (reactive hyperaemia) with pain
   (ii) Dysphagia.
2. *Diffuse scleroderma*, in which skin involvement also involves the trunk and proximal limbs. It usually begins with swelling of fingers due to dactylitis or arthritis. Joint contractures later develop. Raynaud's phenomenon is common. Internal organ involvement is common and the prognosis worse than for limited scleroderma.

Assess severity

This requires a combination of clinical examination and investigations, looking specifically for evidence of:

● Erosive arthritis
● Interstitial lung disease
● Pulmonary hypertension (more common in limited scleroderma)
● Renal failure (more common in diffuse scleroderma)
● Gastro-oesophageal reflux (GORD), gut dysmotility, bacterial overgrowth and malabsorption
● Pericardial fibrosis, myocardial fibrosis, conduction defects and biventricular failure.

Anticentromere antibodies are present in over 50% of patients with limited scleroderma, and antitopoisomerase or antinucleolar antibodies in up to 50% of patients with diffuse scleroderma.

Evidence of decompensation

Tell your examiners that you would:

- Look for the signs of pulmonary hypertension (page 12)
- Wish to know the results of pulmonary function tests
- Be alert to renal crises presenting with severe hypertension and rapidly deteriorating renal function
- Be alert to GORD and possible long-term sequelae (Barrett's oesophagus).

DISCUSSION

What types of scleroderma do you know of?

Scleroderma may be *systemic* (systemic sclerosis) or *localised*:

- *Systemic sclerosis* is usually classified as *limited scleroderma* or *diffuse scleroderma*, depending upon the extent of skin involvement. Both forms involve other organs and the more common multi-organ features are outlined above. A rare systemic form, *systemic sclerosis sine scleroderma*, does not involve the skin.
- *Localised scleroderma* includes *morphea*, which causes plaques of sclerosis, often with a purplish edge, and *linear sclerosis (coup de sabre)*.

Which treatments have been used for systemic sclerosis?

No treatments are curative. Research has recently centred on inhibiting cytokine cascades leading to fibrosis, such as inhibiting transforming growth factor beta (TGF-β).

- NSAIDs can help arthralgia
- Pulsed laser therapy has been used for telangiectasia
- Proton pump inhibitors may help GORD
- Antibiotics may be needed for bacterial overgrowth
- Epoprostenol infusions have been used to treat severe Raynaud's phenomenon, digital ischaemia and pulmonary hypertension
- D-penicillamine may slow progression of skin disease
- Steroids and immune modulating drugs have been used for interstitial lung disease but appear not to help skin disease.

CASE STUDY   9.6 POLYMYOSITIS

Instruction: *Examine this patient's limbs/rash. Discuss your findings, and suggest appropriate further investigations.*

RECOGNITION

There is *weakness* of the *shoulder girdle muscles* (patient unable to raise arms above head) and the *pelvic girdle muscles* (patient unable to rise from chair, stand from squat, climb stairs, etc.).

Fig. 9.21   *Dermatomyositis*

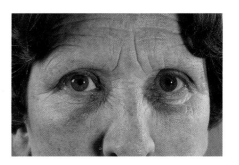

There may be a *heliotrope* (lilac) rash around the eyelids (Fig. 9.21) and on the face and hands, together with *Gottron's papules (MCP and IP joints)* and nail fold erythema (polydermatomyositis).

INTERPRETATION

Confirm the diagnosis

Polymyositis causes progressive, symmetrical proximal musle weakness. It should not be confused with *polymyalgia rheumatica (PMR)*, which causes proximal pain and *marked stiffness* (especially early morning stiffness), but not weakness

Evidence of decompensation

Infrequently, malignancy is associated with dermatomyositis, especially in patients over the age of 50.

DISCUSSION

Which investigations may be used to confirm polymyositis?

- Muscle biopsy (inflammation, necrosis and regeneration)
- Creatinine kinase (elevated)
- EMG (myopathic potentials, fibrillations and complex repetitive discharges)
- Anti-Jo-1 antibodies (may be positive).

In patients with dermatomyositis over the age of 50, clinical examination and/or investigations for breast, ovarian, colorectal or lung malignancy may be appropriate. The threshold for investigating, and what investigations to consider, must be tempered by the fact that only a small percentage of elderly patients with dermatomyositis will have a malignancy.

How is polymyositis treated?

Treatment is with steroids.

What is mixed connective tissue disease (MCTD)?

MCTD is a specific disease defined serologically. All such patients have positive ANAs with a speckled staining pattern and anti-RNP antibodies. Clinically, there is a mixture of connective tissue features. Undifferentiated connective tissue disease is a separate concept, often mistakenly thought the same as MCTD. Undifferentiated connective tissue disease may have inconstant overlapping features of scleroderma, SLE, polymyositis and even rheumatoid arthritis such as telangiectasia, tight skin and a malar rash. In this situation patients should satisfy the criteria for each disease.

What is PMR?

Unlike polymyositis, PMR is very unlikely in patients under the age 50. PMR affects females : males in a ratio of 3 : 1 and causes proximal *pain* and *stiffness*. The ESR is raised, as are other inflammatory markers including CRP and liver function tests (LFTs). Creatinine kinase is normal. Giant cell arteritis occurs in up to 20% of patients. Response to steroids is excellent.

CASE STUDY | 9.7 OSTEOARTHRITIS

Instruction: *Examine this patient's hands and discuss your findings.*

RECOGNITION

There is *bony swelling* of the *DIP joints (Heberden's nodes)* and *PIP joints (Bouchard's nodes)* (Fig. 9.22). There is not usually any evidence of synovitis.

INTERPRETATION

Confirm the diagnosis

Morning stiffness is usually brief, unlike inflammatory arthritis. History, examination and appropriate investigation (X-ray is the investigation of choice but often not indicated) contribute to making the diagnosis.

Fig. 9.22   *Heberden's and Bouchard's nodes*

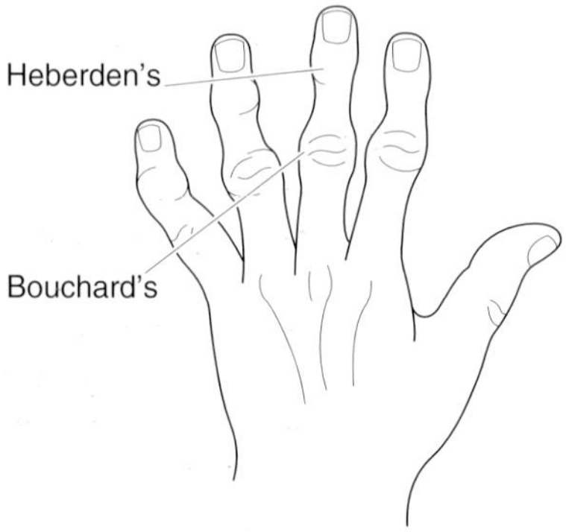

Heberden's

Bouchard's

Look for/consider causes

Other than age or 'wear and tear' induced osteoarthritis, secondary causes include:

- Previous trauma
- Underlying inflammatory joint disease with secondary osteoathritis, e.g. rheumatoid arthritis
- Sensory loss (Charcot's joints, e.g. diabetes)
- Metabolic (e.g. acromegaly, haemochromatosis, hypoparathyroidoism).

Current thinking is that osteoarthritis might be a regenerative process. Primary and secondary causes constitute an insult which, combined with the attempts at cartilage and bone repair, results in the osteoarthritis process. For much of the time a patient will be in a phase of decompensation with symptoms. Eventually there may be continuous decompensation (joint failure).

Assess other systems

Commonly affected are joints in the hands and spine (especially C5, L3, L4), the hips and the knees.

Evidence of decompensation

Complications of osteoarthritis include:

- Pain ● Deformity ● Ankylosis ● Peripheral nerve entrapment
- Cervical spondylosis with cervical myeloradiculopathy.

DISCUSSION

Which radiological features occur?

- Loss of joint space ● Subchondral bone sclerosis ● Periarticular osteosclerosis and osteophytes.

Appearances do not correlate with symptoms. Osteoarthritis is common, but perhaps overdiagnosed in younger patients with chronic pain syndromes who are told they have 'wear and tear' in their joints.

List some treatments

- Education
- Weight reduction
- Physiotherapy
- Occupational therapy
- NSAIDs may relieve symptoms but with the risk of side effects
- Intra-articular steroids may provide good but short lived symptom relief
- Oral steroids are not recommended

- Surgical joint replacement (especially knee) can be life altering
- The use of intra-articular chondroprotective agents and hyaluronic acid derivatives continues to be explored; there is some evidence that glucosamine is of benefit
- Topical capsaicum appears to help symptoms but its place in the hierarchy of treatments is awaited.

Prevention is important. Some types of physical activity are associated with an increased risk of arthritis in certain joints. Previous knee injury, surgery and even occupational or habitual kneeling and squatting can, for example, predispose to knee osteoarthritis.

CASE STUDY | 9.8 PAGET'S DISEASE

Instruction: *Examine this patient's face/legs and discuss any further assessment you would make.*

RECOGNITION

There is *enlargement of the skull*. There is *bowing of the tibia*, and the skin over the leg is warm. There may be kyphosis.

INTERPRETATION

Evidence of decompensation

Important consequences of Paget's disease include:

- High output cardiac failure. Check for the *bounding pulse* of hyperdynamic circulation.
- Neurological compression syndromes caused by bone enlargement such as closure of skull foramina causing deafness. The patient may wear a *hearing aid*.
- Hypercalcaemia, which tends to occur only in immobilised patients.
- Osteosarcoma, although this is rare.

Assess function

Tell the examiners that you would ask about *bone pain*. Other common problems are skeletal deformity, secondary osteoarthritis and an increased risk of fractures.

DISCUSSION

What do you know about the normal composition of bone?

Bone is a dynamic tissue that is remodelled constantly throughout life. The arrangement of compact and cancellous bone normally provides a strength and density that is optimal for mobility. Further, bone is a metabolic reservoir of calcium, phosphorous, magnesium and other ions essential for homeostasis. Bone is also highly vascularised, receiving about 10% of cardiac output.

The *extracellular* structure of bone comprises:

- A solid *mineral* phase, made up mostly of calcium and phosphate as crystalline hydroxyapatite.
- An organic *matrix*, made up mostly of type 1 collagen. The non-collagenous portion contains many types of protein including serum-derived albumin and osteoblast-derived proteins such as osteocalcin.

Of the *cellular* component:

- *Osteoblasts* synthesise and secrete organic matrix. Subsequent matrix mineralisation occurs largely in osteons (haversian systems). Osteoblasts surrounded by mineralised matrix become osteocytes, still connected to their blood supply by a series of canaliculi.
- *Osteoclasts* are responsible for resorption of bone.

What happens to bone in Paget's disease?

Paget's disease is caused by focal or multifocal areas of *abnormally increased osteoclastic and osteoblastic activity* leading to *accelerated but disorganised bone resorption and formation*. Bone in Paget's disease is compact, expanded in size and highly vascularised. Paget's disease generally occurs in elderly patients and is usually asymptomatic.

Do you know of any serum or urine biochemical changes in Paget's disease?

- Raised alkaline phosphatase (reflects bone formation; other causes include hyperparathyroidism, malignancy, growth, osteomalacia and liver disease)
- Raised serum osteocalcin (often normal, however, and not used in practice)
- Raised urinary hydroxyproline and pyridinolone (markers of bone resorption which tend to be used in research).

What are the common indications for treatment?

- Bone pain ● Nerve compression ● Hypercalcaemia.

What is the current treatment of choice for Paget's disease?

A bisphosphonate, the end point of treatment being when alkaline phosphatase levels have normalised.

What do you know about the mechanisms of calcium homeostasis?

Calcium (total serum calcium comprises that bound to albumin and its ionised form) and phosphate homeostasis is maintained by

10. EYES

EXAMINATION: EYES

Introduction

The eye has two separate visual faculties, served by different parts of the retina:

1. *Central vision* is served by the *central retina*, dominated by the *macula* and a super-specialised area of the macula called the *fovea*.
2. *Peripheral vision* is served by the *peripheral retina*.

Unlike a camera photographing images in which everything is reproduced with the same detail, the eye fixes on objects using the central retina and everything in the periphery is appreciated in less detail. Whilst central vision and peripheral vision appear to merge imperceptibly, the *retina's functions are discrete*. This is why it is possible to lose central vision and preserve peripheral vision and vice versa.

Central image perception is dominated by the *cone photoreceptors* in the fovea, particularly sensitive to colour. Peripheral images are perceived by *rods*, particularly sensitive in the dark.

The retina comprises an inner layer of photoreceptors, the *neuroretina* adjacent to the vitreous, and an outer layer of pigment, the *pigment retina*, which receives its blood supply from the vascular choroid beneath (Fig. 10.1).

A normal eye brings parallel rays of light to a focus on the retina. Conventionally, beyond 6 m is infinity. Normal *distance vision* or *visual acuity* (VA) is said to

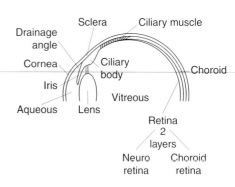

Vertical section through the eye

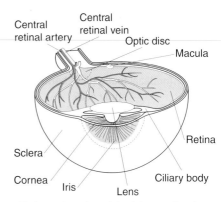

Horizontal section of the left eye, showing relative positions of the pupil, macula and optic disc

Fig. 10.1   *Anatomy of the eye*

be 6/6—meaning that the eye sees at 6 m what it should see at 6 m. 6/24 means it sees only at 6 m what it should be able to see at 24 m. *Near vision* (< 6 m) is made possible by contraction of the ciliary muscle and alteration in the shape of the lens to shorten the focal length. This is necessary because rays of light entering

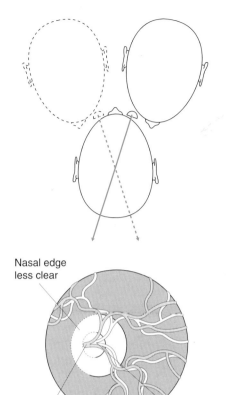

Nasal edge
less clear

Central retinal
artery

Central
retinal vein

A normal optic disc (left eye)

Fig. 10.2 *Fundoscopy*

fields, pupils and ocular movements but you could encounter neuro-ophthalmological disorders at the Eyes Station. Here, we focus on fundal abnormalities.

Fundoscopy (Fig. 10.2)

Examining the fundus is an acquired skill, and useful to incorporate into routine clerkings to appreciate the range of normal appearances as well as recognising abnormalities. Fundoscopy can be exciting! The retina is the only part of the body where blood vessels and nervous tissue are visualised directly.

Fundoscopy is ideally performed in a darkened room. In PACES the Station should be designed for you to assess the fundi as far as the examiners wish, your patient sitting in appropriate lighting with dilating drops instilled unless contra-indicated. Examiners appreciate the limits of fundoscopy and PACES abnormalities are likely to be overt.

1. Approach your patient's right eye from the right side, holding the ophthalmo-scope in your right hand, and vice versa for the left eye (Fig. 10.2).
2. Ask your patient to gaze on a distant object straight ahead at eye level.
3. Check the *red reflex*. The red reflex is attenuated or lost in any condition affecting the transparency of structures in front of the retina (such as a cataract or vitreous haemorrhage), and in any condition affecting apposition of the normally transparent retina with the underlying red vascular choroid (such as retinal detachment).
4. Hold the patient's upper eyelid against their orbit (not against the eyeball!) and approach from 30° to the temporal side. This should ultimately bring the optic disc straight into view. Tilting your head sideways gives both the patient and

the eye have diverged slightly from the parallel, and without refractive adjustment by the lens would converge to a focal point beyond the retina (too long a focal length). *Long sight* occurs when the focal length is too long for the eye. In other words, the eye is too short. *Short sight* occurs when the focal length is too short for the eye. In other words, the eye is too long. Long and short sightedness are merely refractive errors and may be corrected by concave and convex shaped correction lenses respectively.

Chapter 6 discussed eye examination and disorders affecting visual acuity, visual yourself 'breathing space' and enables you to get close to the patient's eye. The closer you are, the easier it is to angle your ophthalmoscope into each quadrant and the bigger your field of view of the fundus.

5. Before looking at the optic disc, focus through the anterior chamber, lens and vitreous as you proceed.

    (i) Find '0' on the ophthalmoscope. West of '0' are negative numbers and east of '0' positive numbers.

    (ii) Dial clockwise so that you start with a short focal length focusing on the cornea.

    (iii) Dialing progressively anticlockwise, through progressively longer focal lengths, will focus through the anterior chamber, lens (detecting any cataract), vitreous and finally onto the fundus.

This takes practice. Remember that short sighted people have long eyes and '0' will focus on the vitreous; long sighted people have short eyes and '0' will come to a focus behind the eye; if a patient is wearing their glasses then '0' will come to a focus on the retina.

6. Now examine the *optic disc*. This full moon like circle is the optic nerve's head. Note its *margin, cup and colour*. If only blood vessels come into immediate view, follow them backwards against the angles of their branches. This should bring the optic disc into view.

7. Be aware of some normal appearances of the optic disc, which confuse many candidates (Box 10.1).

8. Next pursue the four *major vessels* into each quadrant.

9. Remember to look temporally at the *macula*. This can be done by asking your patient to look directly at the light. The macula is found two disc diameters from the temporal margin of the disc and appears as a pale yellow spot on a slightly darkened area of retina. It can be difficult to see (Box 10.2).

Box 10.1   Some Normal Appearances of the Optic Disc

The *nasal margin* of the disc is normally *less sharply demarcated* than the temporal margin, and a *rim of pigment* seen on the *temporal margin* is very common. 'Early papilloedema' and 'retinitis pigmentosa' are often suggested apprehensively by candidates hoping to have seen more overt signs!

The *centre* of the optic disc is normally *paler* than the rim, and the vessels are seen to plunge into it. The *colour* of the optic disc *varies* in adults. Where only the four main vessels are seen on the disc it is normally quite pale. Where the vessels have early branches on the disc itself it appears much pinker. Sometimes elderly patients have very pale discs because of thin vessels.

Box 10.2   Macula, Optic Disc, Central Scrotoma and Blind Spot

Candidates get very confused about the *macula*, the *optic disc* (the optic nerve's head), *central scotomas* and *blind spots*. What especially confuses (and is seldom explained in books) is how disease either at the macula or at the optic disc can produce a central scotoma.

The retina comprises a nerve cell (photoreceptor) layer and a deeper pigment layer, its pigment layer lying over the highly vascular choroid. The nerve fibres from photoreceptors run in an orderly fashion to the optic disc (where they become tightly packed, their millions of converging axons giving rise to the disc's pale appearance) and become the optic nerve. The most important area of the retina is the macula, an area crowded with photoreceptors, whose axons form the most important bundle of fibres entering the optic nerve, the *papillomacular bundle*.

The optic disc, although an area of densely packed nerve fibres, is an area of retina without photoreceptors to receive visual images. The optic disc 'cannot see' and its corresponding visual axis is termed the blind spot (Fig. 10.3). The macula, on the other hand, is an area of densely packed photoreceptors (the fovea being its centre of excellence) and its corresponding visual axis is the area of central vision. Lesions of the macula therefore classically result in a central scotoma (Fig.10.3).

Sometimes it is not just the macula that is damaged but a wider area of receptors and axons situated between the macula and the optic disc. In such cases the scotoma is large, extending between the visual axes of the macula and the optic disc, and this is called a caecocentral scotoma.

Optic atrophy (Case study 10.4) implies damage to and degeneration of axons entering the optic disc. Because the papillomacular fibres are densely packed and thus vulnerable to a heavy casualty rate, central vision disturbance is marked, and can even result in a central scotoma or caecocentral scotoma.

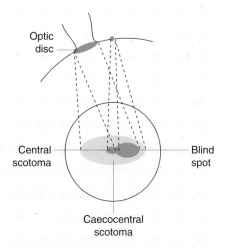

Fig. 10.3   *The optic disc, the macula, the blind spot and central scotomas*

In the early stages of optic disc swelling (Case study 10.3) there is no visual disturbance. Later, retinal oedema may cause blind spot enlargement. Haemorrhages or oedema extending to the macula may cause abrupt central vision disturbance. Chronic scarring resulting from optic disc swelling may cause secondary optic atrophy with a central scotoma and/or progressive visual field restriction as fibres from the periphery entering the optic disc also degenerate.

Arcuate scotomas result from a wide variety of lesions. Arcuate scotomas are scotomas corresponding to damage to a bundle of nerve fibres entering the optic nerve. Primary open angle glaucoma (pages 182–184) causes a special type of arcuate scotoma which radiates from the blind spot. This is because raised intraocular pressure damages nerve fibres at the disc margins.

| CASE STUDY | 10.1 DIABETIC RETINOPATHY |

Instruction: *Examine this patient's fundi and discuss your findings.*

| **RECOGNITION** | |

Diabetic retinopathy (DR) is staged separately from diabetic maculopathy (refer to Box 10.3 for explanations of DR signs).

Non-proliferative diabetic retinopathy (NPDR)

NPDR was formerly classified as:

1. Background diabetic retinopathy (BDR). There are *microaneurysms (dots), blot haemorrhages and leakage ('hard') exudates* (Fig.10.4).
2. Preproliferative diabetic retinopathy (PPDR). There are, in addition to the above, *cotton wool spots (CWS)* (Fig. 10.5) and *large 'blotch' haemorrhages*. There is *dilatation and beading of retinal veins* (sausage appearance).

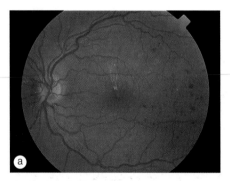 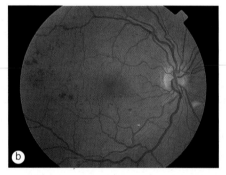

Fig. 10.4   *(a,b) Microaneurysms, leakage exudates and blot haemorrhages. Note that the leakage exudates are close to the macula and that the haemorrhages are of different sizes. Sometimes it is difficult to differentiate between smaller 'blot' and larger 'blotch' haemorrhages (see Box 10.3)*

Fig. 10.5   *Cotton wool spot (see Box 10.3). Note also the small blot haemorrhage at 11 o'clock.*

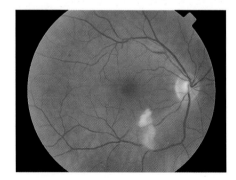

BDR and PPDR have now been replaced by the term NPDR, classified as:

1. Mild (microaneurysms)
2. Moderate (four blots in one quadrant and/or CWS or venous beading or intraretinal microvascular abnormalities (IRMA))
3. Severe (severe haemorrhage in four quadrants or venous beading in two quadrants or severe IRMA in one quadrant)
4. Very severe (any two of severe).

Proliferative diabetic retinopathy (PDR)

There is, in addition to NPDR changes, *neovascularisation* (Fig. 10.6). There may be extensive *laser photocoagulation therapy scarring* (Fig.10.7).

Retinal haemorrhage and retinal detachment

There is, in combination with any of the above features, *preretinal or vitreous haemorrhage* and/or (tractional) *retinal detachment* and/or *rubeosis iridis* (Fig. 10.8). This was traditionally referred to as *advanced diabetic eye disease*, but increasingly the specific lesion is named.

Diabetic maculopathy

There is evidence of diabetic eye disease at, or within one disc diameter of, the macula. This usually takes the form of *exudates* (tending to form *circinate rings*) and *oedema* (Fig. 10.9).

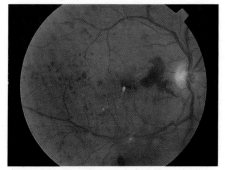

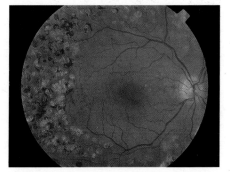

Fig. 10.6   *Diabetic retinopathy changes throughout the fundus with neovascularisation at the optic disc. Neovascularisation (Box 10.3) is also seen notably at 7 o'clock and 11 o'clock (where new vessels have tended to form a loop). Note also the large haemorrhage between the optic disc and the macula.*

Fig. 10.7   *Photocoagulation scars. Note neovascularisation at 8 o'clock*

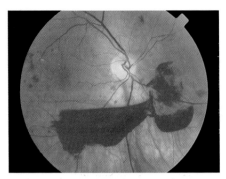

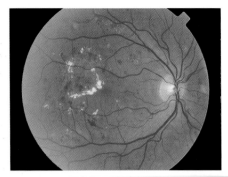

Fig. 10.8 *Subhyaloid (preretinal) haemorrhage in diabetic retinopathy. Blood is in the posterior vitreous space and tends to settle inferiorly and outline the attachment of the vitreous to the retina. The appearance has been likened to a bird's nest. A subhyaloid haemorrhage may also be seen with a subarachnoid haemorrhage. Note how a subhyaloid haemorrhage obscures retinal vessels (Box 10.3; compare with a choroidal haemorrhage in Fig. 10.23)*

Fig. 10.9 *Leakage exudates forming a circinate ring at the macula. Note how bright and crisp leaking exudates are compared to cotton wool spots. Note also haemorrhages of varying size*

INTERPRETATION

Confirm the diagnosis

Diabetic eye disease is usually easy to recognise, the main dilemma being to differentiate it from hypertensive retinopathy. *Microaneurysms* are almost pathognomonic of diabetes, but may occur in venous occlusion. Microaneurysms must be present to diagnose diabetic retinopathy.

Assess other systems

Tell the examiners you would like to:

● Know the level of diabetic control *(HbA1c)*.
● Check for evidence of neuropathy (peripheral neuropathy, mononeuropathy/femoral neuropathy) and nephropathy (proteinuria, serum creatinine)
● Take a history for macrovascular complications such as *ischaemic heart disease* and *stroke*.

Assess severity

Try to grade retinopathy on the basis of the signs. The signs are easier to appreciate when you understand why they occur (Box 10.3).

| Box 10.3 | Understanding the Signs of Diabetic Retinopathy (DR) |

- DR is a microvascular process in which high retinal blood flow induces microangiopathy in capillaries, arterioles and venules, causing vessel occlusion and leakage of plasma contents into the retina itself.
- *Microaneurysms* are bulges in weakened vessel walls and appear as red dots scattered throughout the fundus. Microaneurysms arise as a direct result of capillary occlusion.
- *Leakage exudates* are yellow-white lipid deposits. They represent lipid which has leaked from vessels and been engulfed by macrophages.
- *Haemorrhages* from microaneurysms and weakened vessels appear red but their shape depends upon their site. *Deep haemorrhages* are round (blots) because they are confined by the tightly packed layers of the deep retina. *Superficial haemorrhages* are larger and blotchy as they follow the pattern of nerve fibres.
- *Cotton wool spots* indicate ischaemic areas of retina. They arise because of arteriolar occlusion. To refer to CWS as soft exudates is incorrect.
- *Venous dilatation* is a sign that retinal blood supply is trying to keep up with demand and *venous beading* results from sites of complete vessel closure.
- The term *intraretinal microvascular abnormalities (IRMA)* refers to dilated capillaries. Microaneurysms and IRMAs are best seen as black dots and lines against a green background when the ophthalmoscope's green filter is used to eliminate the redness of the choroid.
- *Neovascularisation* occurs in response to occlusive ischaemia (which stimulates angiogenic factors) and affects veins, not arteries. New vessels are usually 'wild' in appearance. They tend to loop off veins and can look like fronds of seaweed.
- *Subhyaloid haemorrhages* are retained by the hyaloid membrane but may blow into the *vitreous*, threatening vision completely in the affected eye because they are then restrained only by the limits of the vitreous cavity.
- *Retinal detachment* can occur when new vessels exert traction on the retina. *Rubeosis iridis* (new vessels on the iris) may lead to *rubeotic glaucoma*.

Evidence of decompensation

- Sight disturbance (perfect visual acuity may, of course, coexist with sight threatening disease)
- Tell the examiners that worsening retinopathy may occur with rapid tightening of glycaemic control
- Rapid decompensation of eye disease may occur in pregnancy.

Assess function

Tell the examiners that you would *assess visual acuity* and *discuss the impact of any visual loss* with your patient. This is particularly important in diabetic maculopathy with central vision disturbance.

DISCUSSION

Is retinopathy more likely in Type 1 or Type 2 diabetes mellitus?

Diabetic eye disease is the commonest cause of blindness in the UK for patients of working age, and is related to the duration of and level of control of disease. Type 1 diabetic patients generally have 5–10 years of disease before developing eyes signs but eventually nearly all succumb. Type 2 diabetic patients may have eye signs at diagnosis and are more prone to maculopathy.

What do you know about screening for diabetic retinopathy (DR)?

Screening has been shown to prevent loss of sight in 80% of patients with PDR and 50–60% of patients with maculopathy. Routine screening of all diabetic patients is mandatory at least annually. Screening is performed by digital retinal photography.

What are the management principles in DR?

- NPDR with microaneurysms alone requires annual screening with good overall diabetic control. All other grades of NPDR warrant ophthalmological referral (non-urgently except for very severe). In addition to strict diabetic control, a decision must be made about prophylactic laser photocoagulation therapy.
- PDR requires urgent ophthalmological referral for laser photocoagulation therapy, which aims to destroy ineloquent areas of retina (not concerned with vision) and thus attenuate synthesis of angiogenic factors.
- Vitreous haemorrhage is difficult to treat, but requires urgent referral. Advanced microsurgical techniques can sometimes evacuate vitreous blood.
- Maculopathy requires ophthalmological referral. Focal laser therapy may be indicated but must be balanced against potential risk to eloquent tissue.

What other eye complications occur in diabetes mellitus?

- *Cataracts* (early onset age related variety or snowflake cataracts in poorly controlled Type 1 diabetes), or visual changes due to osmotic alteration in lens shape
- Ocular nerve palsies, especially a *sixth nerve palsy*
- Increased risk of *infection* (conjunctivitis, styes, herpes zoster)
- Central retinal artery and vein occlusion are also more common.

| CASE STUDY | 10.2 HYPERTENSIVE RETINOPATHY (HTR) |

Instruction: *Examine this patient's fundi and discuss your findings.*

| RECOGNITION | |

HTR may progress through a number of stages:

1. *Focal arteriolar attenuation and arteriovenous (AV) nipping* represent the presence of arteriosclerosis of any cause. Thickened arteriolar walls appear like *'silver'* or *'copper' wires* (Fig. 10.10).
2. Narrowing of arterioles leads to localised areas of infarction of the superficial retina (*cotton wool spots*) and *flame shaped haemorrhages*. Leakages from these vessels result in *hard exudates* (Fig. 10.10).
3. *Optic disc swelling*, along with cotton wool spots, flame shaped haemorrhages and hard exudates, indicates what has been termed *'malignant hypertension'*. Although defined by disc swelling rather than an absolute blood pressure measurement, blood pressure is often above 200/140 mmHg. *Accelerated hypertension* refers to a recent increase over previous hypertensive levels associated with vascular damage on fundoscopy but without disc swelling.

Beware of diagnosing HTR if disc swelling is unilateral or if it occurs in the absence of other signs of HTR.

| INTERPRETATION | |

Assess other systems

- Ask to take the patient's *blood pressure*
- Be aware of the widespread manifestations of hypertension — cardiovascular disease, cerebrovascular disease, renovascular disease and peripheral vascular disease (Case study 5.17).

Fig. 10.10 *Hypertensive retinopathy. Note AV nipping, the 'wire' appearance of some vessels, leakage (hard) exudates, haemorrhages and blurring of the optic disc margin*

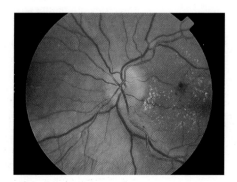

Assess severity

A patient may have other target organ damage with minimal eye signs. The evolving eye signs of HTR are explained in Box 10.4.

Evidence of decompensation

As well as *threatening vision*, hypertension may cause *target organ failure* elsewhere consequent upon poorly controlled chronic hypertension. Additionally, both *central retinal artery* and *central retinal vein occlusion* may occur secondary to hypertension with or without HTR.

DISCUSSION

Explain the signs of hypertensive retinopathy

These signs are explained in Box 10.4.

Box 10.4	Understanding the Signs of Hypertensive Retinopathy

- In childhood, retinal arterioles and venules are of equal width, highly elastic and glisten in the light of an ophthalmoscope. Even normotensive adults lose the sparkling retinal appearances of youth. But hypertension slowly replaces the elastic tissue with fibrous tissue and the glistening disappears. The muscular layer of arterioles is often also replaced and these become rigid. Any remaining arteriolar muscle, still capable of contraction, can give rise to the appearance of *focal arteriolar attenuation*, as the fibrosed segments maintain a static calibre or even dilate.
- *Silver wiring* is an unreliable sign, but *AV nipping* is the natural progression of arteriolar calibre change and the best sign of arteriosclerosis of any cause. It occurs at sites where dilated arterioles cross over or under venules. The 'compression' or 'nipping' is an illusion.
- *Flame shaped haemorrhages* occur in the surface layers of the retina (similar to large diabetic haemorrhages) and *hard exudates* are common at the macula, threatening central vision. They often appear as a *star*, following the line of retinal fibres around the macula.
- *Cotton wool spots*, as for diabetes, indicate ischaemia. They may also be a feature of vasculitis, cholesterol emboli, bacterial endocarditis and myeloproliferative disease.
- *Swelling of the optic disc* implies accelerated hypertension.

What do you know about the British Hypertension Society Guidelines for management of hypertension?

These are discussed in Case study 5.17.

| CASE STUDY | 10.3 SWOLLEN OPTIC DISC AND PAPILLOEDEMA |

Instruction: *Examine this patient's fundi and discuss your findings.*

RECOGNITION

There are many causes of optic disc swelling. Papilloedema, by definition, is swelling of the optic disc as a result of raised intracranial/cerebrospinal fluid pressure. This should be distinguished from other causes of disc swelling.

A sequence of optic disc signs results from evolving swelling (Figs 10.11, 10.12):

1. The veins become dilated and tortuous and capillary dilatation leads to hyperaemia of the disc.
2. The centre of the disc (the *cup*), becomes *pinker than normal* and *less distinct* as it swells. The *vessels seem to disappear* suddenly in the oedema before reaching the cup. The *disc margins blur* (Fig. 10.11) as the nerve fibre layers swell.
3. The entire disc eventually becomes swollen, raised and the origins of vessels completely disappear. At this stage (Fig. 10.12), retinal *haemorrhages, exudates* and *cotton wool spots* may also appear, although any haemorrhages are never as dramatic as in central retinal vein occlusion. *Loss of venous pulsation* implies raised intracranial pressure and is a feature of *papilloedema*. It is difficult to detect and is a normal finding in many individuals. However, *spontaneous venous pulsation excludes papilloedema.*

INTERPRETATION

Look for/consider causes

Tell the examiners that you wish to know the blood pressure. They

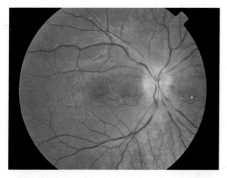

Fig. 10.11   *Swollen optic disc (blurring of disc margins)*

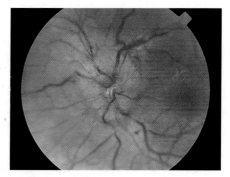

Fig. 10.12   *Swollen optic disc (more advanced case)*

may ask you to discuss possible causes of disc swelling.
Papilloedema is excluded as a cause if spontaneous venous pulsation
is seen, but this can be difficult to detect.

Evidence of decompensation

Check for *enlargement of the blind spot* by visual field testing. Unless
there is also pathology in the optic nerve itself the visual fields are
usually otherwise normal. Chronic untreated hypertension may result
in macula oedema (with macula stars), which can rapidly disturb
central vision.

DISCUSSION

What are the causes of optic disc swelling?

- Papilloedema ● Accelerated hypertension ● Optic papillitis
(page 526) ● Ischaemic optic neuropathy ● Hypercapnia
- Central retinal vein occlusion (CRVO) (Fig. 10.13)
- Hyperproteinaemic disorders (e.g. Waldenström's
macroglobulinaemia) ● Pseudopapilloedema.

What is the pathophysiology of papilloedema?

The pathophysiology of papilloedema remains obscure but involves
transmission of elevated cerebrospinal fluid pressure along the
optic nerve sheath, followed by impaired venous drainage from the
eye.

Papilloedema may take weeks or months to develop, and is
therefore a late sign of raised intracranial pressure. Papilloedema
may be detected in its early stages by fluoroscein angiography.

What is Foster Kennedy syndrome?

Foster Kennedy syndrome refers to optic atrophy caused by
compression of one optic nerve by an intracranial mass, together
with contralateral papilloedema as a result of raised intracranial
pressure.

Fig. 10.13   *Swollen optic disc. Note the
fiery red burst emanating from the optic
disc, often seen in retinal vein thrombosis*

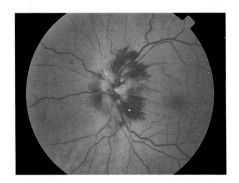

What is idiopathic ('benign') intracranial hypertension?

> This is possibly caused by microthrombi compromising dural venous drainage. It usually affects young to middle-aged females and has been associated with the oral contraceptive pill and corticosteroids. Raised cerebrospinal fluid pressure is a central feature, causing papilloedema and headaches. Treatments include therapeutic lumbar puncture.

What is pseudopapilloedema?

> This is not papilloedema. It occurs in a small, long sighted and often astigmatic eye where the optic disc appears to be crowded by other structures. Apart from the refractive error, there should be no abnormalities, but doubt can be resolved by fluoroscein angiography. Pseudopapilloedema can also result if a disc is raised by drusen.

CASE STUDY	10.4 OPTIC ATROPHY

Instruction: *Examine this patient's fundi and any other aspects of eye examination you think appropriate before discussing your findings.*

RECOGNITION	

> The *optic disc* flashes in to view, *bright, white and crisp*, like a bright full moon in a dark sky (Fig. 10.14) .

INTERPRETATION	

Confirm the diagnosis

> Remember the five features of optic nerve damage (see Box 6.3):
>
> 1. Relative afferent papillary defect (RAPD), the most sensitive and specific sign
> 2. Decreased visual acuity
> 3. Attenuated colour vision

Fig. 10.14 *Optic atrophy. Note how the optic disc is instantly eye catching*

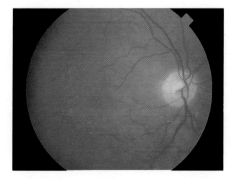

4. Central or paracentral scotoma
5. Optic atrophy.

Optic atrophy is not an all or nothing phenomenon. There are 'shades of white' depending upon the degree of axonal degeneration, and hence degrees of visual disturbance. Patients with multiple sclerosis who have recurrent episodes of optic neuritis develop progressive worsening of the five signs.

Look for/consider causes

If invited, check for other signs of multiple sclerosis (*cerebellar signs, spastic paraparesis, sensory symptoms,* ask about *bladder disturbance*), as this is the commonest cause of optic atrophy in the UK. You will probably be expected to discuss, rather than look for, other causes.

Assess function

Tell the examiners that you would be keen to *discuss the impact of any visual loss*.

DISCUSSION

What are the causes of optic atrophy?

Episodes of demyelinating optic neuritis (retrobulbar neuritis or papillitis) (Box 10.5).

These are by far the commonest cause of optic atrophy in the UK. Whilst a single episode of optic neuritis does not necessarily imply multiple sclerosis, a high proportion (up to 75%) of patients will develop other signs of multiple sclerosis over time. Visual loss during each episode may be subtle, often described as a 'steamed up' sensation and often only noticeable when the good eye is closed. A key associated symptom is pain, especially on eye movement, often preceding visual disturbance. Recovery from an episode of optic neuritis is usual within a few weeks, although even when the field defect resolves, a defect in sharp colour vision persists. Visual evoked potential (VEP) testing usually detects delayed conduction consistent

---

Box 10.5	Optic Neuritis: Papillitis and Retrobulbar Neuritis

In *papillitis,* inflammation is just behind the optic disc, which may be swollen with blurred margins and floridly coloured due to hyperaemia and haemorrhage. In acute *retrobulbar neuritis* the optic disc appears normal because the inflammation is further back along the optic nerve. Papillitis is usually distinguishable from papilloedema because papilloedema is usually bilateral and papilloedema does not give rise to the five signs of optic nerve damage (see Box 6.3).

with demyelination and neuronal loss. Optic neuritis is sometimes treated with corticosteroids, usually intravenously.

Ischaemic optic neuritis

This may be atherosclerotic or vasculitic, notably a complication of untreated giant cell arteritis.

Compression

This may be from tumours, aneurysms, glaucoma or Paget's disease.

Toxic optic neuritis

This may result from chemicals and drugs such as methanol, tobacco, lead, ethambutol, isoniazid, chloramphenicol and digoxin.

Infiltrative lesions

These include granulomatous infiltration of the optic nerve in TB, sarcoidosis or syphilis, and carcinomatous infiltration.

Neurodegeneration

This may occur in *vitamin deficiencies* (especially B_1 and B_{12}), *tabes*, or hereditary conditions such as *Friedreich's ataxia*. *Leber's hereditary optic neuropathy*, a mitochondrial cytopathy, is a rare cause of optic atrophy affecting mostly young adult males.

Retinitis pigmentosa (RP)

RP is associated with severe vessel narrowing, which is thought to be the reason for the frequently associated optic atrophy (ischaemic).

Secondary (consecutive) optic atrophy

The term *consecutive optic atrophy* refers to atrophy due to degeneration of parent ganglion cells and may contribute to the disc pallor in RP, chorioretinitis and central retinal artery occlusion. It also occurs as a legacy of papilloedema due to scarring (gliosis) in the optic disc. The disc margin is not usually crisp as it is in primary atrophy.

What are colobomata?

Colobomata result from persistence of the inferior embryonic cleft of the eyeball which is present during development. A coloboma appears as a white hole in the retina and if in the disc itself as a big white patch. Colobomata occasionally extend into the iris. Colobomata may cause central scotomas or arcuate scotomas.

CASE STUDY | **10.5 CHORIORETINITIS**

Instruction: *Examine this patient's fundi and comment on possible causes.*

RECOGNITION

There is evidence of previous inflammation of the chorioretinal layers. Patches of the normal pink chorioretina have been stripped away to

Fig. 10.15 *Chorioretinitis*

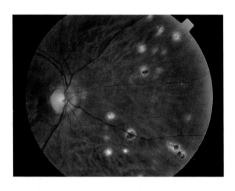

reveal the underlying white sclera. Typically, there are *multiple small white and black patches*, the black reflecting proliferation of retinal pigment (Fig. 10.15).

INTERPRETATION

Evidence of decompensation

Check for scotomas/visual field loss.

DISCUSSION

What causes chorioretinitis?

● Usually idiopathic ● Toxoplasma infection (often secondary to HIV) ● Granulomatous diseases.

CASE STUDY 10.6 RETINITIS PIGMENTOSA

Instruction: *Examine this patient's fundi and visual fields. Discuss your findings.*

RECOGNITION

There are webs of *pigment in the peripheral retina* (Fig. 10.16—if you have seen this once you should not forget the appearance).

Fig. 10.16 *Retinitis pigmentosa*

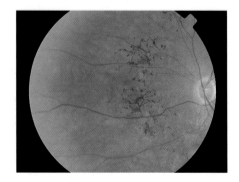

Confirm the diagnosis

Look for *optic atrophy*, which is due to marked narrowing of arterioles and retinal cell ischaemia/loss.

Check the visual fields for *funnel vision*.

Evidence of decompensation

There may be funnel vision (see below).

DISCUSSION

What is retinitis pigmentosa?

Retinitis pigmentosa refers to a group of hereditary, progressive conditions which may be autosomal dominant, autosomal recessive or X-linked and usually begin in childhood.

List some conditions associated with retinitis pigmentosa

● Laurence–Moon–Bledl syndrome (mental retardation, hypogonadism, obesity, polydactyly, deafness and renal cysts)
● Kearns–Sayre syndrome (mitochondrial cytopathy with ophthalmoplegia, ptosis and heart block)
● Refsum's disease (cerebellar ataxia, peripheral neuropathy and deafness)
● Abetalipoproteinaemia (widespread neurological manifestations)
● Usher's syndrome (sensorineural deafness).

What is the difference between 'funnel' and 'tunnel' vision?

Both funnel and tunnel vision refer to the phenomenon of peripheral visual field constriction, with preserved central vision (Fig. 10.17).

Funnel vision results from disease of the peripheral retina. *Tunnel, or tubular vision*, is always non-organic or psychogenic. In tunnel vision, the visual field defect remains the same size (like looking through a tube) regardless of the distance of a target object. This is physically impossible, because a visual field subtends an arc, such that at double the distance an intact field should be doubled in size.

CASE STUDY 10.7 CENTRAL RETINAL VEIN OCCLUSION (CRVO)

Instruction: *Examine the fundi and discuss your findings.*

RECOGNITION

There is *retinal vein dilatation*, together with a flock of *haemorrhages throughout the retina* (an inevitable consequence of the occlusion) and *optic disc swelling*. The overall appearance is like a fiery sunset (Fig. 10.18).

Fig. 10.17   *Funnel and tunnel vision*

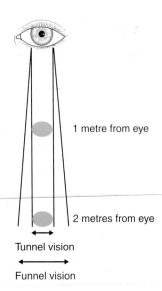

1 metre from eye

2 metres from eye

Tunnel vision

Funnel vision

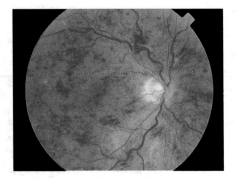

Fig. 10.18   *Central retinal vein occlusion*

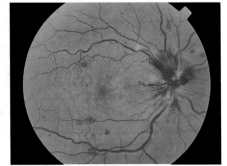

Fig. 10.19   *Optic disc swelling in central retinal vein occlusion (in this case caused by hypertension)*

The picture may be restricted to one quadrant in branch retinal vein occlusion (BRVO).

| INTERPRETATION |

Look for/consider causes

Tell the examiners that you would like to check for *glycosuria* and measure the *blood pressure* (Fig. 10.19).

Evidence of decompensation

Visual loss is *variable*, depending upon macula involvement and the extent of retinal ischaemia.

DISCUSSION

What are the causes of CRVO?

- Arteriosclerosis (ageing, hypertension, diabetes mellitus)
- Vasculitis ● Hyperviscosity disorders (hyperproteinaemias, polycythaemia rubra vera) ● Glaucoma (CRVO only).

CRVO is commoner in eyes prone to primary open angle glaucoma, but glaucoma may also be a complication of CRVO as neovascularisation may extend to the iris in response to retinal hypoxia.

CASE STUDY   10.8 CENTRAL RETINAL ARTERY OCCLUSION (CRAO)

Instruction: *Examine this patient's fundi and discuss your findings.*

RECOGNITION

The *retina is pale*. In the first few days a *cherry red spot* is present at the fovea because the red choroid is visible at the fovea where the retina is rendered especially thin. The entire fundus is otherwise *oedematous* with a *milky appearance*. The *arterioles* are *thin*. Neovascularisation occurs but is never overt, probably because retinal destruction limits the amount of angiogenic factor the retina can produce (Figs 10.20, 10.21).

INTERPRETATION

Look for/consider causes

Tell the examiners that you would like to ask about:

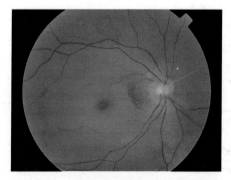

Fig. 10.20   *Central retinal artery occlusion. Note the cherry red spot at the macula, the creamy pallor of the fundus and the wispy appearance of the vessels*

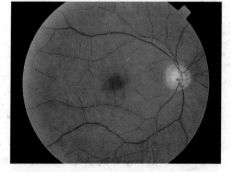

Fig. 10.21   *Central retinal artery occlusion. Note how a deeply pigmented retina (which is normal) can alter the colour and appearance of retinal signs*

1. Symptoms of previous *temporal arteritis* (and look for signs of Cushing's syndrome). Note, however, that visual loss in giant cell arteritis is more commonly due to anterior ischaemic optic neuropathy damaging the optic nerve head.
2. A history of previous *myocardial infarction* (mural thrombus) or *stroke*.
3. Risks factors for atrial fibrillation which may be the source of emboli:
   (i) Coronary heart disease
   (ii) Valvular heart disease
   (iii) Hypertension
   (iv) Thyrotoxicosis
   (v) Alcohol excess.

Occasionally a cholesterol embolus may be visible in a vessel. Cholesterol emboli may occur as a complication of procedures disrupting the endothelium (such as percutaneous coronary intervention). The dislodged emboli may cause visual disturbances, strokes, renal failure or peripheral vascular occlusion.

Assess function

There is usually a history of *sudden painless visual loss*.

DISCUSSION

How does a central retinal artery occlusion differ from a branch occlusion?

The central retinal artery divides into upper and lower branches on the disc to supply a 'half moon' of retina above and below the horizontal meridian respectively. Branch occlusion (BRAO) therefore only causes visual field defects in areas corresponding to the retinal supply of the branch and these are limited by the horizontal meridian.

Which treatments may be considered immediately?

- Aspirin
- Massaging the eyeball
- Lowering intraocular pressure pharmacologically (e.g. with nitrates) to increase circulation.

Rebreathing into a bag to increase carbon dioxide levels and theoretically open up collaterals is a traditional therapeutic measure although its effectiveness may be but a fairytale!

CASE STUDY 10.9 RETINAL DETACHMENT AND VITREOUS HAEMORRHAGE

Instruction: *Examine this patient's fundi and discuss your findings.*

RECOGNITION

The *retina appears opaque* and its reflex is *grey* rather than pink (the normally transparent retina becomes opaque in any profile other than its normal attached position and obscures the underlying red choroid). *Rippling* may be visible if the detached retina folds into hills and valleys as a result of any subretinal fluid.

INTERPRETATION

Confirm the diagnosis

Ask about previous *floaters* or *flashing lights*.

Look for/consider causes

Tell the examiners that you would wish to check for diabetes and hypertension and ask about myopia or previous eye surgery.

Assess function

Checking the visual acuity and visual fields should reveal an area of *visual field loss* or scotoma on an axis corresponding to the area of detachment at the retina.

DISCUSSION

What are the causes of floaters and flashes?

Floaters are usually due to opacities in the vitreous. They may be caused by:

● Vitreous syneresis (degeneration) ● Posterior vitreous detachment (PVD) ● Vitreous haemorrhage ● Inflammatory infiltrates, e.g. in posterior uveitis.

The origin of light *flashes* is less well understood, but they probably result from retinal stimulation by vitreoretinal traction. Flashes are a classic feature of PVD and incipient retinal detachment (see below) but may also occur in migraine with aura.

What is the pathophysiology of retinal detachment?

Retinal detachment refers to separation of the neuroretinal cell layer and its underlying pigment layer. It does not refer to separation of the retina from the underlying choroid.

Posterior vitreous detachment (PVD), in which the posterior vitreous separates from the retina, is the main event predisposing to retinal detachment. As the vitreous collapses, it exerts traction on the neuroretina (with which it is normally in tight adherence) and this may cause a retinal tear, which in turn can lead to separation of the neuroretinal and pigment retinal layers and detachment of the neuroretina. Risk factors for retinal detachment include:

● *Age*: An intact vitreous of normal viscosity is important in keeping the retina in place. With advancing age the viscosity decreases, and the 'fluid vitreous' is capable of creeping behind any small neuroretinal tear that might result from vitreous collapse and posterior vitreous detachment.

- *Myopia*: Here the eye is 'too big' for its retina, which is 'stretched and thinned' and susceptible to tearing.
- *Trauma*: Trauma may cause direct retinal detachment, or produce scarring which can exert abnormal tractional forces on the retina.
- *Cataract surgery*: This can alter vitreous volume or shape.
- *Neovascularisation*: New blood vessel formation in diabetes may alter adhesive forces between the vitreous and retina. Vasculitis can cause similar problems.
- *Congenital retinal abnormalities*: These may sometimes not become manifest until later life.
- *Ocular tumours*: Rarely, pressure from behind the retina such as that caused by a choroidal tumour can cause retinal detachment.

What are the symptoms of posterior vitreous detachment (PVD) and retinal detachment?

PVD may occur acutely, causing *flashes* (vitreoretinal traction) and *floaters* (glial tissue which normally attaches the vitreous to the retina is exposed, and an associated tear in the retina may produce a shower of floaters if specks of blood spurt into the vitreous from torn vessels) or may be of gradual onset with intermittent floaters.

If PVD results in retinal detachment or haemorrhage, visual impairment is very likely, and if the macula is torn or obscured, central vision is abruptly lost. The classic sign of retinal detachment is that of a curtain being drawn across the visual field.

Which patients with floaters or flashes warrant assessment by an ophthalmologist?

Patients with high risk features (acute onset, reduced visual acuity or a visual field defect, previous history or family history of retinal tear or detachment, myopia, previous ocular trauma or surgery, diabetes). Longstanding intermittent floaters are usually benign and caused by vitreous degeneration, and patients with these warrant review if their floaters change or their vision becomes affected.

How is a retinal tear treated?

Laser photocoagulation. Treatment of a detached retina is seldom possible if the neuroretinal layer has become ischaemic and fibrosed.

What are the causes of vitreous haemorrhage?

- PVD ● Proliferative diabetic retinopathy ● Retinal vein occlusion ● Subarachnoid haemorrhage (often limited to subhyaloid rather than vitreous haemorrhage) ● Trauma ● Vasculitis.

Vitreous haemorrhages cause floaters and reduced vision. Large bleeds cause loss of the red reflex (other causes of this include cataracts and, rarely, asteroid hyaline bodies and retinoblastomas).

| CASE STUDY | 10.10 AGE-RELATED MACULAR DEGENERATION (ARMD) |

Instruction: *Examine this patient's fundi and vision, then discuss your findings.*

RECOGNITION

There are *drusen* in the area of the macula, individually or in clusters (Fig. 10.22). These mask the normally transparent retina and its underlying red choroid. There may also be frank *macular atrophy* exposing the white sclera beneath. There may even be areas of *haemorrhage* which mask all underlying structures. The disrupted pigment retinal layer may exhibit areas of *hypopigmentation* or *hyperpigmentation*. The overall appearance of these various changes can be like a *splodge of mixed paints* spilt over the macula (Fig. 10.23). The overall consequence is *loss of central vision*.

INTERPRETATION

Confirm the diagnosis

Visual distortion is a specific and sensitive symptom of *choroidal neovascularisation* seen in 'wet' ARMD (see below).

Assess function

Check the visual acuity and visual fields.

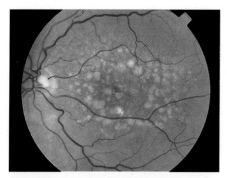

Fig. 10.22   *Typical drusen (heralding age-related macular degeneration)*

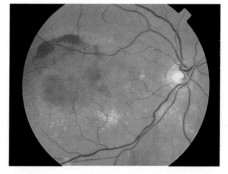

Fig. 10.23   *More advanced age-related macular degeneration with choroidal neovascularisation and haemorrhage. This patient would have marked impairment of central vision. Note that with choroidal haemorrhage, the overlying retinal vessels can be clearly seen (compare with Fig. 10.8)*

DISCUSSION	

What is the pathophysiology of ARMD?

Drusen are early features of ARMD and appear as small, pale yellow deposits on the retina. Their pathogenesis remains uncertain, but they are probably derived from the debris of 'retired' retinal cells. They are commonly detected in people over the age of 65 without other signs of disease.

Visual loss may occur from neovascular abnormalities ('*wet*' ARMD) or non-neovascular abnormalities ('*dry*' ARMD).

In *wet ARMD*, vessels from the choroid layer (which normally nourish the pigment retina) proliferate across Bruch's membrane and into the subretinal space. Visual distortion (e.g. of printed words or grids) is a specific and sensitive symptom of choroidal neovacularisation. Visual loss occurs as these vessels haemorrhage or leak transudate into the subretinal space, the retina slowly becoming atrophic and fibrosed. Large haemorrhages may even cause retinal detachment. Choroidal neovascularisation itself may not be seen on direct ophthalmoscopy, requiring fluoroscein angiography for detection (Fig. 10.24).

In *dry ARMD*, the retina in the areas of drusen slowly atrophies, and visual deterioration is more gradual, often over many years. Visual distortion is not a feature. Dry ARMD is much more common than wet ARMD.

Age related macular degeneration is the commonest cause of central vision disturbance and registered blindness in the UK.

How might you determine if a patient with a cataract has ARMD?

Even early cataracts may obscure adequate fundoscopy. Typically patients with cataracts find that reading is easier when a light is shone directly onto the page. Visual enhancement with such a simple measure suggests that ARMD is not present (of course it cannot exclude ARMD).

Fig. 10.24   *Extensive choroidal haemorrhage*

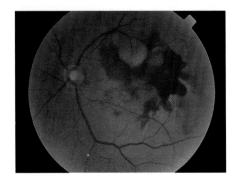

What treatments are available for ARMD?

Laser photocoagulation therapy delivers thermal energy under topical anaesthesia to areas of neovascularisation, but since this treatment also destroys the retina it often cannot be delivered to the areas of greatest need (most patients needing treatment have choroidal neovascularisation extending under the central retina). The closer the treatment to eloquent areas of retina, the higher its risk–benefit ratio. In an attempt to solve this dilemma, *photodynamic therapy* is emerging as a favoured alternative. The principle of this therapy is that a drug which can be photoactivated to destroy tissue locally is given intravenously. When it circulates into the new choroidal vessels, photoactivation is applied.

In addition to regular outpatient follow up, patients with drusen may be taught to screen themselves frequently using such techniques as looking at the fine lines on a piece of graph paper for any black spots or areas of distortion which may indicate underlying neovascularisation.

CASE STUDY | **10.11 ANGIOID STREAKS**

Instruction: *Examine this patient's fundi and report your findings.*

RECOGNITION

There are *dark red trails* or *streaks with irregular edges* (Fig. 10.25). They represent cracks in the retina and Bruch's membrane (page 536) through which the choroid is exposed.

INTERPRETATION

Consider/look for causes

Angioid streaks are uncommon. Many patients with angioid steaks have *pseudoxanthoma elasticum*. They can also be a feature of Ehlers–Danlos syndrome, Paget's disease and sickle cell disease.

Fig. 10.25 *Angioid streaks*

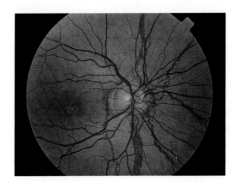

DISCUSSION

The examiners are likely to not know any more about angioid streaks and ask you about something else!

CASE STUDY   10.12   MYELINATED NERVE FIBRES

Instruction: *Examine this patient's fundi and report your findings.*

RECOGNITION

There are *bright white patches with frayed edges* (Fig. 10.26). They can look like an exploding white firework emanating from the optic disc or a bright comet trailing across the retinal sky!

INTERPRETATION

Assess function

There may be visual field defects but frequently myelinated nerve fibres are asymptomatic.

DISCUSSION

How do myelinated nerve fibres arise?

Myelination of optic nerve fibres is normally arrested before such fibres enter the eye. Failure of arrest during development results in myelinated (or medullated) nerve fibres.

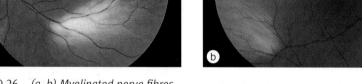

Fig. 10.26   *(a, b) Myelinated nerve fibres*

REFERENCES AND FURTHER READING

Diabetes (diabetic retinopathy) references are given at the end of Chapter 4.

11. ENDOCRINE SYSTEM

EXAMINATION: THYROID STATUS/THE THYROID GLAND

Thyroid disease is much more common in females. Broadly, there are four main ways thyroid disease may present:

1. Hyperthyroidism
2. Hypothyroidism
3. Subclinical disease (index of suspicion or serendipitously)
4. Thyroid lumps.

When you are familiar with the clinical signs of hyperthyroidism (Case study 11.1), hypothyroidism (Case study 11.2) and thyroid lumps (Case study 11.3), a scheme for examining the thyroid makes much more sense. Thyroid disease can affect almost every system but there isn't time for an exhaustive assessment. Many physicians find a head to foot screen useful, such as the following:

1. Ask your patient to sit comfortably at the edge of the bed. Stand back and observe, paying particular attention to the face.
2. *Look at* the *thyroid gland* from the front. Note any *scars* indicating previous surgery.

Box 11.1 Notes on Thyroid Function Tests (TFTS)

Thyroid hormones
The thyroid gland secretes both *thyroxine (T4)* and the *active hormone triiodothyronine (T3)*, whilst T4 is also converted to T3 peripherally. Both T3 and T4 are highly protein bound to *thyroxine binding globulin (TBG)*. Alteration in TBG levels therefore alters the total (but not the free) levels of T4 and T3.

Alterations in TBG levels
- Oestrogens (e.g. pregnancy, combined oral contraceptive pill) and liver disease raise TBG levels.
- Protein losing conditions (e.g. nephrotic syndrome) lower TBG levels.
- Many drugs affect T3 and T4 levels by altering TBG levels or by interfering with conversion of T3 to T4. These include amiodarone, lithium and phenytoin.

You are not to expected to remember which drug does what. Most modern assays measure free thyroid hormones (FT4 and FT3) rendering drug effects mediated by TBG less important

Sick euthyroid syndrome (SES)
This refers to TFT changes in severe non-thyroidal illness. These changes can include decreased conversion of T4 to T3 with normal T4 but decreased FT3 and usually normal TSH (see below) levels (common) and a more extreme fall in FT3 levels probably secondary to decreased T4 production (more seriously ill patients). In very seriously ill patients these changes may be secondary to decreased TSH secretion and T4 may also fall. A rare variant of SES, usually in elderly females, produces raised total and FT4 levels.

[handwritten margin notes: TSH receptor antibodies (Graves') / *thyroglobulin + thyroid peroxidase autoantibodies]*

Most SES is associated with low levels of binding proteins, although the biochemical alterations in SES are complex and multifactorial. Patients are euthyroid.

Thyroid function tests

Tests have been simplified in recent years. The *main tests of function* now are:

- *Thyroid stimulating hormone (TSH)* levels, which are increased in primary hypothyroidism and decreased in hyperthyroidism, assuming there is no pituitary disease.
- *FT4* and *FT3* levels.
- *Thyroid autoantibodies*, including *TSH receptor antibodies* in Graves' disease and *thyroglobulin and thyroid peroxidase autoantibodies* which may be present in any form of autoimmune thyroid disease. Peroxidase is an enzyme needed for thyroid hormone synthesis.

- *Nuclear medicine tests* (either quantitative 4-hour thyroidal radioiodine uptake or pertechnate scintiscan). These tests are not routine but may be used to diagnose hyperthyroidism due to thyroiditis (silent, post partum or de Quervain's) or amiodarone, where uptake is characteristically low in contrast to other causes of hyperthyroidism.

[handwritten: Exophthalmos]

3. Ask if there is any *pain or tenderness*, then *feel the thyroid gland from behind*. Be gentle, because thyroid examination can be uncomfortable for patients. Feel the *isthmus*, which overlies the thyroid cartilage, with your right middle and index fingers, and then feel the *lobes*. Note any *diffuse goitre* or area of *focal nodularity*. Note the gland's *size* and *texture*.

4. Consider asking the patient to swallow a glass of water if your find a goitre, to see and feel if it is readily mobile. *[margin notes: swallow / goitre + water]*

5. Feel for *lymph nodes*—supraclavicular, submandibular, postauricular, suboccipital. If there are palpable nodes, note if they are separate and tender (reactive hyperplasia), hard and clustered together (carcinoma), soft and rubbery (lymphoma), mobile or fixed. *[margin notes: soft + rubbery]*

6. Auscultate the thyroid gland bilaterally for *bruits*.

7. Examine the eyes for:
   (i) *Proptosis* (protusion of the eyeball, best seen from above, standing behind the patient) *[margin: Proptosis]*
   (ii) *Lid retraction* (the upper sclera is visible between the cornea and the upper lid) *[margin: Lid retraction]*
   (iii) *Exophthalmos* (the lower sclera is visible between the cornea and the lower lid)
   (iv) *Lid lag* (move your finger downwards and ask the patient to follow it, whilst fixing their forehead with your other hand. The movement must be quite fast to elicit lid lag
   (v) *Ophthalmoplegia*
   (vi) *Chemosis* (if present, mention that you would consider using fluoroscein to look for corneal ulceration).

8. Observe the *face, skin* and *hair* for signs of hyperthyroidism or hypothyroidism.

9. Feel the *pulse*.

10. Inspect the *palms* for *erythema* and feel for *sweat*. Note any *clubbing*. Note any *tremor* with the arms outstretched.

11. Ask your patient to abduct their shoulders to assess for *proximal muscle weakness*.

12. Look at the legs for *pretibial myxoedema*.

13. Test the *ankle reflexes*.

You will probably discover early in the course of the examination if you are dealing with a thyroid lump, hyperthyroidism or hypothyroidism, directing your assessment accordingly.

| CASE STUDY | 11.1 HYPERTHYROIDISM/GRAVES' DISEASE |

Instruction: *Please determine this patient's thyroid status and discuss the underlying cause.*

| RECOGNITION | |

Look for a triad of possible groups of signs:

1. **Hyperthyroidism** (common). The *hands are warm and sweaty with palmar erythema. Tremor* is often obvious (with the arms extended a piece of paper on the hands detects subtle fine tremors). There is *tachycardia* at rest (usually sinus tachycardia, may be atrial fibrillation). There may be *proximal muscle weakness. A bruit* bilaterally over the thyroid is pathognomonic of Graves' disease. Often the first signs you will see are eye signs (Fig. 11.1).

2. **Ophthalmopathy** (< 50% patients). Lid lag and lid retraction are due to excess sympathetic activity and not specific to Graves' disease. Signs not present in other forms of hyperthyroidism are:
   (i) *Exophthalmos*
   (ii) *Ophthalmoplegia* (due to lymphocytic infiltration of the orbit), often a complex ophthalmoplegia (page 269).

3. **Pretibial myxoedema (PTM)** (rare). PTM is specific to Graves' disease. There are *elevated symmetrical shin lesions* (Fig. 11.2).

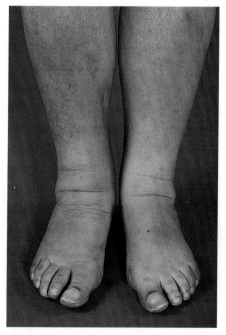

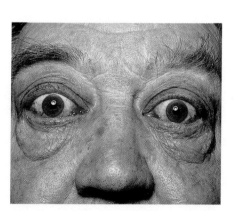

Fig. 11.1   *Hyperthyroidism. Reproduced with permission from M.A. Mir (1995) Atlas of Clinical Diagnosis. W.B. Saunders, London*

Fig. 11.2   *Pretibial myxoedema (also note acropachy)*

PTM may occur at other sites, particularly the forearm. Lesions are *coarse, purplish red or brown*, with *well defined edges*. The *skin is shiny*, with an *orange peel appearance*. These lesions may be asymptomatic or painful. Coarse hairs tend to occur in the vicinity.

Look also for thyroid acropachy (clubbing) and onycholysis (Plummer's nails).

INTERPRETATION

Confirm the diagnosis

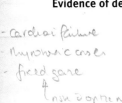

Exophthalmos and PTM are pathognomonic of Graves' disease, and ophthalmoplegia does not occur in other forms of hyperthyroidism. They may run independent courses from hyperthyroidism.

Tell the examiners you would like to ask about symptoms:
- Preference for cold ● Irritability/anxiety ● Weight loss
- Diarrhoea ● Oligomenorrhoea ● A family history of autoimmune disease ● Bone fractures (due to associated osteoporosis) ● Pain or tenderness from goitre (thyroiditis).

Evidence of decompensation

Tell the examiners that you would be concerned about:

- High output cardiac failure
- Thyrotoxic crises (metabolic and haemodynamic instability)
- Fixed gaze (usually painful), a surgical emergency because there is risk of optic nerve compression.

Look for/consider associated diseases

Consider other organ specific autoimmune diseases associated with autoimmune hyperthyroidism, e.g. diabetes mellitus, pernicious anaemia, Addison's disease and primary biliary cirrhosis.

DISCUSSION

What are the common causes of hyperthyroidism?

1. **Graves' disease.** TSH receptor antibodies (IgG) bind to the TSH receptor and stimulate it. Non-stimulatory TSH receptor blocking antibodies may also occur. Both euthyroid and hypothyroid Graves' disease may occur, associated with characteristic Graves' ophthalmopathy. The mechanism of autoimmunity within the orbit is uncertain. The following are known to increase the risk of ophthalmopathy:
   (i) Age
   (ii) Smoking
   (iii) Male gender
   (iv) Radioactive iodine.

Graves' disease is important in pregnancy because TSH receptor antibodies can cross the placenta and cause fetal hyperthyroidism/tachycardia, whilst antithyroid drugs can cross the placenta and cause fetal hypothyroidism.

2. **Toxic multinodular goitre.**
3. **Solitary toxic adenomas.**
4. **Postpartum thyroiditis.** A destructive thyroiditis occurring between 2 and 10 months post partum. It is silent (no pain or swelling) and characterised by a short period of hyperthyroidism followed by a more prolonged but usually self-limiting period of hypothyroidism. Radioiodine uptake (nuclear scanning) is low in the thyrotoxic phase and can confirm the diagnosis. It is associated with thyroid peroxidase antibodies. *(thyroid peroxidase antibodies)*
5. **De Quervain's thyroiditis.** A painful destructive thyroiditis caused by viral infection. Patients may be febrile with a high ESR. There is usually a firm tender goitre. The functional course and diagnosis is as for postpartum thyroiditis. Patients often present with hyperthyroidism because follicles are disrupted and release hormone. Follicle disruption prevents radioiodine uptake. Pain and swelling respond well to steroids. Resolution invariably leads to a period of self-limiting or permanent hypothyroidism ('burnt out' follicles).

What do you know about the treatment of hyperthyroidism? *Se of inflamation & rashes.*

Medical

1. Patients with borderline and unequivocal hyperthyroidism are usually referred to hospital for assessment.
2. If it is unequivocal, carbimazole may have been started by the general practitioner. This will not hinder subsequent radioiodine therapy or surgery. Patients should be warned about symptoms of infection and rashes. The earliest symptom of incipient agranulocytosis is usually a sore throat but fever or mouth ulcers are also common. Patients should stop treatment in this event and seek an urgent full blood count. Neutropenia occurs in between 0.1% and 0.2% of patients taking carbimazole.
3. Carbimazole takes about 1 month to significantly improve thyroid status. Symptom control is achieved with non-cardioselective beta-blockers (e.g. propranolol 80 mg thrice daily, weaning to 40 mg twice daily over 4–6 weeks and then ceased as carbimazole has taken effect) in the interim. Carbimazole may be started according to one of two main regimens:
(i) Reducing dose regimen: 30–60 mg daily reducing as the patient becomes euthyroid, usually to 5 mg daily.
(ii) Block replace regimen: 30–45 mg daily throughout but adding thyroxine when the patient becomes euthyroid.

Treatment is usually continued for 18–24 months, but 50% of patients will eventually relapse when it is discontinued.

Eye treatment

This is urgent if full lid closure is not possible, to protect the eye from exposure keratitis. Fixed gaze and/or visual loss warrants immediate assessment and treatment options include immunosuppression, surgery and orbital radiotherapy. Surgery may be considered electively for less severe disease, but ophthalmopathy often improves significantly over the years with medical treatment.

Radioactive iodine

Contraindications include pregnancy, lactation and active ophthalmopathy. Patients with ophthalmopathy should be offered corticosteroids following radioiodine treatment to reduce the risk of exacerbation of eye disease. At least 50% of patients are rendered hypothyroid after radiotherapy or surgery and will require lifelong thyroxine.

Surgical

Both radioactive iodine and surgical thyroidectomy are very effective treatments and usually result in permanent cure, but with lifelong thyroxine replacement. Indications for surgery in Graves' disease include a large goitre, disease relapse, and where radioactive iodine is contraindicated, unavailable or unacceptable to the patient.

How would you monitor treated hyperthyroidism?

Thyroid function tests (TFTs) should be checked annually if stable, and after 6–8 weeks following any dose adjustment. It takes several weeks for the TFTs to reflect changes in treatment.

CASE STUDY | **11.2 HYPOTHYROIDISM**

Instruction: *Please determine this patient's thyroid status.*

RECOGNITION

You may miss hypothyroidism and think, 'just another little old lady'. Many of the clinical features of hypothyroidism are non-specific and insidious. They include *excess weight* with *myxoedematous facial features (thick and coarse, with periorbital oedema), dry, yellowish skin, and fine, brittle hair with loss of outer eyebrow hair* (Fig. 11.3). There may be *delayed relaxation of ankle and other deep tendon reflexes*. A goitre is unusual.

INTERPRETATION

Confirm the diagnosis

Tell the examiners that you would like to ask about symptoms:

Fig. 11.3   *Hypothyroidism*

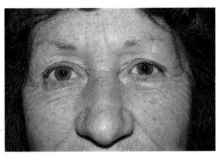

Serous effusions
(pleural, pericardial,
peritoneal, joint)
Carpal tunnel syndrome
Cerebellar signs
Bradycardia / Heart failure
Dyslipidaemia
Depression / psychosis.

● Preference for warmth ● Mood change including depressed mood
● Tiredness ● Weight gain ● Constipation ● Menorrhagia
● Muscle cramps (myopathy) ● Chest pains (myopathic or due to
coronary heart disease) ● A family history.

Evidence of decompensation

Tell the examiners that you would be concerned about:

● Serous effusions (pleural, pericardial, peritoneal, joint) ● Carpal
tunnel syndrome ● Cerebellar signs ● Bradycardia/heart failure
● Dyslipidaemia (raised LDL and total cholesterol levels increase
cardiovascular risk) ● Depression/psychosis.

Look for/consider associated diseases

As with Graves' disease, consider other autoimmune diseases such as
diabetes mellitus, pernicious anaemia, Addison's disease and
rheumatoid arthritis.

DISCUSSION

What are the causes of hypothyroidism?

● Autoimmune Hashimoto's thyroiditis, the commonest cause, in
  which dense lymphocytic infiltration of the thyroid gland may
  produce a diffuse or finely micronodular goitre
● Primary atrophic hypothyroidism
● Post total or partial thyroidectomy
● Post radioiodine
● Graves' disease with TSH receptor blocking antibodies
● Destructive thyroiditis (de Quervain's or postpartum)
● Congenital
● Secondary to pituitary failure
● Iodine deficiency, the commonest cause worldwide.

What do you know about treatment of hypothyroidism?

Young patients, pregnant patients or those patients with evidence of
pituitary disease are usually referred to secondary care. Thyroxine

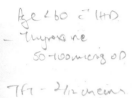

replacement for patients under 60 years without ischaemic heart
disease usually starts at 50–100 mcg daily. A starting dose of 25 mcg
daily is often used in patients with higher cardiovascular risk and
titrated upwards to clinical response.

The TFTs should be checked 2 monthly, aiming for a normal TSH.
Clinical improvement may lag behind normalisation of TSH. Thyroxine
is increased in 25 mcg increments up to 150 mcg daily according to
the serum TSH. Larger doses of thyroxine are seldom necessary and if
needed should alert doctors to question compliance. Daily doses of
thyroxine are sufficient as its half-life is several days.

What is subclinical hypothyroidism?

Hypothyroidism need not be overt to produce a profoundly
debilitating effect. Covert or subclinical hypothyroidism refers to
biochemical changes (raised TSH, normal free T4) with absent or
covert clinical manifestations. It is important because treatment may
enhance wellbeing by erasing hitherto insidious, vague symptoms
and, further, may reduce cardiovascular risk. Dyslipidaemic profiles
frequently portend symptoms.

CASE STUDY   **11.3 THYROID LUMPS—GOITRES AND NODULES**

Instruction: *Examine this patient's neck/thyroid gland and determine their thyroid status.*

RECOGNITION

There is a *diffuse goitre/multinodular goitre/single thyroid nodule.*

INTERPRETATION

Assess other systems

Assess thyroid status as outlined on pages 539–540.

Evidence of decompensation

The key issue is to exclude malignancy with further investigations.

DISCUSSION

What are the causes of a diffuse goitre?

- Graves' disease ● Hashimoto's/autoimmune thyroiditis
- de Quervain's subacute thyroiditis ● Secondary to goitrogens.

What are the causes of thyroid nodules?

1. Single nodule:
   (i) Adenoma
   (ii) Cyst
   (iii) Carcinoma (occasionally lymphoma).

2. Multinodular goitre (the commonest cause worldwide is iodine deficiency).

Thyroid nodules are common, often silent, and increasingly prevalent with age. They may be solid, cystic, mixed (e.g. cystic degeneration within an adenoma) or calcified. The key issue is to exclude malignancy, although this is rare. It is not possible without scanning to determine if a single palpable nodule is part of a multinodular thyroid.

What symptoms may a thyroid lump cause?

- Most commonly an asymptomatic lump (noted by patient, family or GP)
- Most are euthyroid (endocrine glands generally comprise much redundant tissue)
- Pressure symptoms (dysphagia, dysphonia, stridor)
- Pain, especially with bleeding into an adenoma, which sometimes radiates to the ear.

What investigations are used to investigate thyroid lumps?

Ultrasound

- Assesses size and number of nodules (clinical examination is notoriously inaccurate)
- Determines if a lump is cystic or solid
- Guides biopsy.

Fine needle aspiration biopsy

This is the gold standard for diagnosis short of open excision. The histopathological findings may be reported as unsatisfactory, a benign colloid lesion, a follicular lesion, a malignant papillary or medullary carcinoma, or autoimmune thyroiditis. It is not possible to distinguish between a follicular adenoma and a follicular carcinoma on cytology and all follicular lesions should be excised.

Nuclear scans

- Are costly and performed less often these days
- Do not exclude malignancy; malignant nodules may be cold, but most cold nodules are benign
- Are useful in subacute thyroiditis (cold), thyroxine abuse (cold) and toxic adenomas (hot).

What are the indications for surgery?

Most thyroid lumps are benign. Indications for surgery include:

- Concerns about malignancy ● Malignancy ● Large cysts (more likely to be malignant) ● An enlarging lump ● Pressure symptoms (dysphagia, dysphonia, stridor or pain) ● Cosmetic.

CASE STUDY	11.4 ACROMEGALY

Instruction: *Examine this patient's face/hands. Assess any other systems you feel relevant. Discuss your findings.*

RECOGNITION

Classically:

Face (Fig. 11.4)

There are *prominent supraorbital ridges*. There is *prognathism* (protrusion of lower jaw), *soft tissue enlargement* of the *nose, tongue* and *ears*. The *interdentular space* distances are *increased*. There is general *coarsening of features*. The voice may be husky.

Hands (Fig. 11.5)

These are '*spade like*'. The skin is *thick*, often with a rubbery texture and moist.

There may also be gynaecomastia, and other evidence of hypogonadism.

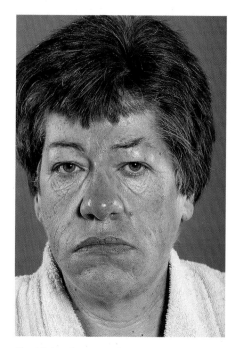

Fig. 11.4   *Acromegaly*

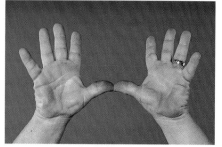

Fig. 11.5   *Acromegaly*

INTERPRETATION

Assess severity

The aforementioned signs are beloved of many textbooks. Some of the terms used, however, are rather old fashioned, even insulting ('spade like hands'), and of little practical value. Recognising acromegaly in PACES is not likely to be very difficult. The examiners will be more keen to hear about features associated with an increased risk of morbidity and mortality (below). Mortality is increased two- to three-fold in acromegaly due to cardiorespiratory disease and malignancy. *×2-3*

1. **Blood pressure**. Acromegaly is a cause of hypertension, cardiomyopathy and increased cardiovacular mortality.
2. **Diabetes/impaired glucose tolerance.** Tell the examiners you would check the urinalysis for glycosuria.
3. **Bitemporal hemianopia**. Ask about field loss and consider visual field examination.
4. **Carpal tunnel syndrome.** Ask about nocturnal paraesthesia and consider Tinel's test.
5. **Obstructive sleep apnoea**. Ask about snoring, excessive daytime somnolence (and accidents), headaches, and poor concentration.
6. **Colorectal cancer risk.** Tell the examiners that you would ask about colorectal symptoms.

DISCUSSION

What causes acromegaly?

Acromegaly is due hypersecretion of growth hormone from a macroadenoma. Other clinical features may arise from hypofunction of the compressed normal pituitary tissue and local tumour pressure effects. Hypopituitary symptoms may include reduced libido and potency. Associated hyperprolactinaemia may contribute to testosterone deficiency.

How would you confirm the diagnosis?

1. Acromegaly develops insidiously and newly diagnosed patients have often had symptoms for years, including increased sweating, increased size in shoes, gloves, rings or dentures and sometimes headaches.
2. Investigations include blood glucose, prolactin, testosterone, luteinising hormone and thyroxine levels. The diagnosis is confirmed by a failure of serum growth hormone to suppress to below 2 mU/L in a prolonged 75 g oral glucose tolerance test and by an elevated insulin like growth factor-1 (IGF-1). *O GTT suppression ↑ IGF-1*
3. When the diagnosis is confirmed, further dynamic tests may be needed to determine the overall function of the anterior pituitary (e.g. insulin tolerance test, thyroid releasing hormone (TRH) test and luteinising hormone-releasing hormone (LHRH) test).

Fig. 11.6   *Growth hormone synthesis*

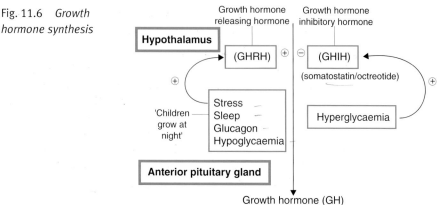

4. Magnetic resonance imaging (MRI) of the pituitary gland is important.

How is GH synthesis normally controlled?

See Figure 11.6.

What treatments are available?

Successful treatment restores life expectancy to normal.

1. Most patients proceed to transphenoidal surgery (transcranial if significant suprasellar extension), by an experienced pituitary surgeon to remove the adenoma. Surgery is invariably complicated by early but transient diabetes insipidus. Larger adenomas are often difficult to completely excise, leaving patients with residual growth hormone (GH) excess. Most symptoms and signs of acromegaly do not regress after surgery, except those of disease activity such as sweating and oedema.

2. Dopamine agonists (e.g. bromocriptine, cabergoline) are generally not very effective at reducing GH secretion and do not reduce tumour size.

3. Somatostatin analogues such as octreotide can be very effective at inhibiting GH secretion, but do not cause significant tumour shrinkage. Octreotide is most conveniently given by monthly depot injection.

4. External pituitary radiotherapy alone takes several years to achieve GH reduction and often ultimately induces hypopituitarism.

Radiotherapy is given routinely post incomplete surgery to prevent tumour recurrence and to reduce GH secretion.

When might growth hormone be administered therapeutically?

Growth hormone has been used in childhood cases of short stature due to growth hormone-releasing hormone (GHRH) deficiency and Turner's syndrome, but is not indicated in constitutional short stature. Adult GH therapy in hypopituitary patients with hypopituitarism may be important in reducing premature mortality. It may improve wellbeing, enhance muscle power, improve bone mineral density, improve the lipid profile and reduce cardiovascular mortality. Unfortunately, therapeutic GH is expensive.

What is ghrelin?

A gut hormone, now known to be a potent stimulator of GH secretion.

What other anterior pituitary tumour disorders do you know of?

There are three main diseases (Box 11.2).

Box 11.2   **Anterior Pituitary Tumours**

The three common secreting pituitary adenomas are:

1. Prolactinomas (usually microadenomas in women, more often macroadenomas in men)
2. Macroadenomas releasing growth hormone (**acromegaly**)
3. Microadenomas releasing ACTH (**Cushing's disease**, Case study 11.6)

Many pituitary adenomas are non-secretory, but may cause hypopituitarism through compression of normal pituitary tissue.

Hyperprolactinaemia

Prolactin release from the anterior pituitary is normally inhibited by dopamine derived from the hypothalamus. Causes of hyperprolactinaemia are:

- Physiological (sleep, stress, pregnancy/lactation, psychogenic nipple stimulation, coitus)
- Drugs (dopamine receptor antagonists (metoclopramide, chlorpromazine, haloperidol))
- Hypothalamic or pituitary stalk disease (granulomas or meningiomas causing 'disconnection hyperprolactinaemia')
- Macroadenomas (e.g. in acromegaly), which may secrete prolactin ('pseudoprolactinoma'), as well as compressing the stalk
- Prolactinomas (most are microadenomas, often producing very high prolactin levels)
- Polycystic ovarian syndrome (PCOS)
- Hypothyroidism (TRH stimulates prolactin as well as TSH)

- Idiopathic, which is likely due a covert microadenoma
- Post seizure

The effects of hyperprolactinaemia are *galacatorrhoea* and ovarian inhibition (*amenorrhoea*) in women. Men may present with hypogonadism causing erectile dysfunction. Do not confuse galactorrhoea, which is always due to prolactin, with *gynaecomastia*, which is unrelated to hyperprolactinaemia and caused by a decreased androgen : oestrogen ratio (puberty, hypogondism, adrenal or testicular oestrogen producing tumours, drugs — oestrogens, cimetidine, spironolactone, digoxin, anabolic steroids).

Prolactinomas may be treated with dopamine agonists such as cabergoline which suppress prolactin secretion and cause rapid tumour shrinkage, even of large macroadenomas. Surgery is seldom needed because of the good response to medical therapy.

CASE STUDY   11.5 HYPOPITUITARISM

Instruction: *Look at and examine this patient. Discuss your approach to further assessment.*

RECOGNITION

Signs of hypopituitarism include *pallor, fine facial skin, decreased axillary/pubic hair, breast atrophy in females and other signs of hypogonadism*, reflecting the fact that gonadotrophins (follicle stimulating hormone (FSH) and luteinising hormone (LH)) tend to be early hormones lost.

INTERPRETATION

Confirm the diagnosis

Tell the examiners that your further assessment would include:

- Blood pressure measurement for postural hypotension
- Visual field assessment for bitemporal hemianopia
- Examination of the testes for hypogonadism in males
- Eliciting a history of amenorrhoea in females.

DISCUSSION

What are the causes of hypopituitarism?

- Pituitary tumours
- Infiltration by granulomatous disease (TB, sarcoid), amyloid, haemochromatosis
- Pituitary infarction.

What are Sheehan's syndrome and pituitary apoplexy?

● Sheehan's syndrome is acute pituitary infarction as a result of hypovolaemia or septic shock, for example in meningococcaemia.
● Sudden pituitary haemorrhage or 'pituitary apoplexy' causes headache, visual loss, diplopia and sudden cardiovascular collapse.

How is hypopituitarism diagnosed?

Diagnosis of hypopituitarism is by combined anterior pituitary function testing, which may include LHRH, TRH, and insulin stress tests with measurement of cortisol, growth hormone, TSH, FSH, LH and prolactin. Therapy is by replacement of the deficient hormone/s (e.g. growth hormone) or more commonly the deficient hormone/s from the target endocrine gland/s (e.g. thyroxine).

What disorders of the posterior pituitary gland do you know of?

● Diabetes insipidus (DI—Box 11.3)
● Syndrome of inappropriate ADH (SIADH—Box 11.3).

Box 11.3   DI and SIADH

DI

DI is due to deficiency antidiuretic hormone (ADH) or resistance to its action. ADH is synthesised in cell bodies in the supraoptic and paraventricular nuclei of the hypothalamus and ultimately released from nerve terminals of the posterior pituitary gland.

Concurrent plasma and spot urine sodium concentrations and osmolalities are usually sufficient to diagnose DI (Fig. 11.7).

Fig. 11.7 *Diabetes insipidus diagnostic pathway*

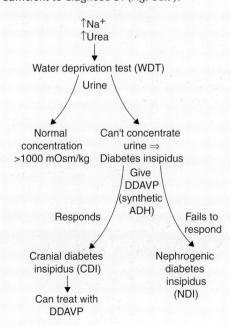

Cranial DI (deficiency)
CDI is usually due to tumours (craniopharyngioma), trauma or sarcoidosis.

Nephrogenic DI (resistance)
NDI is due to renal tubular dysfunction, which may be a primary genetic aberration of the ADH receptor (page 84) or secondary to tubular damage in pyelonephritis, obstruction, sickle cell disease, hypokalaemia, hypercalcaemia or lithium toxicity.

SIADH
Normally ADH responds to elevated serum osmolality by enhancing permeability and water retention at the collecting duct. This increases urine concentration, decreases urine volume and decreases serum osmolality. SIADH is a diagnosis of exclusion. It should not be diagnosed where there is renal impairment, adrenal insufficiency, hypovolaemia or oedema.

Causes of SIADH
Causes include chest disease (especially bronchial carcinoma), intracranial disease (including demyelination) and drugs (phenothiazines, tricyclics, chlorpropamide, opiates, nicotine, vinca alkaloids, clofibrate, NSAIDs).

Effects of SIADH
- Hyponatraemia
- Low urea
- High urine : serum osmolality ratio (> 1) in the face of a low serum osmolality
- Normal or high urinary sodium (> 20 mmol/L)
- Absence of oedema (because aldosterone is generally low and sodium is not retained).

Management of SIADH
This involves:

- Treating the cause
- Fluid restriction
- Demeclocycline, which inhibits collecting duct receptors.

| CASE STUDY | **11.6 CUSHING'S SYNDROME** |

Instruction: *Look at this patient's face and then assess his/her condition further. Discuss your findings and differential diagnosis.*

| **RECOGNITION** | |

As for acromegaly, there are lengthy lists of signs to be found in textbooks, some insulting ('buffalo hump' and 'moon face'), which

Fig. 11.8   *Cushing's syndrome.*
Reproduced with permission from M.A. Mir
(1995) Atlas of Clinical Diagnosis. W.B.
Saunders, London

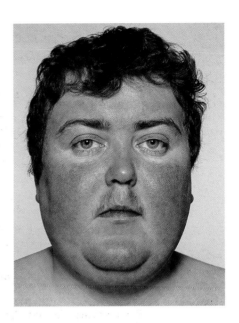

may best be summarised as signs of corticosteroid excess. Again, recognition is often not difficult. The examiners expect more than the following list:

- Centripetal fat distribution ● Supraclavicular fat pads/'moon face' (Fig. 11.8) ● Thoracocervical fat pads/'buffalo hump'
- Protein wasting ● Skin: thin, striae, poor wound healing, easy bruising, hirsutism ● Oedema.

INTERPRETATION

Look for/consider causes

Most patients with such features are on long-term corticosteroids for a chronic inflammatory disease such as chronic obstructive pulmonary disease (COPD), asthma or inflammatory bowel disease, or a renal transplant. Look for/consider these. Otherwise the three causes of Cushing's syndrome to consider are shown in Box 11.4.

Rarely, *pseudoCushing's* syndrome may result from obesity, depression or sometimes alcohol excess.

Assess severity

Consider:

- *Hypertension*—ask to check the blood pressure
- Glucose intolerance/diabetes mellitus.

Box 11.4	The Three Non-iatrogenic Causes of Cushing's Syndrome

1. **Cushing's disease.** This is due to a pituitary microadenoma secreting ACTH. It is by far the most common non-iatrogenic cause of Cushing's syndrome.
2. **Ectopic ACTH.** This is often caused by a bronchial carcinoid or small cell lung cancer. Ectopic ACTH secretion due to carcinoma is usually of rapid onset with *less florid signs of corticosteroid excess but significant weight loss and hypokalaemia* (mineralocorticoid effect due to inhibition of renal tubular 11β hydroxysteroid dehydrogenase—Box 5.8, page 254) and *pigmentation* (co secretion of other peptides). When due to an indolent carcinoid tumour the clinical course can be indistinguishable from Cushing's disease due to a pituitary macroadenoma.
3. **Adrenal adenoma** (and very rarely carcinoma). Some adrenal adenomas secrete cortisol. Adrenal tumours also tend to secrete androgens as well and present with *hirsutism* and/or *virilisation*, e.g. clitoromegaly.

Evidence of decompensation

Consider:

● Osteoporosis/wedge fractures—look for kyphosis
● Immunosuppression and recurrent infections.

Assess function

Examine briefly for proximal myopathy (Case study 6.31).
Tell the examiners that you would also consider the possibility of:

● Depression ● Psychosis ● Amenorrhoea ● Infertility
● Impotence.

DISCUSSION	

How could you determine the cause of non-iatrogenic Cushing's syndrome?

The main point for discussion is usually that of investigating Cushing's syndrome. There are two parts to investigating clinically suspected non-iatrogenic Cushing's syndrome (Box 11.5).

What treatments are available for Cushing's disease?

● Transphenoidal hypophysectomy, complications being CSF rhinorrhoea, diabetes insipidus, hypopituitarism, visual field disturbance, persistent or recurrent disease and death
● Radiotherapy
● Drugs such as metyrapone
● Bilateral adrenalectomy if primary evacuation not possible (which may be complicated by Nelson's syndrome in which ACTH levels rise and cause melanin induced hyperpigmentation).

Box 11.5   **Investigating Cushing's Syndrome**

Diagnosing Cushing's syndrome
Screening tests include:

- *24-hour urinary free cortisol* (normal < 275 nmol/24 hours)
- An *overnight dexamethasone suppression test* (1 mg at midnight—cortisol is normally suppressed and a positive test produces a plasma cortisol > 150 nmol/L at 8 AM the following morning. Dexamethasone is a synthetic glucocorticoid.

More sensitive as a *diagnostic test* is the *low dose dexamethasone suppression test (LDDST)* (0.5 mg qds for 2 days—cortisol is normally suppressed and a positive test produces a plasma cortisol > 150 nmol/L or a urinary cortisol > 275 nmol/24 hours). All causes of Cushing's syndrome should fail to suppress. Normal subjects and those with pseudoCushing's syndrome should suppress.

Assessment of circadian rhythmicity (which is lost in Cushing's syndrome) may be the most sensitive test but requires hospital admission. Normal cortisol levels at 8 AM tend to be in the range 150–650 nmol/L, may be in a range around half that at 4 PM, and can drop to a nadir of < 50 nmol/L at midnight.

Establishing the cause of Cushing's syndrome
The next step is to establish if *ACTH* is:

- Easily detectable (Cushing's disease, ectopic ACTH), or
- Suppressed (adrenal adenoma).

If *easily detectable*, the final step is to determine whether the ACTH arises from the pituitary (Cushing's disease) or from an ectopic site. The best method is controversial. The *corticotrophin releasing hormone (CRH) test* and the *high-dose dexamethasone suppression test (HDDST)* have been widely used. The rationale for the HDDST is that pituitary adenomas to an extent obey normal physiological rules (but with a higher threshold for suppression) and partially suppress. *Ectopic ACTH* generally *does not suppress*, but exceptions are well recognised. Ectopic ACTH sources do not normally respond to CRH.

Imaging is often unsatisfactory because pituitary adenomas may be only a few millimetres wide and undetectable. Equally, 'incidentalomas' are common. Simultaneous bilateral inferior petrosal sinus sampling with measurement of ACTH following CRH stimulation can provide a firm diagnosis and permit hemispheric localisation of tumours (and theoretically permit hemispheric resection and preserve pituitary function). It is not easy.

Are all hormones steroids?

- Thyroxine, triiodothyronine, dopamine and catecholamines are amine hormones.
- Most other hormones are steroids (cortisol, aldosterone, sex hormones, vitamin D) or peptides (TSH, FSH, LH, ACTH, vasopressin, insulin, growth hormone).

Hormones may act intracellularly through nuclear receptors or at cell surface receptors, mediating their effect intracellularly via cyclic AMP and G proteins.

What do you know about non-endocrine disease and pregnancy hormone changes?

As a general rule, 'stress' hormone levels (ACTH, steroids, growth hormone, catecholamines, glucagon) rise in many systemic illnesses, while the others tend to fall. In pregnancy, most hormone levels rise.

What is the value of a suppression or stimulation test in endocrinology?

Many hormones have a circadian rhythm and isolated levels can be difficult to interpret. Most hormone levels are regulated by other hormones or metabolic substrates via a negative feedback loop, and isolated levels should always be interpreted in their context. Where there is difficulty in interpreting isolated levels, dynamic tests can be useful. *Suppression tests* are used for *suspected hormone excess. Stimulation tests* are used for *suspected hormone deficiency.*

CASE STUDY	11.7 HYPOADRENALISM/ADDISON'S DISEASE

Instruction: *This patient (Fig. 11.9) presented with weight loss and weakness. Please assess and then discuss your findings.*

RECOGNITION	

There is *hyperpigmentation*, especially of *skin creases* (*palms, elbows*), the *lips* and *mouth*, and *surgical scars*. There may be *vitiligo*, and *sparse axillary* (and pubic) *hair*. There is *postural hypotension*.

INTERPRETATION	

Confirm the diagnosis

Tell the examiners that you would:

- Ask about nausea and vomiting
- Ask about weakness, fatigue and weight loss
- Wish to know the results of serum electrolytes (tendency to hypokalaemic, hyperchloraemic metabolic acidosis with hyponatraemia, but results may be normal).

Fig. 11.9 *Addison's disease (body).*
Reproduced with permission from M.A. Mir
(1995) Atlas of Clinical Diagnosis. W.B.
Saunders, London

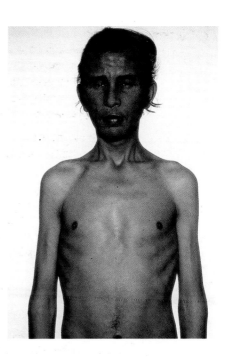

A short Synacthen test would be the next step, to determine whether or not administered synthetic ACTH can stimulate an appropriate rise in cortisol levels to greater than 500 nmol/L. The diagnosis can then be confirmed by measurement of plasma ACTH which is greatly raised.

Evidence of decompensation

Adrenal crises are associated with haemodynamic instability and life threatening metabolic disturbances.

Look for/consider associated diseases

Consider the spectrum of autoimmune disease, as for Grave's disease and hypothyroidism, including diabetes mellitus, pernicious anaemia and rheumatoid arthritis.

DISCUSSION

What are the causes of hypoadrenalism?

- Addison's disease (primary, autoimmune) ● HIV
- TB/granulomatous infiltration ● Amyloid ● Metastatic
- Fungal infiltration (histoplasmosis, coccidioidomycosis)
- Adrenoleucodystrophy ● Waterhouse—Friderichsen syndrome (infarction, e.g. in meningococcal septicaemia).

Hypoadrenalism is common in critically ill patients. Hypotension can be both the cause (hypoperfusion/infarction) and effect of hypoadrenalism in intensive care patients.

Treatment involves identification and management of any underlying remediable cause and adrenal replacement therapy with both corticosteroid and mineralocorticoid.

What do you know about mineralocorticoid excess?

Hyperaldosteronism (Box 5.8, page 254) may be secondary to hyperreninaemia or primary, in which renin levels are suppressed.

Causes of primary hyperaldosteronism include·

● Adrenal adenoma/Conn's syndrome (commonest) ● Bilateral adrenal hyperplasia ● Carcinoma.

Effects include hypokalaemic alkalosis with hypertension, especially diastolic hypertension. Sodium is retained and extracellular fluid volume increases. But there is insufficient water retention for oedema to develop.

Investigations for primary hyperaldosteronism may reveal a *low renin* level and a *low ambulant or erect renin–aldosterone ratio* (screening test). Electrolyte levels alone are a poor screening test. *Aldosterone levels* may *fail to suppress with salt loading*, e.g. saline, salt tablets or fludrocortisone 0.2 mg/day for 5 days. The value of imaging is limited by the high incidence of 'incidentalomas'. *Adrenal vein sampling* may be used to detect hypersecretion of aldosterone from the affected side.

List some endocrine causes of hypertension?

● Cushing's syndrome
● Conn's syndrome
● Acromegaly
● Phaeochromocytoma
● Liddle's syndrome, glucocorticoid remediable hypertension, apparent mineralocorticoid excess (Box 5.8, page 254).

What do know about phaeochromocytomas?

These catecholamine secreting tumours may cause episodic or persistent hypertension, headaches and sweats. Remember the 10% rule:

● 10% are bilateral ● 10% are extra-adrenal ● 10% are malignant
● 10% are familial.

The initial investigation of choice is to check for the presence of excess urinary catecholamines.

Occasionally, a phaeochromocytoma may be part of multiple endocrine neoplasia type 2 (MEN2).

What types of MEN are there?

MEN1

Comprising:

- Pancreatic tumour (especially gastrinoma or insulinoma)
- Parathyroid adenoma/hyperplasia ● Pituitary tumour.

This is autosomal dominant and may also include adrenal and thyroid adenomas

MEN2

Comprising:

- Phaeochromocytoma (bilateral, extramedullary) ● Parathyroid adenoma/hyperplasia ● Thyroid medullary carcinoma/C cell hyperplasia.

This is autosomal dominant and is associated with the ret 2 protooncogene. MEN2b comprises the features of MEN2 and a marfanoid phentoype, mucosal neuromas, myopathy and skin pigmentation.

CASE STUDY | **11.8 HIRSUTISM AND POLYCYSTIC OVARIAN SYNDROME (PCOS)**

Instruction: *Look at this patient. You may ask her a few questions. Tell the examiners how you would proceed with your assessment.*

RECOGNITION

There is *hirsutism*, or excessive hair growth, particularly over the face and limbs. There may be *acne*. There may be other *signs of virilisation*.

INTERPRETATION

Confirm the diagnosis

- The diagnosis of PCOS rests on a combination of symptoms, clinical findings and biochemical abnormalities which you should aim to discuss. In addition to hirsutism, common associations are *acne, obesity, male pattern hair thinning, subfertility and oligomenorrhoea or secondary amenorrhoea* (hyperplasia of ovarian thecal cells and multiple cysts).
- Always consider the possibility of a virilising adrenal tumour causing Cushing's syndrome in your differential diagnosis.

Assess other systems

Tell the examiners that you would check for glycosuria.

DISCUSSION

What is meant by the terms hypertrichosis, hirsutism and virilisation?

- *Hypertrichosis* refers to excess body hair.
- *Hirsutism* refers to excess hair in androgen dependent areas (male pattern).
- *Virilisation* refers to male pattern hair loss and other physical changes including voice change, breast atrophy and clitoromegaly. Hirstutism and acne are invariably present.

Hirsutism may be constitutional, or it may be due to adrenal or ovarian disorders, such as androgen secreting tumours in either of these organs. It may be caused by congenital adrenal hyperplasia (CAH). It may also be caused by drugs. One of the most common causes of hirsutism is PCOS.

What is PCOS?

The pathophysiology of PCOS is incompletely understood. It is a condition of androgen excess, characterised biochemically by:

- Raised testosterone and androstenedione levels
- A raised luteinising hormone : follicle stimulating hormone (LH : FSH) ratio with an abnormality in the usual pulsatile secretion of gonadotrophic releasing hormones
- Normal or elevated oestradiol levels
- Mild hyperprolactinaemia
- Low sex hormone binding globulin (SHBG) levels
- Low HDL cholesterol
- Insulin resistance with hyperinsulinaemia.

What is congenital adrenal hyperplasia (CAH)?

These are a group of disorders, all autosomal recessively inherited, the commonest defect being 21-hydroxylase deficiency. There can be a spectrum of clinical manifestations from mild, late onset signs resembling PCOS in females, to ambiguous sexual differentiation at birth. The enzyme defect results in a deficiency of glucocorticoids or mineralocorticoids leading to hyperstimulation of the adrenal gland which can only respond by producing excess hormones from unaffected pathways—testosterone precursors and testosterone. CAH may cause precocious puberty in males and female virilisation.

What are the causes of testosterone deficiency?

Testosterone deficiency is becoming increasingly recognised, and is not uncommon. It may be a result of a specific hypogonadal disorder or age related decline. It can present in many ways, most commonly as:

- Sexual dysfunction
- Reduced muscle mass

- Reduced bone mass with an increased risk of osteoporosis
- Reduced facial, body or pubic hair
- Small testes
- Tiredness, depression or non-specific cognitive changes such as poor concentration.

It may be hypergonadotrophic or hypogonadotrophic:

1. Hypergonadotrophic hypogonadism refers to primary testicular failure, often with elevated FSH and LH levels. Acquired causes include mumps, trauma, torsion, surgery, radiotherapy, drugs (spironolactone, chemotherapy, marijuana) and myotonic dystrophy. Congenital disorders include Klinefelter's syndrome (XXY, tall stature, small testes, azoospermia, raised gonadotrophins, gynaecomastia) and 5α reductase deficiency (androgen resistance).
2. Hypogonadotrophic hypogonadism is gonadal failure secondary to hypothalamic/pituitary disease, usually with low or normal FSH and LH levels.

Systemic disorders including chronic renal failure or liver disease, and sickle cell disease can also cause testosterone deficiency. Chronic alcohol excess is a common cause.

What are the features of Turner's syndrome?

Turner's syndrome (45X0) causes primary amenorrhoea, short stature and delayed puberty. There may be a webbed neck and widely spaced nipples. Sometimes there is a horseshoe kidney or aortic coarctation. Oestrogen levels are low with raised FSH and LH levels.

Appendix. 100 tips for passing PACES

Before PACES

Timing

1. Many candidates feel that MRCP exams should be sat (and failed) as often as possible in the belief that passing will be the reward of negative but repetitive experience! With the right preparation you can easily pass PACES. Take it when you feel ready and don't listen to pessimistic colleagues.

What the examiners are looking for

2. The examiners want to be satisfied that you are a safe, competent doctor, suitable to enter specialist training.
3. They are not looking for specialist knowledge.
4. They are not looking for the next Professor of Medicine.
5. They want to know that, as your general medical consultant, they could have a sensible discussion with you about the care of a patient.
6. They want to know that, as your consultant, they could entrust the care of their patients to you when away from the wards.
7. They respect a friendly and confident manner, but not arrogance.
8. Many candidates adopt 'victim mode' with head down and victim posture throughout PACES. This concerns examiners, who wonder how a nervous candidate might cope in an emergency. Examiners are likely to be more impressed by the candidate who stands with an upright, confident posture, hands by sides or behind back, and makes good eye contact.

It's in your hands!

9. Passing PACES is well within your grasp.
10. The idea that passing is in your examiners' hands is a negative one.
11. It's in your hands!
12. You can pass with the right preparation. A short text such as *PACES for the MRCP* as an adjunct to seeing patients on the wards is ideal preparation.
13. Success is about discipline and desire. You must work to pass, and want to pass.
14. Passing is easier than you think and you probably need to know less than you think. Reading larger textbooks are not a good use of time. Seeing patients is.

Practise

15. Most candidates are competent enough to pass PACES by the exam date. Invariably lack of confidence is the problem. The aim of practise is to build a natural confidence into your already adequate competence.
16. Practise your examination technique for each system at every opportunity (whenever possible in front of senior colleagues).

17. Practise the history taking skills taught in this book with patients at every opportunity.

18. Practice your communication skills at every opportunity. As well as discussing management and ethical dilemmas with patients and colleagues, some candidates find it helpful to form discussion groups.

19. Be alert to any topical issues in the news and in general medical journals that could be examined and discussed.

20. Read widely. Reading strengthens your communication prowess.

21. Practise does not automatically make perfect. Perfect practise does!

22. When you go into the exam you should appear as though you have performed your examination of each system hundreds of times before, ideally because you have!

ON THE DAY OF PACES

Some formalities

23. PACES requires sustained energy and you must not be so tired through stress and studying as to lose momentum on the day. Meerkats get plenty of sleep each night to be alert and vigilant each day! Try not to work continuously in the run up to PACES. Have some early nights and avoid caffeine and alcohol.

24. Dress professionally.

25. Arrive at the exam venue in good time.

26. Take your stethoscope. Other equipment should be provided but you may prefer to carry your own ophthalmoscope, tendon hammer and red pin. A case of 'James Bond' gadgets will not impress examiners.

27. Thank your patients and examiners after each case.

At the start

28. Keep in mind that there should be nothing particularly rare and therefore nothing to be particularly scared of throughout the five stations. However, even good candidates find some cases much more difficult than others. A few poor performances can still mean an overall pass and you should be determined from the start to put any difficult cases behind you and give the next one, with different examiners, your best shot.

The patients are more important than the examiners!

29. The patients are your prime concern. Thinking that the outcome of the exam is in the hands of the examiners is not helpful. The examiners will pass or fail you on the strengths and weaknesses of your performances with patients. Focus on your patients and the exam will take care of itself.

30. Do not hurt patients on any account! This is one of the easiest ways to fail PACES.

31. Be considerate to patients. This is one of the easiest ways to pass PACES. It may seem obvious, but the notion of treating other people as we would like to be treated ourselves is a remarkably effective guiding principle in PACES as it is in medical practice.

Examiners

32. Examiners come with the full range of personalities. The best advice is not to worry about what sort of examiners you get. Focus instead on doing what you do as well as you can do it.

33. The examiners are not trying to catch you out but want to find out what you know.

Examining patients

34. Be nice to patients! This is worth reiterating. Treat them with respect at all times. A considerate (but not obsequious) approach to patients is the single biggest determinant of success.

35. Ask each patient for permission to examine and if they are in any pain.

36. Ensure that each patient is positioned correctly before you begin.

37. Observation is a vital part of examination!

38. Don't wait for the examiners to keep telling you what to do. Do it spontaneously, using the *Recognition– Interpretation–Discussion (RID)* sequence.

39. Don't look for feedback from the examiners. You won't get it, and looking for it will unnecessarily unnerve you. A good candidate, without appearing to rush, will elicit signs and gather information considerately, swiftly and spontaneously.

40. Remember that you are 'on stage'. Let the examiners see your performance. As in a driving test, your actions should be natural but clearly visible.

41. Remember that from the examiners' perspective you do two things in each case. Firstly you *examine* your patient. Secondly you *present* your findings. From your perspective, you are doing much more. Whilst examining, you are looking for signs, deciding how best to interpret these and thinking about how you are going to present your findings. A structured approach is essential. The examination schemes in this book can be performed automatically with practise, allowing you to concentrate on recognising and interpreting signs and to use this same framework for presenting.

42. At the end of each case ensure that your patient is comfortable as you found them.

43. Don't forget to thank them.

Examining and presenting

44. Avoid the 'running commentary' approach. Many candidates wonder if they should 'talk as they go' or 'present their findings at the end.' Some candidates believe the running commentary a way of scoring points— such that even if their final diagnosis is incorrect, they may at least have reported some correct findings. This is risky.

45. A running commentary slows you down and fragments the smooth flow of your examination. Examiners don't want to be told that you're examining the pulse to check whether or not it's collapsing. They want to *see* you doing it. Examiners are human and easily bored. They will forgive you for omitting things here and there but may be irritated if you don't 'just get on with it'. Constant stops and starts are more likely to draw the attention of examiners to mistakes. Conversely, candidates with competent examination skills who 'get on with it' tend to impress examiners, often lulling them into a sense of security—switching them from hawk to dove mode and blinding them to mistakes.

46. Talking whilst examining interferes with your *rapport* with a patient. You may think rapport is something you can't develop within a few minutes. But patients in PACES generally have a very good idea of how well a candidate performs, simply because what impresses patients is what impresses examiners —a natural, considerate and considered approach. Be attentive to your patient,

not the examiners, whilst examining. Be completely absorbed by your patient. Tell them what you are doing as you are doing it, smile, look and listen for the subtle cues of cooperation, and above all show that you care. Rapport will come naturally and your examiners, at this stage, should fade into the background.

47. The 'absence' of the examiners allows you to pool all of your mental energy into the case, and should reduce anxiety.

48. The opposite applies when presenting your case. Be decisive in finishing your examination and politely turn away from your patient to give your undivided attention to the examiners. At this point, some candidates are so relieved if they have a diagnosis that they blurt it out and wait for feedback—'Graves' disease!' Talk through the *Recognition–Interpretation* sequence instead.

49. When presenting, avoid lots of 'ums' and avoid reporting lists of negative findings.

50. Conversely, if you have elicited a sign, mention it. Candidates surprisingly often fail to mention signs they have clearly elicited. Do not assume the examiners know that you have elicited a sign.

51. Never make up signs to conform to an anticipated diagnosis. It is a sure way to fail.

52. If you know the diagnosis, state it and then give the relevant supporting findings.

53. If you do not know the diagnosis, describe what you found.

54. The key to impressing examiners is in ever striving 'to go further'. Examiners prefer candidates who spontaneously present their findings and thoughts.

55. Candidates who lack confidence often look back at their patient when presenting or asked questions as if the findings or answers will magically appear. Try to avoid this.

56. Avoid uncomfortable silences (where no marks can be awarded) by saying something intelligent. For example, if you find a mass in the left upper quadrant and are not sure if it is a spleen, you could describe findings you might expect in support of it being a spleen and findings you might expect in support of it being a kidney. You could also suggest an ultrasound scan to resolve the uncertainty.

57. The key is to try to keep talking, and saying sensible things.

When the diagnosis is not clear

58. Don't always expect a full house of signs. Patients are not from textbooks and examiners frequently disagree about signs before the exam starts. Try to keep calm. Simply blurting out a diagnosis about which you are unsure is hazardous. Remember that describing your findings, even if your diagnosis is incorrect, will allow points to be awarded.

59. There will always be cases where the diagnosis is not clear. Report your findings, telling the examiners which other signs you might have expected to find in support of the important differential diagnoses and what else you could do to resolve the uncertainty. Examiners seldom fail candidates who can demonstrate logical approaches to dilemmas. What often happens is that candidates fail themselves by 'going blank' when they are uncertain.

60. *PACES for the MRCP* has tried to strike a balance between structure and flexibility. It provides a framework for diseases likely to be encountered in PACES, but every patient is different.

The same disease is exhibited in different ways in different patients and its impact is individually determined. You should tailor your knowledge to specific patients. *PACES for the MRCP* is not a substitute for seeing as many patients as possible on the wards, and *Recognition–Interpretation–Discussion* is not something to which you need always adhere. It is simply a map to guide you through cases and bring you back on course if things go wrong.

61. Remember that 'common things are common'. You will have seen most things before.

62. Remember that double pathology can occur.

63. Diagnoses can be difficult. Many candidates struggle especially with neurology and heart valve cases. In cases where you are unsure:

(i) Describe what you found. Be honest. Never make up signs.

(ii) Tell the examiner two or three differential diagnoses.

(iii) Describe what else you might have expected to find in support of these.

(iv) State some things you could do to help resolve the issue, e.g. dynamic auscultation, arrange echocardiogram.

64. Before this point, many candidates have failed themselves, believing the signs too confusing and their diagnosis to be wrong. Practice often falls far short of theory.

History taking skills

65. Use the history taking skills described on pages 103–110.

Communications skills

66. Awareness of the history taking and communication skills described in this book allows you to further improve your history taking and communication skills.

67. Watch good communicators at work. See how they handle situations.

68. Try to bring discussion with examiners to life. Add sparkle by appearing enthusiastic and interested in the topic for discussion.

69. Watching politicians and debate programmes on television is a way of seeing negotiation at work. You don't have to like the politicians or agree with their arguments. But take an interest in how they communicate. They are usually effective speakers.

70. Remember that we are all more similar to each other than we are different. We share the same molecular ingredients, separated only by a twist of the genetic kaleidoscope! It is never hard to imagine ourselves in other people's shoes. If all the lessons you have learnt seem hard to remember, then one guiding principle should ensure that you never stray from the right ballpark—that of asking yourself what you would want if you were in your patient's situation.

Answering examiners questions

71. Listen to the question!

72. Answer the question asked!

73. Try not to repeat the question asked!

74. Take a moment or two before answering it.

75. Look at the examiner and not at the floor. Eye contact is very important.

76. Try to appear confident, yet reflective, giving a well structured answer. Your examiners will be as impressed by your communication skills as your knowledge.

77. Speak clearly and succinctly. Try to avoid speaking too quickly, and rambling.

78. Some candidates speak very quietly. It is unusual for candidates to speak very loudly. Unless you are one of the latter,

it may help to speak up slightly, more *authoritatively*.

79. Do not think of the examiners as examiners. This is easier said than done. But try to think of the examiners as colleagues with whom you are discussing interesting ward cases. Some candidates find it helpful to imagine themselves on a ward round.

80. Curiosity keeps us alert. Let your enthusiasm, curiosity and interest shine through.

81. Difficult questions often reflect a good performance. Examiners will challenge and probe and sometimes make you feel uncomfortable or inadequate.

82. Be confident if you think you are right, but never argue!

83. Be confident, not arrogant.

84. Avoid casual phrases and abbreviations.

85. Avoid emotive words like 'tumour' in front of patients.

86. Do not be afraid to retract statements you feel are wrong.

87. If you don't know the answer to a question, be honest in your ignorance.

88. Above all, avoid saying anything that would pose a danger to patients.

89. Remember that examiners' questions are often not predetermined but built around what you tell them—'Would you like to explain that?' You have some opportunity to take control of the areas to be discussed.

Answering examiners' questions at the communication skills and ethics station

90. Don't be too dogmatic. It can be dangerous to go down one route when discussing ethical dilemmas. It is wiser to state the broad range of issues an ethical dilemma creates, and that there are often numerous viewpoints to consider.

91. Remember that you are not expected to have all the answers. Examiners may be impressed by a mature attitude of self-awareness and a need to discuss an issue further with colleagues, a medical defence organisation and so on. Willingness to communicate with colleagues is considered a strength.

92. Whilst there is often no right or wrong answer, you can state what you think is the best course of action. Examiners may challenge you but it doesn't mean that your argument is flawed. Provided you feel that your argument is 'safe', run with your convictions. The examiners are usually checking for consistency of your argument, ensuring that it is genuinely your belief, and that you can justify it.

93. Sometimes examiners' questions will be hard! They may be searching, probing and uncomfortable. Again, this does not necessarily mean that you are doing anything wrong. It may mean that you are performing well.

94. Try to be 'patient centred' in your responses.

When you think things are going badly

95. Do not expect feedback from your examiners. They do not give it. This said, a confident, respectful and competent candidate with a friendly but not overly familiar manner is someone examiners warm to immediately.

96. Difficult cases may be genuinely difficult to all candidates (and to examiners!).

97. Difficult questions often reflect a good performance!

98. Examiners may play on your nerves and ask 'Are you sure?' in response to your answers. Often, they are simply testing your confidence and your answer is correct.

99. Each station and case is marked separately. Try not to lose hope if you feel you have performed badly in a particular case. Examiners allow numerous mistakes (provided these would not have overtly dangerous clinical consequences) and a poor performance does not necessarily result in overall failure.

AFTER PACES

100. Most candidates who pass do so despite a few weak performances. Many candidates are convinced they have failed until they receive the 'Pass' envelope from the College. Now is the time to put PACES behind you, watch a movie and relax.

INDEX